Pregnancy ~
Four Trimesters!?

Expert Tips & Doula Tricks

Kim Turton Palmatary

First Published in Canada in 2023 by MyDoula Publishing.

Illustrated by Sandy Thynne Nelson.

Pictures taken of the model for Hip Squeeze are by Christine Germano.
The model for Hip Squeeze is Agnes Turton.

Disclaimer

This book was written for informational purposes only, to encourage and educate pregnant people and partners on the birth choices for their babies. I have intentionally written to be inclusive of all gender-neutral birthing individuals. I specifically did not change any language in Dr Jack Newman's chapter on feeding the baby, as I respect that the entire chapter was written specifically for this book. I apologize if I have missed the mark. Thank you for your understanding.

Please note that I am not a professional medical authority. The information in this book is intended to be used for general information only, and should not replace consultation with health care professionals. Always seek medical advice from your own healthcare provider.

I *mention* procedures and technical terms in this book. Please, do your own due diligence by asking your care providers, what they mean, and how they may relate to YOU. If I attempt to explain more in-depth, I will be out of my scope of practice; a Doula does not give medical advice.

Praise from Clients

Kim's experience and guidance really helped during Mia's labor experience. Thanks Kim!

M & M July 2019

We are doing great. The baby loves to sleep and eat. I'm also recovering well. We can't thank you enough. You made our experience so enjoyable, from the communication with the nurses and midwives, to making me feel comfortable and at ease. I couldn't have asked for a better doula. You even put up with my husband's dad jokes.

Elana & Chadwick, 2nd baby, Born Sept 2021

It meant so much to hear your comforting words and to have you dry my tears while we talked. Cesarean delivery

Y & M, June 2022

Kim was our doula during a challenging labor and emergency c-section. We will never forget her wisdom, compassion, sense of humor, and support during the scariest and also happiest day of both our lives. So lovely.

J & N Sept 2022

My Definition of Doula

A popular definition of a 'Doula' is a Greek word referring to an experienced person who helps other birthing persons. It has become a term used for a person experienced with labor and birth that provides continuous non-medical support to the birthing person and their family before, during, and after the birth.

I Define a doula as someone you can trust that will educate you, assist *all* persons in the delivery suite, encourage you, and communicate with care providers on your behalf regarding your concerns, questions, or wishes. To maneuver stressful moments, reassure and comfort both emotionally and physically, and be the constant at your delivery. Doulas should never replace the partner, only enhance their participation during the whole birthing experience. Doulas can help the birthing person, the partner, and the baby with prenatal care, labor, and postpartum care.

I define a care provider as a medically trained professional that has the title of doctor, midwife, nurse, anesthetist, and more. I believe it is the doula's job to support everyone at the delivery, primarily the birthing person.

A Personal Note to My Readers

My wish for you is to have enough information with these *Tips and Tricks* to guide you to your best birth.

~ ~

I know that a baby makes a family.
I know that a baby can bring extreme joy and love.
I know that a baby does not always live through the birth process.

~ ~

The mystery of labor will always be just that, but if you are lucky and have good care, and enough information, birth can be a very normal and exciting journey.

For all Earth Angels

I dedicate this book to all earth-bound angels.

Treat every baby with the utmost respect.

I believe we can never love a baby too much, especially in the first year.

And to my twin nieces that are watching us from heaven.

*****

I wish you love, joy, and laughter while raising your baby.

Acknowledgments

I live in Vancouver, Canada, where we have an amazing medical system that offers very good prenatal, birth, and postpartum care for birthing people and their babies.

Most people deliver at a hospital, but many also deliver at home. Sometimes they pull over at the side of the road and have a baby on the seat of the car as well. Labor and birth can be spontaneous, or it may take its very sweet time; I have seen *almost* all of it.

My heart tightens when I hear of the tragedies here and in other countries where birthing people or their babies do not have successful birthing results. I have seen loss, and it is heart-wrenching, thus the impetus for writing this book. I am blessed to have contributions from some amazing professional experts, and with my wisdom and experience as a doula, I hope to encourage discussions and bring better results for you and all births.

I outline doula techniques for a faster and easier birth. I know when a birthing person has help from someone they know and trust, their labor and delivery is more successful. When a baby is positioned in the most ideal way, it makes for fewer interventions. The benefits are that the baby is not stressed, the birthing person is more effective, and the partner participates more effectively.

A successful labor, and a healthy baby, with support for the birthing person, before, during, and especially after delivery, will ensure a very successful life for the family and our community.

You will find that your child (biological or not) will bring you a very unique life experience. They will give you more joy and love than most other people ever can.

***

Please note that most of the information in my book is written with the assumption that you are having a single baby; twins or more babies are usually born earlier than their due dates. They involve more prenatal care and usually have more complications attached to the pregnancy, labor, and birth.

I wish you all an easier and shorter labor. The journey doesn't define you; it is a means to the end result, your *baby*. I wish you and your baby, health and happiness.

May this book bring a better understanding for you to understand the magical experience of birth!

Thanks to My Family

My husband, Kevin, is my rock. He loves unconditionally and has more patience than anyone I know. I am so blessed to have such an amazing human in my life. Kevin encourages me while I work long, crazy 'on-call' hours, and takes care of me with strong arms to hug me, or an ear to bend when things sometimes go sideways.

~~

My 5 adult 'children' have taught me to listen. They are all strong, healthy adults, and a very important part of my life, and I can not imagine living without them.

~~

The love for your children is the strongest bond that a person can find.

So much love to all the generous and very talented people that have contributed content and/or their time to help me with this book. I am SO VERY thankful to you all.

Sandy Thynne Nelson: Sandy is the primary illustrator for this book, including the cover and most of the images inside. She also helped with some pre-edits. Born and raised in Victoria, Sandy is a graphic designer, currently living on Saturna Island with her husband, Don. She is a mother, grandmother, avid reader, Nordic knitter and a student of Norwegian and Scots Gaelic languages. She is a member of the Society for Canadian Artists and the Southern Gulf Islands Arts Council.

Feeding Baby Chapter was written exclusively for this book by **Dr Jack Newman** IBCLC. Their clinic is based in Toronto, Canada. I call Dr Newman the GURU of chestfeeding! I have used and taught their techniques by using their videos and CDs over the years. *I have not altered the chapter by changing the use of gender or terms*. I hold so much respect for the work their clinic does.

www.DrJackNewman.com **ibconline.ca**
(**http://ibconline.ca/breastfeeding-starting-out-right/**)

Doula **Jalana Grant**, AdvCD (DONA), DONA International Approved Birth Doula Trainer, Director Doula Programs, LCCE, Doula, South Community Birth Program as Doula Co-ordinator, Instructor. As my mentor, Jalana truly knows and understands the challenges of being a full-time doula. She is a wise person and a great sounding board, especially when birth goes sideways or when I need to talk about birth or decompress from a tough day at work. A big hug and much love to this person.

Kim Vopni is a self-professed pelvic health evangelist and is known as 'The Vagina Coach.' Kim is a certified fitness professional who wants to end the suffering associated with pelvic floor dysfunction. Kim is a published author, a passionate speaker, and a women's health educator. Kim is the founder of 'Pelvienne Wellness Inc,' a company offering pelvic health programs, products, and coaching for people in pregnancy, parenthood, and menopause. Find more about Kim at **www.vaginacoach.com** and on social media '@vaginacoach'.

Noriko Ishibashi is a colleague and an amazing doula. Noriko has been instrumental in helping me write content for the birth tricks. Noriko also works at the South Community Birth Program, and has a thriving private practice in Vancouver, Canada. Contact at:
DoulaMatch.net

Huge love and respect for my friend and Midwife **Michelle (Entwhistle) Bergot**, helping edit some medical jargon for me. I have had the pleasure and privilege of working with so many midwives in my career. Midwives are truly special people!

Paula Jaspar MEd, RMT, published Author. Owner of Family Center Therapeutics in Vancouver, Canada. The very talented Paula is the author of *Massage for Birth Techniques.* These should enhance your birth experience and can be used daily to decompress with your new baby. **vanfct.com**

Kim James, owner of 'Doula Match. Find your *ideal* Birth or Post Partum Doula for your birth in North America.'
www.doulamatch.net

Genevieve Howland for the use of 'One Icon' to show you how easy it is to make a one-page visual birth plan, downloadable from their site: **MamaNatural.com**
www.mamanatural.com/visual-birth-plan/

SIDS, Sudden Infant Death Syndrome, from **canada.ca** website. I have used some parts of their fact sheet.

Mrs Dhillon's Kitchen: I can not bake, so I defer to Mrs Dhillon. This is all over the internet and social media with labor cookie recipe and SO very much more. **mrsdhillonskitchen.co.uk**

Nadia Hawkins: BScN RN IBCLC, Hand Express for Colostrum **MoreMilkSooner.com**

Purple Crying I have referenced this in *Quick Guide Feeding, Pooping & More.* I find this to be a valuable site to learn more about why a baby cries and why we need to be extra gentle, and Not Shake a Baby. **www.dontshake.ca**

Thank you to the model Agnes Turton (pictures of Hip Squeeze)

Thank you to the Photographer Christine Germano

Birth
It is not easy
It always changes
It is not predictable
It can have bad outcomes
It is *the* most important day of your life

***

My Wish is to educate you to achieve an easier and shorter labor.

I have seen scary times when we (care providers) didn't think the baby would make it.

I have seen when a baby didn't make it.

I wish you much joy, laughter, and love as you raise your child(ren).

Contents

Chapter 1: Birth, Back in the 1940s

Back in 1945, my mother-in-law delivered the first of her four babies at Vancouver General Hospital VGH. The expectant parents were given a booklet, with specific instructions on how to care for their infants and exercises after 'confinement', which meant the time after having your baby, which we now refer to as Post Partum or the 4th Trimester.

My husband had kept the instruction pamphlet from his older siblings' birth, and it was fun to read. I can not imagine doing some of the required 'instructions'. Thankfully we have better information and a different set of 'instructions' today. I had my first baby at VGH, but *many* years after this booklet was published, thankfully, I was never given any of this information. I probably would have thrown it in the trash.

I have shortened the entire read. Here are some of the 'fun facts' that popped out to me on raising an infant 'back in the day':

- Faithful observance of the instructions and reports to the doctor will prevent many complications and difficulties.

- A specimen of your urine should be sent to your doctor once a month for the first 6 months and every 2 weeks thereafter. Collect in a clean gallon receptacle or any other container that will hold all the urine you pass in 24 hours.

- Dress and underskirts should be comfortably made and should hang from the shoulders after the fourth month (pregnant). Tight-fitting clothing, which is suspended from the waist, should not be worn. Avoid round, elastic garters, tight-fitted belts, collars and shoes. As soon as the abdomen enlarges, "perceptible refrain" from highly lacing your corset. A fitted maternity corset gives the expectant mother satisfaction and comfort and can be worn throughout pregnancy.

- Care of Breasts: After the 4th month, a secretion frequently forms at the nipples and dries, causing the nipple to crack. This is what has been suggested:

- Breast Tray; includes Castile Soap - small bowl - Jar of cotton balls - Mineral Oil. Be sure to scrub your hands and have all utensils thoroughly cleaned before caring for the nipples. Do not handle the Breasts. Keep the nipples and breasts scrupulously clean but wash with soft soap and water daily. After washing, anoint the nipples with liquid petrolatum or mineral oil to keep them soft.

The document goes on to give one paragraph for each of many topics like sleep, diet, bathing and exercise.

- (Cloth) diapers must be scrupulously clean; they should be placed in a container of water as soon as removed. When convenient, they are washed in the hottest suds; boil them if possible, and rinse thoroughly (3 times) to remove all traces of soap.

- Wear a surgical mask if you develop a cold. Most folks with colds take themselves off the visiting list. Be diplomatically firm that the baby is not in view to those with colds or other infections. And if baby must be kissed, the back of the neck is best - but never the mouth.

Some Don'ts: I can not imagine this was ever considered, but I found it a good laugh:

- Don't forget to 'bubble' your baby after a feed.

- If you feed the baby out of a silver mug, be careful that the cup is not too hot.
- Don't give the baby tea, coffee, beer, or wine of any kind, fried foods, pickles, pie, lollypops, any sort of candy, nuts, pancakes, berries, ice cream, decadent cakes, puddings or meat gravies.
- Don't buy bedding or clothing which can not be laundered satisfactorily.
- Though they cry, don't pick your baby up if they are well; a good lusty cry is an excellent exercise.
- Don't allow play after feeding hours.
- Don't wash out your baby's mouth unless your doctor tells you to.

After the confinement of six weeks, report to the doctor to determine if the pelvic organs are in good condition. Do not neglect this.

There are specific times to feed your baby, precisely every 3 hours.

The Vancouver General Hospital suggests feeding Milk Formula.

Use pasteurized or certified milk when fluid milk is ordered. 4% butterfat milk is usually certified milk pasteurized with none of the cream removed. Shake the container the milk is in to 'distribute' the cream evenly. 3.25% milk is standard whole milk, pasteurized. Mix well before using. Add sugar or syrup and boiled water.

As fun as it is to reminisce, I find living in this time, where chestfeeding or formula feeding is much easier. You will be tired enough to get through the first few months.

'After Care' or baby checks with your care provider last 6 weeks, it is a great time to ask the care provider any and all questions that pop up during early Post Partum for the baby and you.

Today in the Vancouver area, we have two hospitals to birth at; St Paul's Hospital is downtown, and they are waiting to move into a beautiful new maternity hospital a few miles away. Women's Hospital, where I work, is a maternity hospital, and Children's Hospital is connected to it with NICUs for all different levels of care.

Chapter 2: Journal Ideas; Pregnancy and the First Year

There is a common saying that pregnant people have a 'placenta brain', not literally. However, it feels like most of your brain power is being zapped away as you grow this baby in your tummy. It happens to every person, and it makes you feel like you are losing a bit of your mind as you become very forgetful. But do not worry, it comes back sometime around twelve months postpartum.

The idea of journaling or keeping a diary for pregnancy and for the first 18 months after the baby is born is so you can look back at the time this person was first in your womb and then arrived into your life. A simple truth, you will forget most or all about your pregnancy, labor, delivery and the first few years of their life.

A fun way to remember this time is to start journaling, buy a writing pad or make notes on a calendar or use the calendar on your phone or on your computer. This makes it easy to print and store/keep the document. Decorate and personalize your journal/diary to post on your fridge door or desk in your office or frame the special event and give to your child, now an adult, when they graduate from school or are getting married or have their own baby.

Here are some examples to get you started. Ask yourself the following questions for your journal/diary:

- What made me think I was pregnant and document that date, the date I confirmed I was pregnant?
- What was my first reaction when I found out I was pregnant?
- What am I doing in my life now – before the baby?
- Who and when did I tell I was pregnant, and what was the reaction the first time I heard my baby's heartbeat?

- Write down your weight and body measurements (all through pregnancy). Write down appointments and what was said.
- What cravings am I having?
- When did I first feel the baby move? What did it feel like?
- When was the first Ultrasound? Did I record the heartbeat with my phone during an Ultrasound? Did they tell me the sex of my baby?
- What am I doing in my life right now?
- What do I imagine the baby will be like? i.e., happy-go-lucky, the next leader of my country, more like me or the other parent.
- What was labor like?
- What was my first thought when I delivered? Any other important thoughts?
- Have some fun decorating your diary. Draw on it or paste pictures of the baby (ultrasounds). Keep notes short.
- What was going on in the world the day my baby was born? How much has the baby changed over each new year?
- How has that changed our family dynamics?
- Momentous occasions, 1st food, Crawl, Walk, First birthday.
- Start taking pictures of yourself in a mirror, track the growth of your belly and body.
- Make a collage cutout pictures of advertisements in the newspaper or advertising, i.e., the price of bread or a car, Who was popular in the news or media. What were the news headlines during this time? Picture of the Ultrasound of the baby, first pictures at delivery etc.

Pregnancy Journal/Diary:

My Estimated Due Date is _____________

I will be pregnant for 40 weeks or 10 months.

Week _______ My weight _________ Date_____________

I feel

____

____

____

I am supposed to

____

____

____

The World today is

____

____

____

What do I need to add to my routine this week

____

____

My next scheduled appointment is

____

____

My concern right now is

____

What do I want to ask my care provider

____

____

I noticed that something has changed

____

____

How big is my baby

____

What have I been dreaming about

____

____

Birth Journal:

I always write notes at a client's birth. I go over my notes the next time they call when they are having another baby. I have written many birth stories from these notes. It makes a beautiful memory of your baby's birth, and truth be told, your birth experience will fade quickly, and along with your pictures, and the journal, you can bring back your special day.

Have paper or a notebook for your partner - or an extra person at your delivery that can make notes of the time for everything that happens. Many times I have been asked questions, What time did the water break (the rupture of the amniotic fluid)? When did I get an epidural?

Suggested ideas to make notes on:

The name of the hospital you delivered at, or if you delivered at home Doctor or the Midwife names that delivered your baby

Who else was at your birth - Doula, Nurse, Anesthetist, anyone that left a positive impression and went the extra mile to ensure you felt safe and cared for

In Early labor, what time did contractions start, how long and how often were they? When did contractions start to pick up frequency and get stronger and more often? When did you or your partner realize you are 'not tolerating the contractions anymore'? Then as labor progressed, how did contractions change?

** This is an excellent tip for telling your care provider what time contractions started and then changed, and any other notable progression.

Write the time when you had a SROM - Spontaneous Rupture of Membranes and the color of the water.

Note when you had a AROM - Artificial Rupture of Membranes. When did labor pick up?

Was there an induction? If so, what and when did things start, i.e., was it Cervidil? I always note when a vaginal exam (VE) is done.

What coping skills worked best in early labor, AND then what worked best in active labor? When your labor got really hard (active) and what time did you ask for help or some relief from the pain, i.e., gas, epidural, massage, water wither tub or shower, ball

When did you start to push, and when was the baby born? What were your favorite positions during the pushing stage? How long was the labor (note times start to finish)

How long was your pushing time? Note when you started to push until your baby was delivered. What time was the baby born?

***Please do not forget to take a picture of the time the baby was born. Were you in the OR for Forceps or C-Section?

Who caught the baby, i.e., did you or your partner 'help' catch the baby, or did the doctor or the midwife or nurse catch the baby who cut the cord?

How much does the baby weigh at the 1-hour check-up?

Was there anything 'extraordinary' that happened when the baby was born, i.e., was there a cord around the baby's body? If so, how many times? Was the baby holding the cord, or did the baby have its hand at its face? When was the baby's first poo and first pee?

First thoughts about your new baby - did you fall in love immediately? Who did the baby look like (or if the baby is IVF)

Come up with any of your own questions.

Birth and Post Partum Diary / Journal

Baby _______________ comes home today __________________

Baby's parents are

____

Grandparents /Other Family

____

Animals in our house

____

My Baby is now ______ weeks old

Today's date _____________ they rolled over, smiled, tried to touch my face, tried to touch a toy or our pet

TODAY they weighed _____________

Chapter 3: 1st Trimester

1st Trimester, it's all new; you are officially pregnant! The growing baby inside your tummy may become the head of government, cook a meal in your favorite restaurant, or drill a cavity in your mouth. It is up to us to love unconditionally, nurture, and guide our babies to be the best they can be. Enjoy your pregnancy, the birth, and your baby. You are contributing the most important thing to this beautiful world that we all share. A healthy and loving human being.

Always be kind to your wee baby angel. They may have come here unexpectedly or after a long time of waiting. This baby feels your emotions and hears your words in utero. Your life and future is about to change forever, and meeting your baby will be the single most important day of your life!

Do you think you are pregnant? Have you missed your menstrual period? You may be feeling some common symptoms, more tired, or your breasts are tender or a bit swollen, you may feel bloated, or you are nauseous, or you are possibly going to the bathroom to pee more often. If you suspect you are pregnant, your body will have secretly been going through a lot of change. You might use a home pregnancy test or go see your doctor to confirm a pregnancy.

At the first appointment with your doctor, they will confirm your pregnancy, and they will ask you to have some blood work done at a lab. They will ask about any family history of any genetic disorders. They will do a physical exam, including a cervical exam and a Pap smear. Then they will calculate your expected due date, from your last menstrual period, on a small cardboard 'Pregnancy Wheel'. There will be many tests recommended by your care providers that are for your health and well-being to ensure the baby is healthy and growing inside your tummy.

Your care provider will pre-register you at the hospital, where they have privileges, where they deliver babies. They will guide you with any other tests or requirements as needed throughout your pregnancy.

A 'Primip', short for Primipara, refers to a person who is having their first baby. The labor may be long and complicated because, at first, the baby has to 'forge' the way through the birth canal.

A 'Multip', short for Multipara, refers to a person who has delivered one or more babies. If their first baby was a vaginal delivery, the multip or subsequent deliveries usually are faster and with less complication than the first birth. If, with your first baby, you went into the OR for a cesarean section, then you may be offered a VBAC.

In VBAC, Vaginal Birth After Cesarean, you are having another baby with the intention to have a vaginal birth this time, and quite often, this is very successful. You will have a 'trial' of labor, and this happens if all circumstances with labor are amenable. You would have discussed this with your care provider to see if you are a good candidate. Where I work, you are expected to have at least 18 months between your deliveries. If there is any reason the delivery is not successful, you will have another cesarean section, and it is suggested that no more than 3 cesarean sections are advised. There are times a VBAC is not successful, but it is really good for you and the baby to do a trial of labor with the outcome of having a vaginal birth, even if you know a Cesarean is inevitable. There also may be specific reasons you will be told it is not advisable to have a trial of labor.

Fun Fact: Ovulation is when the sperm and egg join together. The sperm can live for five days, and the egg can live for 24 hours after it is released from the ovaries. The window of opportunity to become pregnant is approximately 5 days each month.

Your team of doctors, midwives, doulas, and birthing places should be filled with people you are comfortable with and trust, and who can give you the care you want and may need.

Care providers may be a doctor, midwife, obstetrician, anesthetist, paediatrician, nurse, ultrasound technician, or other people who will routinely see you for prenatal checks during pregnancy, labor, and birth. They attend your labor and delivery, and they will follow the baby for six weeks postpartum, but after delivery, your postpartum care will be transferred back to your general practitioner. The first or second prenatal visit will be filled with questions about your health history and family history. The care provider will do a physical exam, including a pap smear, and weigh you. Your baby is developing and growing quite quickly, and the hormones in your body are preparing for big changes. The following are routine at a visit with your care provider:

- Care Providers will check your weight at all visits to keep track of your weight gain throughout your pregnancy.
- Blood pressure is checked.
- The baby's heartbeat is noted.
- Your belly and the feel of the baby from outside of the tummy are measured in later months.
- A chance to ask questions (make a list of questions to take to your care provider).

You should be seeing your care provider every four to six weeks until week 28, then every two or three weeks until week 36. In the last month, you should see them weekly until you deliver.

Doctor or midwife - hospital or home. If your doctor delivers babies, then you can stay with them for prenatal care, labor, and delivery. They may or may not attend home births, but they definitely attend hospital births. Your doctor will ask you your thoughts about choosing either hospital or home birth, and who you want to deliver your baby with, a midwife or them? If your doctor does not deliver babies, they will transfer care for your pregnancy, labor, and delivery. You can ask for guidance and referrals for a practitioner that will deliver in your community. All practitioners that deliver babies have a similar practice; they offer prenatal care for you and your baby during pregnancy, which keeps you and your baby healthy. Their office will set up regular appointments and all tests and ultrasounds needed at the appropriate time. You may already have a preference regarding where you want to deliver your baby, at a hospital or at home.

Your care provider will pre-register you at the birthing hospital, where they have privileges to practice, especially when you are planning a home birth. This ensures that if you need to transfer to a hospital from home birth, all your information is there for you.

Obstetrician - OB may have a private practice and/or work with a group of doctors at a hospital that specialises in complex and high-risk pregnancies. They will consult with your doctor or midwife to assess why the labor is not progressing or why the baby is not tolerating labor. It could be you or your baby having complications; you have high blood pressure; your cervix is not progressing; the baby is having a high heart rate or having dips in the heartbeat. They may want to try to rotate or turn the baby that is not in the most ideal position, or an emergency, where you might need help with an expedited delivery in the delivery suite, or you need to go to the OR (operating room) for forceps, vacuum or Cesarean Section. To prevent problems in a long delivery, they will try options that can help you dilate and vaginally deliver your baby. They might suggest an augment or induction.

Midwifery care is unique, and they are fully qualified to deliver babies. The training includes natural ways and the latest techniques for you to have a healthy pregnancy and delivery. They also uphold the same professional standard of care as doctors. They offer prenatal care during pregnancy, but allow a longer time for each regular appointment, which gives you more time to ask more questions and get to know each other better. They specialize in home deliveries, but if a problem arises in labor, for you or the baby, they transfer you to the hospital, where more options for helping your delivery are available. They attend both home and hospital births.

Fun Trick: When you go to any care provider appointments, and they listen to your baby's heart rate, record that on your cell phone.

Importantly if there's anything out of the ordinary, for example, if something feels different to you, or you are feeling itchy, you may or may not have a rash, you are in discomfort, it may be on your hands or the soles of your feet, and/or other places. The itch may be worse at night and bother you so that you can not get any sleep; this most likely is Cholestasis. If your vision is off, or you are stressed or anxious, then call your care provider, either talk to them or go in for a visit.

Vitamins & Medications: Your care provider will ask you to start taking prenatal vitamins to help with the growth and development of your baby. Vitamins in your diet that contain calcium, iron, and folic acid enhance the baby's brain development in the first days and weeks of conception. You may be eating foods with this in them, but taking a daily supplement helps you to get enough to prevent major birth defects in the baby's brain (anencephaly) and spine (spina bifida).

Before taking aspirin, ibuprofen, or other drugs (i.e., medication for a cold), ask your care provider about what to take that is safe for the baby.

Tests: There are many routine labs and screening tests that your care provider will ask you to take all throughout pregnancy. These will help them to know that you and the baby are keeping healthy. In your first appointment, you will be given a requisition for blood work;

to find out your blood type and the RH (rhesus) factor, screen for anemia, check for immunity of rubella and test for hepatitis B, syphilis and HIV or other STDs, all done at a lab.

An ultrasound will be booked for approximately week 8 of pregnancy. The first ultrasound/sonogram appointment is fairly easy. You lay down on an exam table, and the person doing the procedure will put gel on your tummy and take a handheld wand that they can easily slide across your baby bump. It shows up on a screen as a black and white ultrasound picture of inside the placenta where your baby lives until born.

The technician will take measurements of the fetus, and you can listen to the beating heart and see your baby on the ultrasound machine for the first time. The baby's size will confirm your due date, and more importantly, the technician will confirm if you are having a single baby or twins, triplets, or more. They check to see whether the organs are developing properly or not.

NIPT Test, or Non-Invasive Prenatal Screening Test, taken around week 10, is an elective test as an option to help identify if the baby is at risk of any genetic abnormalities, such as chromosomal disorder. They can determine the risk of disorders like Down syndrome and other conditions caused by missing or extra X and Y chromosomes. The test can also tell the gender of your baby.

Fun Facts: With any pregnancy, but especially with your first, it is normal to be worried or anxious. You wonder if your baby is okay, growing in your tummy. This feeling lasts until you hear your baby take its first breath and cry! Then you will truly relax.

Being excited and terrified is an understatement, but falling in love immediately with your baby is inevitable.

The full moon and new moon are baby magnets; we have more babies born around these two times of the calendar month. I have read that a baby born at a full moon is an old soul, and a new moon is a new soul.

Birth Tip: Do not tell your family and friends your exact due date. Not many babies are born on the actual due date; they deliver between week 39 to week 41, simply because every person's cycle is different. For example, if your estimated due date is May 19, tell everyone the baby is due mid-May. Your loving and concerned family and friends will be texting or phoning daily near the end of your pregnancy, and it can make you more anxious. You will doubt yourself that you will ever go into labor. The last few weeks of pregnancy should be about you doing your 'birth tricks' and staying *stress-free*. Start learning how to relax now!

Practice breathing. I get that you might think this sounds silly; however, this is a fabulous way to calm yourself at any moment, more importantly, while raising your beautiful children. There are many different practices that teach breathing, and this is effective and easy to learn. Slowing our breath allows us to let go of anxiety and stress in our bodies, and helps us navigate and control our minds so we do not *overthink* our contractions or other life issues. Start now and practice daily. Learn how to relax yourself throughout your pregnancy, and you will breathe amazingly during your labor and the push.

Take a big slow, long breath, pause, and exhale big. Repeat, repeat, repeat…

If, at any time, you have a strong painful headache; visual problems; or any discharge that is clear or bloody; severe pain in your tummy, or something that does not feel right, contact your doctor immediately. You can easily over-exert yourself just by doing regular activities, long work days, and playing extreme sports. Experts say that you should be able to do what you normally did before becoming pregnant, but try to use common sense. If you tire more easily, start *now* to learn how to take some rest, stay hydrated, and put your feet up. Find some natural therapy practitioners that can help keep you relaxed, possibly yoga, shiatsu, acupuncture, homeopathy, and, later on, prenatal massage, to mention a few.

You will gradually and gently gain weight over the next 36 weeks due to the changes and growth of your baby. Your body will change a lot; your breasts will become bigger, and your back may give you some pain because of your growing tummy. You can expect to gain 25 - 40 pounds for an average single pregnancy, but less or more weight might indicate something else is going on in your body. They monitor your weight for a variety of reasons, so you stay healthy and the baby does not get too big.

Your taste and sense of smell, your nose and tongue perceive things differently, and you may notice that you taste and/or smell foods much differently. You may no longer tolerate certain scents or cooking smells. You may start to have cravings for something that you would never normally eat. Cravings can be a factor in weight gain, which will be difficult to lose after the baby arrives because, with a newborn, you will not have very much time to work off your baby weight. The taste and scent issues should all resolve themselves soon after the baby delivers.

Vision Changes: Vision changes, blurred vision, and dry eyes may be common in pregnancy. It is important to tell your care provider, as it may mean something else a bit more serious could be going on. Your vision usually goes back to 'normal' or the way it was after giving birth.

Eating and staying hydrated during pregnancy, labor, chestfeeding baby, drinking lots of water, eating fresh, healthy, and organic foods, and exercising. It may be beneficial to start eating smaller portions more often during the day, especially if you have some morning sickness.

Dietary Options: It is recommended that you stay as healthy as possible by choosing healthy options for the food you eat and your beverage intake. Avoid processed foods, caffeine, and nicotine. You may not have 'cravings' yet, but they definitely can compromise your intention of eating a healthy diet during pregnancy.

The first trimester is SO important in the baby's development, where body structure and organ systems develop. Choosing a balanced diet in addition to exercise will help keep you healthier during pregnancy. It can be a challenge and cause other problems, like gestational diabetes later on. You will have an easier pregnancy and delivery if you can make changes earlier on.

Healthy choices; proteins, fresh vegetables, and fruit. Drink healthy beverages, and stay away from liquor and other caffeine or sugar-filled beverages and candy. Water is always best. This healthier diet change should last from when you are trying to get pregnant, OR the time you find out you are pregnant, until you finish chest feeding your baby.

A misconception in pregnancy is that we can eat whatever we want. You run the risk of being overweight, which is harder to take off after the baby is here or leads to other complications in pregnancy. If the baby gains more weight, that could lead to a possible cesarean delivery. Always check with your care provider regarding what *not* to eat. Cravings feel real in pregnancy but can do more harm than the satisfaction it brings in the moment.

Consult your care provider for the safety of eating raw or undercooked meats, fish, chicken, or other foods. They need to be cooked at specific temperatures. A food thermometer should be placed in the thickest part of the food.

I live in Canada, and it is recommended NOT to eat raw sushi when pregnant. Please follow the guidelines in your country and from your care provider.

The following food should be cooked to at least these temperatures:

Meat	- at least 145 degrees F or 63 degrees C
Ground meat	- at least 160 degrees F or 71 degrees C
Poultry	- at least 165 degrees F or 74 degrees C
Fish	- at least 165 degrees F or 74 degrees C

Fish or shellfish, ceviche, sushi, and sashimi should not be eaten raw, and it is not recommended during pregnancy. Smoked seafood can have Listeria. For fruit and vegetables, they should be peeled and/or washed thoroughly.

Make sure when preparing all the above, you clean the cutting boards and knives thoroughly, so you do not cross-contaminate bacteria.

Avoid unpasteurized products, such as juices or cider, raw milk, soft cheese, and other raw milk products. They may contain E.Coli or Listeria.

If made with pasteurized milk, you may eat hard cheese, cheddar, Parmesan, Brie, feta, Camembert, and Roquefort, to name a few.

Uncooked eggs can contain Salmonella, so make sure you cook eggs thoroughly.

Do not eat the following homemade items, hollandaise sauce, eggnog, raw batter, salad dressings, and ice creams.

No to pre-made deli salads - ham, chicken, seafood salads, or pates.

No to hot dogs and luncheon/deli meats or poultry, cold cuts, or dry sausage.

No to raw sprouts, radish, mung bean, or clover.

The foods mentioned below contain folic acid and are good for you to eat:

Asparagus - Avocado - Beans - Beets - Bread - Broccoli - Brussel Sprouts - Cauliflower - Carrots - Celery - Cereals - Citrus Fruits - Corn - Eggs - Leafy Green Vegetables - Lentils - Okra - Oranges & Orange Juice - Pasta - Peas - Rice - Seeds and Nuts - Squash Liver - Whole Grain Products.

Foods that contain Calcium and are good for you to eat:

Dairy, and I do not mean ice cream, unless in moderation. Milk - Cheese - Yogurt. This will obviously not be eaten if you are lactose intolerant. Your care provider will suggest healthy alternatives.

Foods that provide calcium and other vitamins to our diet for a healthier baby:

Legumes, which are plant-based and contain fiber, protein, iron, and folate, are Lentils - Peas - Beans - Chickpeas - Soybeans - Tofu - Peanuts - Sweet potatoes - Cooked eggs - Broccoli - Dark leaf greens - Salmon, and other seafood - Lean meat.

Great food additions for your diet:

Berries fresh and dried - Fish liver oil by capsule - Avocados - Whole grains - AND WATER; you can drink as much water as you can, from the start of pregnancy, during labor, and afterwards when you are chestfeeding. Every day!

Foods that contain Iron:

Dark left vegetables - Dried beans & peas - Dried fruit - Egg yolks - Fish - Liver - Meat - Nuts – Poultry.

Foods that contain Magnesium:

Cocoa - Dried beans & peas - Nuts - Seafood - Whole-grain products.

Foods that contain Vitamin B6:

Liver - Meat - Whole-grain products.

Foods that contain Vitamin E:

Eggs - Cereals - Fish - Leafy vegetables - Milk - Meat - Vegetable Oils.

Foods that contain Zinc:

Dried Beans & Peas - Milk - Meat - Nuts - Seafood

Bad Habits: We know what is bad for us; drugs, cigarettes, liquor, and unhealthy eating, i.e., fast food and pre-packaged foods, because they have a lot of preservatives and calories.

I hope that your partner will honor this time by eating in solidarity with you to help and encourage you to eat healthy.

Many over-the-counter cough syrup, pain, and sleep medications contain alcohol and aspirin. Ask your care provider before taking anything.

Give up or reduce coffee and black tea, and switch to herbal tea. Chocolate and some energy drinks have more caffeine than we realize, which is not good for growing a baby. It is advised by health organizations that we eliminate or drastically reduce our caffeine intake. Consider abstaining for the 40 weeks and the chest feeding time to ensure your baby grows as healthy as possible. This gift of health to your baby will last their whole lifetime.

Everything that you put into your body will go through the umbilical cord and into your baby.

Things to Avoid During Pregnancy: Baths and Showers *are* very good for relaxing. Although, the water should be kept at a comfortable temperature, not too hot, as it can be harmful to the fetus as they are already in warm fluid in the amniotic sack. Sauna and hot tubs can easily raise your body temperatures too high and can cause serious problems or loss of pregnancy.

At work or in your home, be aware of airborne chemicals that are used to clean. If you can breathe it in, or your body can absorb it, by being close, then take extra precautions to prevent exposure while pregnant. The human you are growing will get small amounts of anything that is breathed in or absorbed by you. If there is smog in the area where you live, wear a mask.

If you're pregnant and you own a cat, there is a possibility that your outdoor cat has been infected with a toxoplasma parasite that passes through its feces. It is best, when you are pregnant, to avoid cleaning the litter box. If you have to clean the litter box, make sure you use gloves and wash your hands very well afterwards. There is the chance that if you were to pass it to your unborn baby, later in the baby's life, it may cause blindness or mental disabilities.

Morning Sickness or Nausea: Not everyone gets morning sickness, but it is very common, and it can start around week six and last into week fourteen. However, it knows no time. Some people have a milder version. It may be uncomfortable, and sometimes you feel like you can not keep anything down. Crackers Crackers Crackers! Soda crackers and ginger ale or water are usually suggested to be consumed in small amounts but frequently. You can squeeze fresh ginger into your food or into camomile tea, water, or ginger snaps. Sniff lemons or squeeze them into your water.

Also suggested for the morning to help subside nausea is that you get out of bed and gently move about your home.

When it is severe, you may feel nauseous and will vomit most of the day and into the evening. The lack of fluids will dehydrate you, and the lack of food can compromise your pregnancy. You may lose weight, and you will not be meeting the nutritional needs of you and your baby. You should seek help from your care provider and discuss what medications might help tame your tummy at this time. This miserable part of pregnancy will, at some point, slow down and phase away.

Heartburn, also called indigestion or acid reflux, is common and can be uncomfortable during pregnancy. Your body is going through hormone changes, and the shape of your body is changing with the growing baby. Usually, your food moves slower throughout the intestines and the stomach and is compressed by the uterus as it grows and moves higher into the abdomen. It may help if you eat smaller portions more frequently. Talk to your care provider about what dietary changes you can make and what possible antacids or natural remedies might help. I have had many clients that are still having heartburn during labor.

Constipation: With so much change happening to your body and the growing baby in your uterus, there will be changes in your bowels. If you have constipation, irregular bowel movements, or hemorrhoids, basic care would be to hydrate with lots more water. More high-fiber food, fruits, vegetables, beans, and whole grains.

At week 18 (approximately), your care providers will set a long appointment for an ultrasound, for which there are many reasons why; to take measurements of the baby's limbs and the head circumference; to check the chambers of the heart, and the heart is beating normally; also including the brain, stomach, kidneys, skull, and genitals. This information is vital, so your care provider knows that the baby is growing and the organs look healthy. If there is a concern, then a more detailed ultrasound would be booked. People usually ask about the sex of their baby, but even at this ultrasound, the technician may get the gender wrong, and so they usually decline to tell.

Exercise: If you do not have a regular exercise routine, now is a good time to start something that is sustainable during your pregnancy. It can help with the labor and pushing, and you can slowly work up to a regular routine by the end of your pregnancy. Walking is a great start; dance around your home, and do some gentle stretching. Yoga or pilates is a very gentle way to keep your body and muscles limber and stretched. Start practicing at least two or three times a week or daily for your entire pregnancy. There are many yoga positions specific to pregnant people.

Hot yoga *is not* recommended while pregnant.

Swimming is a great activity, especially when you float in the water, and it takes the pressure off your joints from the weight of a growing baby. Read in the 3rd Trimester chapter, for more information, if you find that you have a breech baby.

Where I live, we have a strenuous hike called the 'Grouse Grind.' It is on Grouse Mountain and is a serious workout in itself. I have had several clients that have kept up their routine of hiking several times a week, up until the day they have gone into labor. Their labors were quicker, and the push was faster.

Exercise definitely makes a difference in labor, and it can give you the will and stamina to get through both labor and the pushing stage.

Changes Inside and Out: Your body will start changing in many different ways. Your monthly period/menstrual cycle has stopped. Your uterus starts to grow; in an upwards motion. Eventually, when the baby is bigger, you will notice you can not eat as much as before, and you may experience indigestion. The sack baby is in, is getting bigger, and sits next to your bladder; this will cause you to urinate more frequently. All pregnant people complain about going to the bathroom every two hours, all night long.

Your chest is making unique changes; they may feel tender or sore, one of the first signs that might have made you suspect you were pregnant. In early pregnancy, the hormone progesterone is released, helping with the growth of the milk ducts and forming lobules (milk-producing glands in the breast) for milk production. The area around the nipple, the areola, is usually light brown or pink and starts to change to darker brown in color. They also become bigger in the early stages of pregnancy and then bigger as your milk comes in after birth.

Body Changes (what an understatement): Weight gain and water retention are quite common. Changes can start early, but the most visible should start around week 32 and last until you have delivered. Fluid/water retention and the changes in your body, with increased blood circulation, will show in aches and swelling in your face, hands, legs, and feet. As the weeks pass by, practice relaxing with your feet up on a pillow, on your couch, or in bed.

Body Weight: An average weight gain is 25 - 35 lbs or 11 - 15 kg during your pregnancy. A baby's average weight at birth is 7 - 9 lbs or 3 - 4 kg. Many factors affect how much weight you will gain over 40 weeks of pregnancy. If you have 'morning sickness,' trying to keep food down may be a challenge, or you may have a sensitivity to the smell of some foods. So you might lose weight, or if you have *cravings* and can not stop eating the yummy and fattening foods filled with sugar, fats, and starch, you may gain too much weight. Staying within the standard weight gain helps make your pregnancy easier and the weight loss afterwards much easier.

Your sleep can be compromised by hormone changes, your growing baby, and anxiety and worry. Getting up to the bathroom every couple of hours, and having trouble getting back to sleep, is normal. Your sleep pattern will change over time during your pregnancy. *Learn now to rest or nap!* It will serve you well all through pregnancy and especially during the postpartum time.

Sleeping on your back and positioning yourself to stay comfortable in bed may get more difficult as your belly grows, especially as you get closer to the 2nd and 3rd trimesters. Most or many people prefer one side of the other to sleep on. Most times, we simply do not pay it much attention. If you are a tummy sleeper, you will change that up very soon; it simply does not work to have a growing baby in that position.

Practice now! Sleep on your left and your right side, and change every other night. I would suggest props, a rolled or folded blanket that fits under one side of your back so you are not lying flat. Care providers suggest that you do not lay flat on your back in bed as you progress in your pregnancy. After week 20, the weight of your uterus can compress a major blood vessel. This can disrupt the blood flow to your baby and can make you nauseated, dizzy, and short of breath.

The earlier you start to make a change, the easier it is to do. By the third trimester, your baby will get themselves stuck in your pelvis on the side you favor. It can be difficult to encourage them to move, and it can lead to a longer and more painful labor. Props can be blankets, pillows, or a longer body pillow. I have seen a pillow that wraps from the foot up to the head and backs down to the other foot. It curls right around the person. You will need extra support as the baby starts to grow and is eventually uncomfortable in your tummy.

Put the blanket or pillow in between your knees; behind your back to support yourself. To relieve the hip that you are lying on, put a small folded hand towel under the lower foot that rests on the bed.

We tend to have a favorite side, and as your baby grows inside, it will sleep on that side as well. They get their head lodged in the pelvis, and moving it can be difficult the larger they grow. By the third trimester, we want the baby to move into the most ideal position for delivery, so you have a shorter and easier time in labor.

Once your baby is born, sleep is even more important. Feeding every 3 hours, a diaper change, and then trying to put the baby to bed will only leave you a very short period of time to take your rest. After 9 months pregnant, then the first month or two with your newborn, you will be exhausted!

Learn to sleep in an ideal position and how to rest or nap

Music and Meditation are very good ways to help you relax.

Feeding Baby (see Dr. Jack Newman's full Chapter): I respect everyone's choice to use their own pronouns. For this chapter, I respect Dr. Newman's choice and have not changed any words. He has graciously sent me a lengthy chapter that should answer ALL your feeding questions. I encourage you to read and re-read this chapter, so it will be easier to go back and review when your baby is here. If you have questions, Dr. Newman has a link to his website for more information.

Birth Tip: No one believes it when they are told, "You lose your memory during pregnancy and get it back around the baby's first birthday". But don't laugh; it is true.

You have no control in pregnancy, labor, and birth. Find a team of care providers that you trust and are comfortable with. Stay positive and healthy. Seek as much information, to prepare for this amazing life-changing experience.

Chapter 4: How Big is my Baby, Now?

- Week 1:
- Week 2:
- Week 3:
- Week 4: Baby is best known as a Zygote and the size of a poppy seed.
- Week 5: Looks like a tadpole or as big as a peppercorn, and the brain, spinal cord, heart, and blood vessels are developing.
- Week 6: Size of a pomegranate seed starts to develop arm buds.
- Week 7: Size of a blueberry; arm buds now look like paddles.
- Week 8: Size of a cranberry or bean, length 1.6 cm; weighs 1 gram; hands and feet have webbed fingers and toes.
- Week 9: Size of a cherry, length 2.3 cm; weighs 2 grams.
- Week 10: Size of a Kumquat, length 3.1 cm; weighs 4 grams.
- Week 11: Size of a Brussel Sprout, length 4.1 cm; weighs 7 grams.
- Week 12: Size of a Passion Fruit, length 5.4 cm; weighs 14 grams. Fingernails, Toenails, and toes are forming, and a fine layer of hair covers most of the body.
- Week 13: Size of Lemon, length 7.4 cm; weighs 23 grams. Vocal cords are developing.
- Week 14: Size of a Nectarine, length 8.7 cm; weighs 43 grams, the start of the 2nd trimester. The internal organs are formed and will now mature until born.

- Week 15: Size of an Apple, length 10.1 cm; weighs 70 grams, the brain now controls all muscles in the body, and is able to move and do somersaults.
- Week 16: Size of Avocado, length 11.6 cm; weighs 100 grams, they can suck their thumb.
- Week 17: Size of a Pear, length 13 cm; weighs 140 grams. The baby can hiccup, fingernails are developed.
- Week 18: Size of a Peach, length 14.2 cm; weighs 190 grams; fingers have their unique fingerprints.
- Week 19: Size of a Mango, length 15.3 cm; weighs 240 grams, legs are longer than arms.
- Week 20: Size of Artichoke, length 16.4 cm; weighs 300 grams, thin eyebrows, and some hair on the head.
- Week 21: Body is as long as a Carrot, length 27.7 cm; weighs 360 grams, the skin responds to touch. If you put pressure on your belly, the baby will move or push back.
- Week 22: Size of a Papaya, length 27.8 cm; weighs 430 grams; lungs are developing rapidly and will begin making a protein called surfactant, which will help them breathe independently once they are born.
- Week 23: Size of an Eggplant, length 28.9 cm; weighs 501 grams. Brain and hearing are more developed, and the baby starts to recognize your voice.
- Week 24: Size of an ear of Corn, length 30 cm; weighs 600 grams, nostrils are open, and they do some practice breathing; they inhale amniotic fluid.
- Week 25: Size of an Acorn Squash, length 34.6 cm; weighs 660 grams, develops a firm grasp and may reach and grab the umbilical cord, can stick their tongue out.
- Week 26: Size of a Zucchini, length 35.6 cm; weighs 760 grams, eyebrows and eyelashes are now defined, also some more hair on the head.

- Week 27: Size of a Cauliflower, length 36.6 cm; weighs 875 grams, they can distinguish between your and other people's voices.
- Week 28: Size of Kabocha Squash, length 37.6 cm; weighs 1005 grams, beginning to open eyes and blink.
- Week 29: Size of large Butternut Squash, length 38.6 cm; weighs 1153 grams; skin is wrinkly, but fat accumulates so baby will fill out.
- Week 30: Size Large Cabbage, length 39.9 cm; weighs 1319 grams, has cycles of sleep and wake; you are feeling more kicks.
- Week 31: Size of Long Bunch of Leeks, length 41.1 cm; weighs 1502 grams, will start gaining approx. 23 grams per week till birth.
- Week 32: Size of a Napa Cabbage, length 42.4 cm; weighs 1702 grams. The last taste buds are developed and may acquire a preference for the food 'you' eat because they are swallowing amniotic fluid.
- Week 33: Size of a Pineapple, length 43.7 cm; weighs 1918 grams, lanugo, the fine hair that covers baby's body to keep them warm, is starting to disappear.
- Week 34: Size of a Cantaloupe, length 45 cm; weighs 2146 grams, Bones are fully developed now, and baby can turn its head and move the body from side to side.
- Week 35: Size of a Honeydew, length 46.2 cm; weighs 2383 grams. They should be head down in the uterus in preparation for birth.
- Week 36: Size of Canary Melon, length 47.4 cm; weighs 2622 grams, their wrinkly skin is starting to fill out with body fat.
- Week 37: Size of a stalk of Swiss Chard, length 48.6 cm; weighs 2859 grams. The baby starts to fill all space and is mostly stretching and wiggling.

- Week 38: Size of stalk of Rhubarb, length 49.8 cm; weighs 3083 grams. Connections are forming in the brain that help to swallow and sleep better once born.
- Week 39: Size of a Watermelon, length 50.7 cm; weighs 3288 grams. Vernix has mostly shed itself, it is the creamy white substance.
- Week 40: Size of a Pumpkin, length 51.2 cm; weighs 3462 grams.
- Week 41: length 51.7 cm; weighs 3597 grams.
- Week 42: length 51.5 cm; weighs 3685.
- Week 43: Never heard of having to wait this long.

Size and weight are average; it usually depends on the parents.

Chapter 5: 2nd Trimester

Welcome to the 2nd Trimester. This is such a fun and transitional time. Around weeks 16 - 20, your body starts making big changes, and you can almost watch your blooming baby bump! Some people may still have morning sickness, but it should be gone by now or very soon. There will be many more routine tests to ensure both you and your baby are healthy and growing as expected. More importantly, you will be halfway through your pregnancy soon, and then you get to meet your baby!

You may be making plans for where in your home the baby will have a space. You will need a bassinet and change table for starters; a crib is only needed later on when they are several months old. Many people tend to think big because of the expanding family, and start renovating or packing up and moving to a bigger home. These next weeks will be filled with birth preparation, organizing life for when this new person arrives, and all the things you need for them. It is an exciting time because you are starting or increasing your family.

Exercising: If you have a regular exercise routine, it should be easy to keep up with for as long as it makes sense and there is no harm to the baby. Your care provider may ask you to slow down or stop if they are concerned. Some of my clients that are used to a strong workout routine seem to have an easier labor and a faster push for their delivery. It appears they seem to have more reserve to push the baby out.

As the baby grows, especially in the last two months, some activities may not be safe or may give you discomfort, so reduce or stop them. I have had clients that refuse to stop riding their bicycles, but there is the possibility that your balance may be compromised, and the size and weight in your tummy can throw your sense of balance off, and you may fall.

If you have not been exercising, then please start gently now and slowly increase every week. Fresh air, stretching, yoga, and walking, for starters, will make a big difference in your well-being. Read and do all of the birth exercises from birth tricks.

When to slow down on some exercises: With my first baby, my doctor asked me to refrain from water skiing, snow skiing, or horseback riding as the pregnancy gets farther along. Your equilibrium becomes compromised as your body changes and grows, and it is directly caused by the hormone progesterone, as it is elevating quickly in your body. Your body and balance change weekly, and the chance of falling while doing sports or other regular day-to-day routines should be avoided or toned down. For instance, climbing up a ladder or riding a bike. The best practice is to check with your care provider regarding when you should slow down or stop.

Client's Story: With permission, I am telling you a client's story, told to me during labor; it made me laugh out loud! My client and their friend, both pregnant at the same time, often spoke very candidly to each other. They mentioned to the friend that they would 'leak' from time to time, especially when they would cough or laugh. The client told me the story of getting up to buy a drink while watching a game at an arena and leaked. They started to text crying face emojis and more to each other for support when they leaked. They went fairly deep with this 'newfound issue' that the friend told my client when they go grocery shopping, they tuck a small glass jar with fluid in it, into their pocket, so if they were to 'leak' down an aisle, you let the jar fall, on the floor and say "oops sorry it dropped." Over time, they realized that this was a part of pregnancy, and they wished someone had told them that it is common to 'leak' while pregnant. They formed the '*Pissy Pants Support*' club; it is anonymous - but you can start your own branch where ever you are. It is assured that all pregnant people will have some uncontrollable bladder issues.

This is very common during pregnancy, though, because the growing baby can put pressure on the bladder, and it is common to carry into postpartum. Take extra care to read the chapter on Pelvic Core Health by Kim Vopni for helpful suggestions.

Pelvic Core Health: It is such an important topic these days and is sometimes hard to access. Thanks to a colleague, Kim Vopni, who is a self-professed pelvic evangelist known as 'The Vagina Coach,' has written a full chapter on pelvic floor health. There are visuals and a lengthy description about how pregnancy and labor can change our body and then how to get your body back to pre-pregnancy.

Yoga: It is a popular way of exercising your body and soul. It is more than exercise; it is a philosophy and way of life. You can practice it everywhere, in studios, online, and on social media, for example, Youtube, in the comfort of your home. There is specific instruction for pregnant people, which includes all 3 trimesters and postpartum. Any practice that teaches you to breathe and, releases stress and anxiety, increases strength and flexibility is a must-have for your birth preparation. A huge part of labor is breathing big breaths and relaxing, then when pushing, holding your breath and using all your strength to push.

With the baby growing inside, they may put pressure on your body, so try to find ways to relieve your sore and tired body. Go for body treatments and massage, or have someone at home give you a rub. Start Yoga or gentle stretching techniques, and learn about taking a bath or shower for the simple task of relaxation. Raise your feet on a couch more often and listen to music.

Acupuncture and Acupressure: It applies the same principles to promote relaxation and wellness and to treat disease. Traditional Chinese medicine theory describes special points that lie along the meridians in our body. It is believed that through these invisible channels flow vital life force energy, called qi (ch'i). Also, the 12 major meridians connect specific organs, or networks of organs, that organize a system of communication throughout our body. The meridians begin at the fingertip, connect to the brain and then connect to an organ associated with a certain meridian. When one of these meridians is blocked or out of balance, we have an illness, and we can have physical, mental, and emotional conditions that give us discomfort.

The goal is to restore health and balance to the body's energy channels and to regulate the Yin and Yang forces in our body. The practice of using very thin needles for acupuncture or pressure by a finger or thumb for acupressure on the same and specific parts of the body to release blockages so our internal pathways of energy can be corrected and flow again. This is very effective in relieving morning sickness, anxiety, heartburn, constipation, insomnia, and hip/pelvic pain. As you get further along into your pregnancy, positioning the baby most ideally, helping them turn from the breech or posterior position, cervical ripening, sciatica, and back pain can give you grief.

The most important and specific pressure points on the body to help prepare for labor and birth can be found in ***Acupressure Points & Double Hip Squeeze;*** *this is in its own chapter.* If you happen to go in for a treatment, watch closely or ask where exactly they put the needle so you will know where to touch by fingers/hand pressure at the same spot. You should be able to feel the release and effects of the pressure very quickly.

Routine testing at your care provider appointments will monitor that you are staying healthy and not gaining too much weight and have your blood pressure taken. They listen to the baby's fetal heart tones and measure your tummy to make sure the baby is growing inside. They will ask how you are doing, if you have any complaints or if you have questions. Use this time to ask about what to expect until the next visit.

Baby's Heart Rate - Intermittent Auscultation: Auscultate means 'to listen' to the internal sounds of the body. Your care providers will listen to the baby's heart rate during all regular visits, at home births and in labor. It is a quick and easy way to know that the baby is healthy and tolerating pregnancy and later on during labor. They use a stethoscope, or a Doppler fetal monitor, which is a hand-held ultrasound transducer; it has a volume switch that you can turn up to hear the baby's heartbeat. They put a thick gel on the end of the wand 'transducer' that goes on your tummy. They find the best place to hear the baby's heartbeat and then listen for one minute as they count the beats. This allows you to be very mobile during your labor or have time in a shower or tub. Midwives use a pin horn, a type of stethoscope that is a hollow device made of wood or metal, approximately 20 cm long. The midwife will hold the wide end against your abdomen and their ear at the other end. They can also use this to find fetal positioning.

Electronic Fetal Monitoring: You will lay on a hospital bed, and the care provider will wrap two stretchy belts around your body, midsection around your tummy, the first one near the waist and the second belt between the waist and pubic bone, to listen to baby's heart rate. They will attach one small round monitoring devise onto each of the belts that have wires attached to a plug that goes into a machine that has a screen to watch and record all data. The information shows on the screen and provides a paper copy. This information tells the care provider when the contraction starts and ends and gives them *an idea* of how strong the contraction might be (the monitors are not too efficient at advising the strength of the contraction). They apply the gel on the monitor, which is against the tummy, to receive a better pick-up, when listening to the baby's heart rate.

There are down falls with this system, it can be hard to move around, or bounce on a ball, and have the monitors stay in place.

You may be asked to lay on the bed and not move, so the pick up of heart beats is heard.

This monitoring tells the care provider how the baby's heart rate is responding to the contractions. If the baby is not tolerating, then the care providers can keep close attention to the baby, in the event they need help, by having a faster delivery.

Both Auscultation and EFM will become very familiar, as they will be used up until your baby is delivered. It does give one comfort to listen to their baby's heart rate.

At weeks 18 - 20, you will have a 'detailed' ultrasound/sonogram appointment. The procedure will be much longer, up to an hour. Care providers want to compare the growth of the baby's limbs and body length from the first ultrasound. There are many images taken of all parts of the body; face, spine, chest, legs, feet, arms, hands, brain, heart, kidneys, stomach, diaphragm, bladder, genitals, and the umbilical cord. They measure the size of the fetus and the amount of amniotic fluid, and look to see where the placenta is lying.

You will see a bigger version of the baby, and the practitioner will give you a picture or two of the baby. Have the record button ready on your cell phone to listen to your baby's heart beating. It will be very hard to see the gender of the baby because the images are grey and blurry. It is very nice to watch on the screen the movements of your baby; they may be moving or making faces, or sucking their thumb. If you ask about the sex of your baby, they usually decline to say, for good reason; they are often not correct.

Around this, it is important to know that the baby is still moving and active. You may be asked to count the movements made by the baby in a two-hour period. As they grow, it will be more obvious and easier to feel their movements. If the baby is having a nap, they may not be moving. If you are not feeling these movements in the recommended time frame, contact your care provider. In a few months, you will be wishing they were not so big! As they get bigger, you realize you actually have a baby growing in your tummy. For fun, consider talking to your baby as they can hear you.

Author's True Story: My very good friend worked in the radiology department. When the technicians had a few moments free, they would have a look at my friend's baby in her tummy. For two pregnancies, the technician told her the wrong sex, and her partner was not impressed. It is the biggest reason why the technician will not tell you the sex of a baby; it is not definitive.

Baby moves and hears in your tummy: Their movements will become visible from the outside of your tummy and make it very evident that your pregnancy is progressing and now feels more real. It may be a bit uncomfortable as they continue to grow, you may get a foot up and under your rib cage, or you may not be able to eat as much as you used to because your baby is pushing up into your stomach.

Around week 18, your baby will be able to hear sounds in your body, like your heartbeat, then at week 27 to 29, they can hear outside sounds, music, and voices. Then at full term, they should be able to hear the same as an adult. If you have not yet started, you can start talking to your baby through the tummy. They will get to know your voice over the next months of your pregnancy. It is fun to read books out loud, sing to them and listen to music. Babies fussing around in your tummy can be soothed by listening to your voice or music. They also can hear the tone of an angry voice, and that can cause them confusion and stress.

I love to watch when the parent talks to the baby within that first half hour of life. The baby tilts their head up to match your face to the familiar voice. Soon their movements start to become restricted by their size, so you feel more arms and legs move and kick around. If the baby is head down, you get kicks up under your ribs, and what seemed like a thrilling time, becomes uncomfortable as they grow more. You will also have movements that make you jump, and your sleep might start becoming even more uncomfortable.

As long as you give permission, it is okay for other people to put their hand on your belly to feel the kicks and movements.

Screen for Gestational Diabetes to determine if you might have this type of diabetes during pregnancy, a result of your body not being able to produce enough insulin, to keep the sugars in your blood at their proper levels. The test is given between weeks 24 and 28, and involves you having a fizzy and unpleasant flavored drink, then waiting an hour and having your blood drawn to measure the blood sugar levels in your body.

After the diagnosis of gestational diabetes, you will either be put on a diet, or if that does not control the blood sugar levels, you will also have to take insulin. You will be given a home kit to test yourself daily and then administer a shot of insulin.

If you are not diagnosed but have gestational diabetes, it raises the risk of you having high blood pressure and preeclampsia, both of which are serious complications of pregnancy that can threaten both you and your baby.

Often it can mean you will have a bigger baby, which may lead to a longer and harder labor and an unsuccessful push, where you may end up in the operating room for a Cesarean section.

Gestational Hypertension is diagnosed when blood pressure readings are higher in a person who had normal blood pressure prior to 20 weeks and did not have proteins in their urine. It can progress into pre-eclampsia.

Pre-eclampsia is diagnosed with someone that has sudden higher blood pressure and has proteins in their urine. People that have this are at risk for heart complications, bleeding, stroke, and blood clots.

Decreased blood flow to the placenta means your baby gets less oxygen and fewer nutrients. This can result in lower birth weight and premature babies.

Placental abruption Preeclampsia increases your risk of this condition, where the placenta separates from the inner wall of the uterus before delivery. It would cause bleeding and can be life-threatening for you and the baby.

Hypertension could result in the baby having a slow or decreased growth. Poorly controlled hypertension can result in injury to your brain, lungs, heart, kidneys, liver, and other major organs and can be life-threatening.

Premature delivery because of high blood pressure, you may have to have an early delivery, and that can bring on complications with induction and having the baby born early.

Age 35 seems to be the threshold for many people to have more screening tests for birth defects or if you have any family history of birth problems. Placentas may not be as effective, especially as the birthing person is 35 years and older and/or you go past Week 38. Your care provider may ask you to deliver a few weeks earlier via induction of labor. They will advise and explain why this is so important. Ask many questions about the procedures, benefits, process, and what effect that might have on the baby or you.

The amniocentesis test is fairly common for prenatal diagnosis of chromosomal abnormalities and fetal infections, but mainly for genetic disorders, like Down syndrome, and can determine the sex of your baby. The procedure involves inserting a very long thin needle into the abdomen and then into the amniotic sack to retrieve some of the amniotic fluid for testing. This test was highly suggested for me to have done when I was 38 years old and having my last baby. I was frightened to have the test done because it might have resulted in a possibility of miscarriage. I did the test, not worried if my baby had Down syndrome, but I fretted until I got the results back.

Blood tests for MSAFP (maternal serum AFP) screens for open neural tube defects. Open spina bifida (or open spine) and anencephaly. Neural tube defects are malformations of the central nervous system, the spinal cord, and or the brain.

Pregnancy Hormones are essential in helping us with the development of a healthy pregnancy and growing a healthy baby in utero. Our body is working hard, and hormones are changing very quickly in the 40 weeks it takes to grow a baby. It has a huge effect on the pregnant person. You will be affected by all or some of them: mood swings, lack of sleep, random throwing up, 'morning sickness'. It does not know time. You can be sick around the clock; have deficiencies in diet; gain or lose weight; lose sleep (especially as a growing baby makes it difficult to get comfortable), and simply not feel like yourself. Take all of the prenatal vitamins a care provider asks of you. Eat and drink small amounts of healthy options in your diet, keep up with or start a gentle exercise routine, and get out into nature!

After birth, it is normal for your body to take up to a year for your hormones to get back to their pre-pregnancy state. Never again will you gain and then lose weight so fast. What happens to our brains, appropriately called 'placenta' brain? It seems all of our usual common sense, focus, and memory, goes into the amazing organ that we grow during pregnancy that feeds our baby! From experience, it seems that we do not get 'our' full brain back until the baby is approximately one year old. It means we can break down in tears at a diaper commercial, cry when we see a romantic movie, want sex, or want to stay far away from our partner in the same week. We seem to be all over the map during pregnancy, yet we do not have a clue we have changed because we have forgotten already! Hormones can make us feel happy or sad or bring on anxiety or depression, and sometimes we just do not know what we want. It seems we experience everything much *more* during pregnancy; the highs and lows seem exaggerated. (Do not tell a pregnant person that, *in the moment,* or you should duck).

With the uptake of hormones, our hair and nails tend to grow faster, and often we are complimented on how lovely our skin and hair look. Take time to center yourself and sit in nature to help calm yourself. The practice of being calm will befit you both throughout your pregnancy and in labor and your postpartum time. Some of the crazy hormones that are coursing through your body will make you feel nauseous and cause vomiting or give massive heartburn. *There is so much going on in your body; take care of yourself.*

Relaxin is a hormone produced by the ovaries and placenta during pregnancy. It will help relax the ligaments in the pelvis to soften and dilate the cervix, preparing our body for labor and delivery. In the early months of pregnancy, it relaxes the ligaments, which can make our muscles and joints feel pain or uncomfortable if we over-exert ourselves. It will be beneficial to listen to what your body is telling you and take time to rest so you do not have an injury.

Cortisol is a stress hormone, and it helps the development of the fetus. It regulates our metabolism and controls blood sugar levels. You may experience redness in the face, stretch marks, or problems with blood pressure.

Human Placental Lactogen (HPL) This hormone is secreted from the placenta, and is associated with insulin resistance in pregnancy, called gestational diabetes. If too much HPL, it can lead to a bigger baby.

Prolactin is a hormone made by the pituitary gland at the base of the brain. It causes the breast to grow and make milk during pregnancy and after birth, and is normally high during and after pregnancy. It will begin stimulation in chest tissue to get ready for lactation and the start of colostrum, which is called the first milk that comes in before the regular chest milk.

Oestrogen helps support your baby until the placenta takes over. It helps the development of the baby's organs and the correct function of the placenta. It can be the culprit that causes some nausea. It also may relax or soften the ligaments that put pressure on your lower back and pelvis. These levels should peak around week 32. It also enables your uterus to respond to oxytocin in labor.

Oxytocin and Estrogen: The combination of both oxytocin and estrogen helps release prostaglandins. They soften the cervix in preparation for labor. Oxytocin also produces contractions in our body, and the expelling of the placenta after delivery. It is called the 'love' hormone; we release it when we chest feed the baby or cuddle our baby, giving us feelings of love and deep bonding.

Estrogen: The placenta also produces estrogen and raises hormone levels. The higher levels of estrogen allow the uterus and placenta to create new blood vessels and transfer nutrients to the baby. This rapidly increasing hormone, may contribute to why you might have nausea in the first part of pregnancy. Both estrogen and progesterone levels peak around week 32

Progesterone is a hormone that is naturally produced in the ovaries, the placenta, and the adrenal glands during pregnancy. It helps the implantation of the fertilized egg. It helps the chest get ready to produce milk. Progesterone levels become very high throughout the body. This is what helps to relax and loosen ligaments and joints that help with delivery. Although you have to be careful not to overwork your body, it could result in you having strains and /or sprains. Please ask your care provider when you are in doubt about YOUR body health.

Dietary Changes: You are truly eating for two; you are growing a human being, so eat fresh and healthy options. Cravings for sweets and/or carbohydrates will add to your and your baby's weight gain, meaning you will have a bigger baby to push out! Pushing out a big baby may cause you to have an assisted birth, either forceps or Cesarean section.

If you must eat unhealthy foods, try to do it in moderation.

Eating: Have you gained too much weight? Now is not the time to go on a diet. Possibly you are under the weight of what is expected. There may be a variety of reasons that your care providers can help you with.

Eating properly and not binging on ice cream and chocolates is so important when your labor starts. *What* we eat, also goes to your baby. The bigger the baby, definitely relates to our baby fitting into the Pelvis and being birthed vaginally. If the baby does not fit, you will have a longer labor and possibly have a vacuum, forceps, or Caesarian Section.

At this point in pregnancy, your consumption is less due to the baby growing, and you literally have less space. This will also increase moving into the third trimester. However, eating to grow a healthy baby means it is time to be diligent about what you are putting into your body. They are taking more than ever from you through the placenta, so be aware "you are literally growing a healthy baby".

Eating fresh means taking vitamins, staying away from carbs and sugar, and drinking plenty of water. You may find that there are some foods that you have given up. Your desire to eat and drink certain favorites can go away till after your baby has delivered.

Contact care providers: If at any time in your pregnancy, when you experience the following or are concerned about something, get in contact with a care provider. Early detection can alert them that something may be starting in your pregnancy that requires extra attention. It is essential for them to know, sooner than later, about:

- Vaginal bleeding
- Swelling in the face or fingers
- Severe abdominal pain
- Leak or gush, trickle or continuous fluid from the vagina
- Big chance of baby movements - or lack of movement
- High fever or chills
- Vomiting - or unable to keep food or fluids down
- Blurry vision
- Painful urination
- Headache that won't go away
- Severe headache
- Fall, accident, or injury from a fall or accident.
- Or go to the hospital if you have:
- Severe pain in the abdomen
- Blood loss or fluid loss from the vagina
- Fainting or Dizziness

Visualize your 'Peaceful' Birth Place. Discuss with your birthing partner before the labor about any special considerations or traditions for labor. For instance, a sacred knife for cutting the cord, having an elder present for a blessing. Where you would like to labor, outside in nature, at home, with family or friends helping and encouraging you, or just your partner present until the birth care providers attend. Discuss where you would like to birth. Whether you want a water birth or not, at home or at the hospital?

Visualization is a very effective laboring technique that is done with your birthing partner's help and can be used all through labor and pushing. It helps you to relax and visualize memories of favorite places from your travels or a wish of somewhere you would like to go or something you really like doing or spending special time with. Your birthing partner will start a dialogue in early labor at home and carry this on at the hospital. The dialogue can be kept simple so as not to overstimulate the birthing person. Discussion and practice at home before labor, so you can learn to relax quickly when your labor starts. Practice by sitting or laying in a quiet place, on a chair or on your bed, or in a tub with or without your favorite relaxing music. See, with your eyes closed, when your partner starts to explain your special place, that can make you feel at ease and quickly relax. Practice bringing this vision to your mind in a few minutes. For example, a warm white sandy beach, with crystal blue warm water that laps at the shore, while you lay on a comfortable lounge chair and have the warm, gentle breeze caress your body, making you float and relax. An ideal place to relax is lying in a tub with warm water, low lighting or candles and gentle music to feel your peace and listen to your partner's story.

The dialogue will change with pushing, and become more of a 'cheering squad, helping the participates in a race to finish'. Then, the dialogue would be more expressed. Some ideas might be, 'You are almost there!' 'Go strong!' 'You are Doing This!'

To remind yourself and start being more confident, put notes on walls or mirrors, kitchen cupboards, and any place that you walk past daily, at home and at work, and in your car. The notes should be positive and encouraging, short messages to yourself about your labor and delivery. For example, I can easily birth my baby.

Breathing: A deep, long breath in; hold for a moment, and release that breath fully. And repeat, repeat, repeat. This is the single most important part of breathing for your labor. You can start to practice now, and be very good by the time labor starts until you are 10 cm and your body is ready to push. This is also a valuable tool; when you feel a bit anxious or concerned, practice breathing. Now try and add your favorite music in the background. Pick music that can soothe your soul for the times you want or need to relax AND music that makes you want to get up and dance for the times you need to be more active in your labor.

Author's Birth Trick: A funny note, while my client was pushing, their partner put on the theme from Star Wars, and it was fairly loud, but it was the person's *push music*. They pushed very well, and it was repeated many times. We, in the room, got a bit weary of hearing it, but it was all about the client and their wishes.

Have your partner reminisce about places you both have enjoyed or where you want to go for your next vacation or special events. With a gentle voice, they can encourage and distract you during labor. You will need encouragement at many different times, and your partner can reminisce and remind you about your favorite things - or future hopes, plans, and wishes you have for this baby.

Another great way to distract the birthing person; my client's partner started to talk about the times that they were on a lake, in a rowboat, the sun shining, and only a gentle breeze, and the gentleness of the water that barely moved. It was very moving to watch the client delve into a relaxed state while listening to their true adventure.

Do these relaxing techniques often so that you are very familiar with releasing into calm and peace. I come across many people that can not do the simple act of relaxing! This not only serves you well in labor, BUT in life. As you will find out soon, if you can take 5 minutes every day (as many times in a day as needed) to ground and calm yourself, with the techniques above, you will find you can be a better parent and a better partner.

Prenatal Classes should be booked by the end of this trimester; they often fill up. Your care provider may be able to recommend classes. They may be offered at hospitals, community centers, private and online, to name a few. You need to understand all procedures that may come up before and during labor and postpartum, know what your options are and how to cope. Group classes provoke lots of questions and more answers that you may have never considered.

There are many different techniques, philosophies, and ways to labor, do some research and find the one that feels best for you. Here is a short list of a few of the more popular ones offered; Lamaze, Kopa Birth, Alexander Technique, Bradley Method, Hypnobirthing, and Birthing From Within.

A lovely bonus to attending classes is meeting other people that are in your community who are due at the same time as you, which can make for unique ways to meet new friends. Many people now are making network groups with cell phone chats, which are informing, empowering, and comforting. When feeding the baby at 4:00 am in the morning, you can text each other or talk or ask a question. It is a way of feeling like there is someone else doing the same as you, in those first tiring months. It is nice to ask the group quick questions about feeding or feelings of loneliness and isolation.

The class should give you an overall basic idea of *what to expect,* in early labor, active labor, and delivery. Prenatal classes are of such benefit to you and your primary support person that will be with you at your delivery. With internet access, you should be able to compare each one, for times of class times offered and cost. There may also be VBAC classes, introduction to new baby classes, or feeding classes.

I appreciate you reading my book; thank you! There are also many books that you can read, I have read most of these books and met some of these authors, and they all have something different to contribute to birth. Some names that come to mind are Penny Simkin, Ina May Gaskin, Sheila Kitzinger, Pam England, Rob Horowitz, Dr Sears, Dr Keppler. There are SO many wonderful authors that have added to the collection of books on pregnancy, labor, and delivery.

Chest Feeding classes are harder to find. I have been extremely blessed that the renowned Canadian Chest Feeding Guru, Dr. Jack Newman, has written *for you* an entire chapter on feeding a baby, including pictures and what a good latch looks like. Dr. Jack Newman explains why it is best to chest feed. Their website is where you have a chance to ask questions about feeding. There are also links to other sites for all of your feeding and storing questions.

I have always used their DVDs, which are full of feeding information produced by his clinic, to help prepare my clients for feeding babies. I believe there is pretty much all that you need to understand regarding the dynamics of feeding your baby.

*I have not altered the chapter that Dr Newman has written and *their* use of pronouns, so please forgive me for this one chapter.

Sleeping: As your body changes and gets bigger, it may be an idea to acquire a body pillow (if not already) and or start using pillows. A prop under your belly while sleeping can help you achieve a more restful night. Doctors prefer us not to sleep flat on our backs because it can restrict blood vessels that run down our backs. So use a small wedge from a blanket or pillow to incline to one side or the other.

Sleeping is hard to achieve as the growing baby inside gets further along in your pregnancy. Be creative, and try to be kind to yourself while trying to get comfortable.

Meditation, as a precursor to your bedtime routine, will not only help in the earlier stages, but also help during labor. It is also important to nap or rest, as you will need to do this after the baby is born.

Advantages of hiring a birth doula: We are there for you! All the care providers in the delivery suite at a hospital or at a home delivery are there for the medical side of labor and delivery. Some midwives have been doulas in their early years and wear two hats.

They might do some things like massage and pressure points but are primarily busy with the medical side and charting. Even if partners attend prenatal preparation classes, they should not be expected to know the hospital protocols or when to change up the birthing person's positions for maximum effectiveness of the contractions. Nor should they be expected to know what the care providers are talking about, with all the medical language.

Doulas are with you, for one-on-one support, for anything that happens or changes during labor, arriving earlier in your labor and staying for the entire labor and delivery. Then after birth, for approximately 1 to 2 hours, to make sure you are comfortable, make you tea and toast, and help with the baby's first feeding. They specialize in encouraging, enhancing, and guiding the partner and help if the partner has needs, like taking a break.

Doulas are on-call for you weeks before and after your due date. They will have a backup doula in case there are two conflicting births at a time or if they are ill. They are available for you via telephone or text any time of the day or night, if you have questions or you think your labor is starting. They leave what they are doing, to come and be with you, any time of the day or night. They have ways of helping you cope with pain and changes in your labor.

My Doula Philosophy

I am present, to enhance your birth experience,

I will try all my tricks to help you have a vaginal birth

to guide your partner, so they can encourage and support you;

while keeping you on task, breathing, and being as comfortable as possible.

Doulas can suggest what to do and how to encourage the partner, to better support the laboring person, or the Doula will just do what is needed; wiping a much-needed cool cloth on your face, back, neck - remind you to take sips of water throughout labor - encourage you in all stages of labor - guide your partner to touch, hug and kiss, even when you are at the 'do not touch me' time - pressure points and help your partner to do the points on you - lower the lights - make sure unwanted people are not allowed in the room, i.e., family members - rub or massage i.e. feet hands - remind you to relax muscles or suggest music or tv for distraction.

I have had many people stare into my eyes while I was counting down contractions (from 10 down to 1), and then without me losing eye contact, tell them to breathe slowly as they gently grunt baby out.

As a *thank you* to my clients, I take birth pictures; they can decide either above the waist or below. Below means they want pictures of the delivery and the moment you see your baby for the first time. These are moments you will never get back, and I can promise you this, you will forget all about the labor during your postpartum period.

Author's Note: **Vulnerability and Anxiety from Trauma:** I have helped many clients that have had some form of trauma in their past. It can come from an experience that was negative and unexpected. The experience can come from people, a place, things, attitudes, words, or silence, and can emerge in pregnancy and comes up in their labor. In labor, it is very important to make sure the client's needs are met with respect and privacy.

A birthing person can feel vulnerable and have anxiety as their bodies are draped in flimsy hospital gowns, or they are pushing a baby into this world. You may want to take advantage of relaxing in a tub during your contractions, but hesitate. If you have had any kind of trauma or abuse in your life, memories can come back, which can stall labor. It is paramount that the care providers, Doulas, especially, need to have a *wee* bit of information, even the acknowledgment that there was a trauma, so they are aware you may have triggers, but more importantly, they will know to be extra sensitive in the best way they can help you. Past memories can stall a labor at any time.

Reminder to Breathe Be Calm - Relax - Ground - Positive Attitude.

Post-Partum Doulas: Now is the time to consider hiring a postpartum Doula. They are professionals that come to your home and help with many things. For example, meal preparation for you and your partner, tips for feeding the baby, teach you how to diaper and bathe the baby. Light cleaning, tidying, laundry, looking after other siblings, running errands. Allowing you to nap or shower while they watch your baby. Going on a walk with you and baby, or help with taking you and baby to doctor appointments.

You set up the hours you feel work best for you. They may work 4, 6, or 8 hours for a day shift, and overnight is usually an 8-hour shift. Look into what they offer and what your needs might be. Do the research before you have your baby. You can usually find a PP Doula after you are home, but if you know you want a PP Doula, then pre-hire them so they are ready to come and help you when you are home with the baby.

"I work closely with postpartum doulas. They are badass healing warriors. They walk into the midst of a family in transition and plant themselves firmly, giving everyone something to hold on to. They are there to mother the mother, and having one in your home can lower the incidence or severity of postpartum mental illness. They are trained. They are professional. They change the lives of families every day (and night). They deserve more than this. So do moms. So do dads."

Unknown Author

To Hire a Birth or Post Partum Doula in Canada or USA, go to the website and start your search in finding a Doula www.doulamatch.net for tips regarding what to ask and what Doulas may do for you, go to my Document, **Doulas for Labor and Post Partum.**

Author's Fun Facts:

The birth partner can show signs of pregnancy if they have cravings, start to put on weight, and have some nausea.

The baby swallows its amniotic fluid and pees it out.

Your baby can hear outside noises. They can hear voices, music, and other loud noises; choose the right music and gentle voices - without anger.

You should be able to stick to your regular diet, unless it is not so healthy.

You are growing a baby that we want to be an average size, so you can push them out with little or no complications.

Chapter 6: Twins, Triplets, or More

Multiple Babies at Once: If you are pregnant with twins or more, congratulations comes to mind. Then my next thought would be, *goodness, you will be busy!* I always wanted twins for my first pregnancy, but after going through labor with a singleton, I was so very happy that there was only one. Having twins, triplets, or more can come with many more complications because you have more than one human growing in your belly. Then raising multiples will be a challenge and a lot more work. But eventually, everyone gets through, and then you have so much more joy and love!

The baby appointments will increase exponentially, and pregnancies will be considered high-risk. Doctors will keep a close eye and make sure that all babies are growing similarly in size and approximate weight, that one is developing at the same rate as others, and *where* they are positioned in your tummy. The care providers will keep close attention on all the babies by doing non-stress testing and monitoring the body movements and the amount of amniotic fluid in the sack(s) for starters.

You are at a higher risk of gestational diabetes, high blood pressure, pre-eclampsia, and more which can affect the pregnancy and the baby's health. There is a possibility of one baby growing bigger than the other or one not developing as quickly. There is a risk of babies delivering early, or you may be encouraged to have an induction of labor, or possibly have a planned Cesarean section. Some complications may occur with having multiple babies; premature delivery is common, but sometimes there might be ways to slow down or stop labor if it is too early in your pregnancy. You may have to be on bed rest or stay in the hospital to stave off labor while techniques are administered to keep you pregnant.

If you have a general practitioner or midwife, they may be able to do a 'shared care' or will transfer care to an obstetrician that specializes in delivering multiple babies. You will be given guidance and education to understand changes to expect every new week in pregnancy. It may be suggested that planning a hospital or birthing center birth might be a safer option for babies to have paediatricians and delivery doctors, and nurses that specialize in multiples.

You may need some guidance on restriction in some regular exercises and routines, and I would ask if you are doing any of the labor tricks that you consult with your care provider. Your body will grow bigger during the pregnancy period, and it may be evident that part way through, you may need to take time off work or slow down your daily routine. You will need guidance, with special attention, on how to take care of YOURSELF and what your body will need to keep babies healthy and growing at the correct pace. Your body will quickly change with more than one baby, especially as babies get farther along in pregnancy.

It is common that one baby is in a breech position, meaning your baby is bum first and comes through the vaginal canal or possibly a footling breech; the foot would come down first or head down. Positioning is key when figuring out the way you will deliver, and you may be given a trial of labor or asked to have a Cesarean section. We might assume that if the first was breech and was smaller and weighed less than a single baby, it should be easier to push out. The logistics can be surprisingly unstable when more than one baby is trying to be born.

These births are well planned out, and there will be many people to help at the delivery. Present at the delivery, will be either one paediatrician (or doctor), at least one but usually more, nurses for each baby, and each baby will go into their own baby warmer for care and monitoring straight after they are delivered. You may be allowed a trial of labor, if you have had a fairly straight forward pregnancy and babies are healthy in utero, and the doctor deems it to be safe. Any birth can have complications, especially with each extra baby that you are carrying, from the confines of the space in which they are in, to the stress it can cause them or the logistics in which way they are laying, the chance of a vaginal birth can change without notice. The care providers will be monitoring each baby's heart rate externally very closely during labor, and best plan to deliver each baby. There are many situations that can occur for each baby and/or the birthing person. The health of one or more of the babies can change very quickly, that will make changes to the birth plan and you may be advised to have a scheduled Cesarean section. This is to ensure a healthy birth for all babies and the birthing person.

I have been witness to many scenarios where sometimes, you may be able to have a vaginal birth in the birthing suite without complications. However, at any time, with two or three humans in your tummy, they may not be able to tolerate labor. If, while monitoring, the baby's heart rates are not normal or if there are any other indications that the baby or the mother is not tolerating labor, it can become very chaotic when something is *not ideal.* Then, there is no choice but to race to the operating room and get the baby delivered quickly via a Cesarean section.

The difference that I 'see' in a delivery suite is the volume of staff. There are more people in the operating room; two doctors performing the Cesarean section, a staff of approximately ten nurses, and two anesthetists for the birthing person.

There is one bassinet per baby being born, with a crew of a few, or up to 12 people from NICU staff, paediatricians, and nurses per baby, monitoring the baby and how they respond to being born, they could have breathing issues and more.

When things are considered an emergency, a noise rings through the halls to advise that certain personnel are needed 'stat' to the OR.

All care providers race to the operating room for an emergency C-section and race to help one or both babies recover quickly. It may be necessary for one or more of your babies to need extra help during labor or delivery, and they will be taken quickly to the NICU (Neonatal Intensive Care Unit), where they are equipped to deal with highly specialized care for one or more babies that might be in distress at delivery. Time will be of the essence for proper care.

The surgeons doing the Cesarean section, several anesthetists and nurses will be taking care of you. It feels like you are in a bee hive, and it can be a bit of a scary scene, especially for the partner. Firstly, you are usually exhausted from the labor, and your care providers are usually busy watching the surgery. I find it helpful to communicate with our care provider for an update and reassure the birthing partner about some of what is going on; it helps them to relax (a bit), so they can reassure the person on the surgery table.

Multiple babies rarely get to 40 weeks

Having more than one baby is overwhelming, and you will definitely need extra help for the delivery and when you come home, especially if you already have a child or children. Prepare to double the baby basics; diapers, bottles, and formula. Although you can learn how to feed twins, check out Dr Jack Newman's chapter. Then separately look into car seats, strollers, or carrying pouches, clothing, blankets, and baby pillows. All for the many beautiful babies you will soon meet.

Gather your helpers, family, or friends, or hire a postpartum doula for when babies are home early for your peace of mind. It is common that multiples often deliver much sooner than 40 weeks gestation; an average for multiples can be from 32 - 38 weeks or earlier. It is common to be extra tired with multiples. My postpartum calendar can come in very handy to organize your helpers for when you come home from the hospital.

After some time, you will have so many fun and exciting times with your growing children. Whether its one or more babies, the first few months are tiring, no matter how you look at it.

*I do **NOT** recommend you do the exercises in the Birth Tricks with two or more babies and going into labor earlier than possible. It can be a challenge to keep them in your tummy until week 38.*

Chapter 7: Home Births

There are so many wonderful reasons to labor and birth at home; if you are having a low-risk pregnancy and are having one baby, not twins or more; if you and the baby are healthy and the baby is not breech. Your home can become a very special and intimate home-birthing space. You may have a large bathtub at home, or you can rent a birthing pool to give birth in. You can choose your team, which includes midwives, a doula, friends, and family members.

You can labor in a birthing pool in the middle of your living room, with curtains closed, listening to your favorite music, or watching a funny movie. Back and forth, in and out of the tub. You may want to burn candles or have low lighting, essential oils, or aromatherapy in the room, all the while having a close group of support hand-picked by you.

People often labor and deliver in the middle of the night. If you already have children in the home, you may not have options to drop your children off or do not know anyone that you are comfortable having come to your home; it is a huge convenience to have a home birth. There is a possibility that your other children may sleep through your labor during the night. You may want your child/children present when their sibling is being born as a family bonding moment. Being in your home, where you are comfortable, the option of delivering at home can be very satisfying.

Midwives specialize in attending home births. In my city, they are totally equipped with everything needed to deliver your baby if it indicates that it will be a straightforward delivery. They even bring a small portable container of nitrous oxide or 'gas'; it is very easy to use and can be very effective for a portion of your labor. Gas, in combination with being in a bathtub or birthing pool, is even better.

Midwives also have privileges at a hospital in or near your neighborhood, where you will be pre-registered in the event you have to transfer to the hospital. It makes for an easy transition to the hospital if there are any complications that the midwife suspects are starting. For instance, while monitoring the baby's heart rate, it might be creeping up, which would indicate that the baby is not tolerating labor contractions. Or if you or your baby show signs of needing extra help at delivery, then you will be transported to a hospital. They may suggest the partner drive you to a hospital, or if dire, an ambulance will rush the birthing person to a hospital, and the partner and team follow.

Having a doula that will come to your home when you are transitioning from early labor to active labor is very helpful. The doula can communicate with your midwife in early labor, then arrive for belly checks and blood pressure checks, and when you are in a more active stage, the midwife will come and stay. When you are getting closer to delivery, a second midwife will come and stay to help the primary midwife until after your delivery. Everyone together makes a unique and continuous care team. They all specialize in ways to help with natural pain relief and encouragement that will get you through your labor.

Water Births: A birthing pool is one of the best ways to get through all stages of early, active labor and delivery. If you do not have a big enough bathtub, you can rent a birthing pool. Being in the water helps de-stress you, takes the pressure off of your body, and reduces the sensations of labor pains, allowing you to float through contractions. It can be a perfect place to have a gentler delivery. Water births are safe and quite magical.

Advise your support team, family, or friends when you are in early labor. They can prepare for when you need them to come to your home. Ahead of time, advise all of your team where spare linens, towels, tissues, items in your kitchen cupboards, tea or coffee, mugs, and sugar and cream are, what you prefer to drink during your labor, how to turn off/on or lower music or tv, and where the light switches are.

Have a list with the information for times your children need to be picked up from school or activities; have someone to come and get them for their stay with family or friends. Have someone advise the Doula that it is time to come to your home. The midwife may be in to check on you, or the doula can relay how you are doing in early labor. The midwife may come and check in with you and do 'vitals' for the baby's heart rate, your temperature, then may leave if labor is still early. When they have reason to believe that you are getting more active, they will stay at your home. Later on, when you are close to delivery, they call in a second Midwife to help with the delivery. In Canada, we have 2 Midwives present at birth.

TENS Machine: If your midwife or doula does not have a TENS machine, you can rent one, or you can buy one at stores or online. The machine can be used during your labor but can also be used afterward with other family members that have sore muscles.

Read the **Birth Wishes Plan** section to help you put together a home birth plan.

If the venue for delivery has to change part way through labor, and you need to transfer to a hospital for any reason, a backup hospital-birth plan is essential. Many times for a lot of different reasons, people have to change the place the baby will be born. Understand the change of venue is in the best interest of the baby and/or your health.

You can tuck that in your packed hospital bag. You need to write both birth plans, in case labor starts to change, where you or the baby are showing signs of distress, or not tolerating labor. If the midwife advises that you need to transfer to the hospital, it will be fast.

It will be beneficial for the midwife and the hospital staff to know your wishes for delivery. You may be going to the hospital for monitoring and an assessment as to the best way to deliver, *or* you may be going straight to the operating room for forceps or Cesarean section birth.

Pre-arrange and have someone that can come into your home to take care of the mess from your home birth when you are transferred to the hospital. They can drain and take down the birth tub; feed and tend to the care of pets; put birthing laundry in the washing machine; get rid of garbage, and change the sheets on your bed. They can also look after any children that are in the home. It will be really nice for you to come back from the hospital to a clean home.

Supply List for a Home Birth: Purchase the following items by week 36. It is less stressful if you go into labor early, knowing you have all your birth preparation done. Most likely, your midwife will have their own list for your home birth

Rent a Birth Pool: It usually comes with all the below-mentioned items in the rental fee:

Birthing Pool

Disposable Pool Liner

Plastic Sheet for under pool that extends a couple of feet.

Air Pump to inflate the pool

Submersible Pump to deflate the pool

Tap Adapter

A hose that attaches to your tap to fill and then drain the water (one-time use only).

Thermometer: To keep the water at body temperature and not overheat it.

Small fish net (3 x 3) to scoop out 'bits' that come from the laboring person.

If you choose to buy a child's pool, you will need everything on the above list. You will be sending everything to the dump afterwards. You will not be able to buy a pool liner as the pool is going to be a one-time use only.

The Plastic Sheet or Plastic Shower Curtain: A thermometer and fish net can be bought at a dollar store, but you will probably throw them away after delivery. Everything else you will need, you will buy separately from a hardware store.

Some things to consider if you're thinking about laboring and delivering in a bathtub or birthing pool, a bathtub should be large and deep enough to hold both you and a second person; otherwise, you can rent a birthing pool. Space around the outside of the tub is needed that allows people to have access to you on three sides. If you do not have a big enough bathtub, then I suggest renting a birthing pool, or you may be able to buy a child-size pool that is deep enough to submerge in.

In the Birthtub for your Delivery?: Your partner and the rest of your team need to be close for encouragement, massage and pressure point techniques, and to allow the midwife to do belly checks, while you labor in a tub. Having easy access to 3 sides is essential.

Where to set up the Birthing pool for your delivery?: Consider a place that ensures privacy, so not in front of the living room window and sheer curtains. The midwife needs space to catch your baby from any angle, and the second midwife will also be present. Your support team will need room to be around you (on stools or a birthing ball) for massage, comfort, placing water on your belly and anything else that you wish or need. You will want your photographer to have access to take perfect pictures of the delivery. The birthing person may want to walk around naked and have easy access to a bathroom. If we need to get the birthing person to a bed to complete the delivery, that should be fairly close.

VBACs can try for a home birth when you know why the first baby was a C-section, and it is deemed safe by the care provider. To labor at home with the expectation to deliver at home can be empowering.

Preparing for your Home Births: Your care provider will most likely have a list of all the necessary items that you would need to buy and have in your home by Week 36, in case you deliver early:

- 2 sets sheets & pillowcases. So you can birth on one set and have a change of sheets to sleep on after the birth.
- Plastic cover for mattress - large plastic tarp or shower curtain
- 6 - 8 Large cotton towels - 3 or 4 to mop water off the floor from getting in and out of the tub/pool. Buy cheap ones from a thrift store; you may throw them in the garbage at the end of the birth. An additional 3 - 4 towels for you when you get out of the tub/pool; people tend to get in and out several times during labor.
- 8 face cloths
- 8 receiving blankets
- 2 long t-shirts or gowns that cover up to the knee but are open and flowing. A bathing suit is too awkward to get out of when wet.
- Heating pad, plug-in or microwaveable, for your tummy or back in labor.
- Gravol (use in early labor)
- Liquid calcium - magnesium (for early labor cramps)
- Tylenol bottle 325 ml

- Ibuprofen bottle 200 mg
- Ibuprofen or acetaminophen - for afterpains
- Bucket (to throw up in)
- Large garbage bucket and several large plastic bags for all garbage
- Large plastic bags to put dirty towels that are in need of laundry or to be thrown out.
- 4 Maternity Maxi Pads
- Hydrogen Peroxide 500 ml
- 2 - 3 mesh panties or oversize panties
- Container to drink from, with a straw that can bend
- 1 squeeze bottle - to rinse perineum after delivery (approx 500 ml)
- Flashlight with good batteries
- Hand Mirror, so you can see when pushing
- 1 plastic sheet or shower curtain on a mattress with the sheet on top
- 2 fitted sheets (something that you do not have to wash - throw away)
- Hot water bottle, microwaveable heating pads or rice packs (for your back/tummy)
- Epson Salts
- 12 4x4 gauze pads
- 24 blue pads (23 x 36), similar to puppy training pads
- 4 large black garbage bags
- 1 large ‘Ziploc’ bag (for the placenta)
- Inflatable bath pillow or ‘donut’ shape cushion, for ease of sitting on afterwards.
- 1 digital thermometer
- Box of newborn diapers - or cloth diapers
- 2 newborn ‘Hats’
- Medium pot with a lid

- Camera or Video equipment or Phone (film, batteries, charging cords)

Food & Beverages for Labor:

Lots of water, and for a change, 'Labor Aide' drink (see recipe) other fluids, like clear juice or Emergen-C powder. You can make yourself popsicles or ice cubes or buy them from a store. All of this is to keep yourself hydrated or if you need a bit of sugar for energy.

The container you will use to drink out of should not be too big for you to hold but should have a lid and a bendy straw, which makes it easier for you to drink from when you are lying down or are in the tub.

Early Labor: You may eat small portions of food that easily digest in your tummy. Frozen fruits like grapes and high protein fruit or chocolate are good.

Active Labor: You lose the sensation of hunger. You may only want popsicles, jello or clear soup. At some point, you will 'forget about eating food'.

After the delivery, you may be hungry, something small in the first hour, then you should be able to eat and drink what you want. Have something from the freezer that can be warmed up, or order in a meal to your home.

Food and beverages for your TEAM. Tea or Coffee, especially in the middle of the night, juice, and small items that they can snack on and keep them going. Many times people bring their own but can run out of their own snacks. It is a special treat to be offered something. I have had clients ask me if I have allergies or if I am a vegetarian. Keep it simple.

Baby in the first few hours of birth

- 6 Receiving blankets
- 1 Diaper
- 1 undershirt
- 1 Sleeper
- 1 Pair socks
- 1 Cotton knit cap or bonnet
- Thermometer
- Cord care
- Q-tips
- Hydrogen peroxide or alcohol
- Rosemary, arrowroot or goldenseal
- What your midwife should bring
- Your chart - now online, probably on their cell phone
- Fetoscope or doppler
- Blood pressure cuff & stethoscope
- Thermometer
- Sterile gloves, water-soluble jelly & butadiene solution
- Sterile birth pack - includes hemostats, scissors, cord clamp or tie 4x4 gauze pad
- Amnihook - to break water
- Bulb & DeLee suction for the baby
- Pitocin & Methergine, drugs to stimulate uterine contractions 'Oxytocin shot.'
- IV bag, tubing and catheters
- Oxygen
- Ambu bag - if baby needs help breathing
- Sterile suture material, drapes, scissors, needle holder & medication to numb a tear that needs repair
- Sterile catheters - to drain the bladder
- Antibiotic Eye ointment and Vitamin K for baby

- Baby scale to weigh the baby and measuring tape to measure the length and head circumference

Early Labor: You should do all the labor tricks; see the early labor section, but enjoy listening to music, dancing, watching movies, and stay hydrated. Call your team to tell them you are in early labor, or to have it confirmed that it is early labor. Often when animals are in the home, people either shut animals into a separate room or someone comes to take them away. Animals are especially sensitive while you are in labor, and it can confuse them, making them anxious, and, in turn, you get anxious. Your children and animals may not cope well with you in labor. They may also need to eat, play, walk, or need to go to bed, so having people that can accommodate their needs will help you progress in labor.

After Delivery:

Perineal Wash - Homeopathic Arnica: Witch Hazel on a pad is a gentle & effective healing agent that heals soft tissue cuts. Prepare by putting fluid on a pad, wrapping them and keeping them cold in the fridge. Use them for the first 1 hour intermittently on your perineum; they calm swelling and bruising from pushing. Mother's milk tea, 2 - 3 bags of sitz bath with special herbs, bought from many wellness and organic stores selling herbs and teas, and on the internet. Ingredients might be lavender flowers, red raspberry leaf, comfrey leaf, plantain leaf, yarrow flower and calendula flowers, just for one mixture.

Chapter 8: VBAC Birth

VBAC Vaginal Birth After Cesarean section is when your prior birth would have been in the operating room for a Cesarean section, and now, you are hoping to avoid another operation. My first baby was by Cesarean section, then I had 3 VBAC deliveries, and in my career, I have helped many clients have successful VBACs. I understand how satisfying it is to deliver vaginally, but more importantly, the recovery time is easier and faster, as you already have a child(ren) running about and keeping you busy at home.

TOLAC for VBAC is when you are having a **Trial of Labor After Cesarean**. The recovery from a successful vaginal delivery, with a repair of the perineum, is vastly easier than a Cesarean incision. Your recovery is shorter, with very little risk of infection and less blood loss. Your stay at the hospital may be from 6 hours to 24 hours, and not the 3 days from a surgery.

You will have early labor at home, then after coming to the hospital and being admitted, your nurse will site an IV (Intravenous) into your arm or hand, for ease of giving fluids and medications directly into a your vein or if you need pain medication or if you need to go to the operating room in a hurry.

The benefits of it are; no other scar on the uterus, which could make subsequent pregnancy riskier; less pain after delivery; recovery at home is easier and shorter; lower risk of infection; and most importantly, you can be more involved with your baby and other child(ren). Your trial of labor will start. You will labor, then push the baby, and then they are put straight to your chest for skin-to-skin bonding, which is best for both you and your baby.

During a vaginal birth, many hormones are released into our body. The biggest advantage for a baby coming through the birth canal is having the natural squeeze that puts pressure on the baby's chest to push fluid out of the lungs, esophagus, nose and throat.

Babies born vaginally have higher APGAR Scores. They can come to skin-to-skin contact faster with the parent - which encourages chest feeding and bonding. During labor, you will be closely monitored for any signs of a uterine rupture during labor; it is very rare but necessary.

A Few Facts:

- Your doctor will advise if it is feasible to try a VBAC.
- Sometimes, a VBAC is not successful.
- It is not recommended to have more than three Cesarean sections.
- If you want a successful VBAC, you need to be diligent at doing the birthing tricks.
- There is always a possibility with a VBAC of uterine rupture when the cesarean scar on the uterus breaks open (this is rare).
- Your care providers will monitor your trial of labor very closely for any issues that might creep up.

Many times the baby may not be in an ideal position, which may cause many complications and a long labor, leading you to have a Cesarean section. If you are unsure about having another Cesarean section, your care provider can explain both pros and cons of having a VBAC delivery.

Standard practice in Canada is to wait for at least 18 - 24 months or more before you deliver again. Care providers do not recommend more than three Cesarean sections for any one person, as it can be dangerous for the health of your uterus. I have been with a few clients where when there are signs of a rupture in the uterus, the care providers watch to confirm something is not right, and then you are taken to the operating room very fast!

Many of my clients have felt the loss of not getting through their labor and feeling like they have failed in pushing the baby out. If you have feelings of this kind, it would be beneficial to talk with postpartum groups that have experienced the same. There are many VBAC support groups on social media. The way you deliver your baby should not have anything to do with your expectations that you have failed, and you should not carry that burden. As long as **you** and your **baby** are healthy, then you've had a successful delivery!

Author's note: I have been at many deliveries where the shape of the pelvis does not allow a baby through the pelvis. It is a heart shape, and its nickname is 'Lucy' or 'Australopithecus afarensis.' No baby can come through this particular shape. There is no way of knowing this beforehand, it is only found out when a surgeon is delivering a baby by Cesarean section and they notice the bones of the pelvis.

There is a diagram of Lucy in Cervix & Vaginal Exams

Chapter 9: Birth Wishes Plan, Home/Hospital

Birth Wishes Plan is an essential part of your labor. It is your way of expressing your specific wishes, hopes and desires, the true essence of what you want in your labor and delivery. The capacity to make decisions or tell anyone your wishes in labor will be impossible.

You will need to let go of distractions and focus on your contractions, and allow your team to advocate for you when labor changes. It allows your care providers to know how to help more efficiently during labor and when change happens. Your dream of how your baby's birth will be should not be set in stone, mind that the baby and labor may dictate otherwise.

Discuss and write your birth wishes plan around week 36 with your partner or main support person, and share it with people expected to be at your labor and delivery, i.e., doctor, midwife, nurse, doula, family or friends.

When arriving at the hospital, you are taken to an assessment room, for tests and decide if you are in an active labor. If so, you will be admitted. Then when you are taken to the delivery suite, the partner will give your nurse the Birth Plan, and they will put it in your chart, where your medical history and test results are kept.

Any traditions or birth ceremonies? I have seen many times a special knife brought in to cut the cord, putting a drop of 'sweet' like honey on the baby's tongue, the first thing baby tastes in life.

Author's Story, a Tradition: I was at a birth in early 2022. During labor, my client brought a jar out with what looked like a shriveled-up weed floating in the water. I was told it is called Anastatica hierochuntica, also referred to as 'Kaff Maryam,' and is native to the Middle East and a part of the client's Muslim birth customs.

My clients had used it during their first baby's birth, then dried the plant and kept it for several years until this birth. It is known to be dried out for a long time, but then when needed for another labor, it will blossom again when put into water.

As things progress, the Anastatica 'listens' to the birthing person's body and opens as the laboring person's cervix dilates. I was told they would know when the person was fully dilated by watching the plant become fully open, and it would help facilitate an easier labor, so the baby would 'flow like water'.

Confused, I watched the plant over the next few hours. It indeed became a vibrant and lush plant, and once fully open, it was obvious that the labor was reaching the end. The birthing person then drank a small amount of the water, and the baby was soon born. It all worked as described, much to all of us in the delivery suite that witnessed this! Then an hour or so after delivery, I looked at the jar, and the plant had already started to shrivel up. I found this fascinating.

Two years after the Anastatica birth, I was hired for another birth. My new client started to talk about this 'plant' that a friend of theirs was allowing them to use for their birth. I was happily surprised to find out it was my past clients.

My present client was having prodromal labor (taking several days). The client had prepared the plant in water, and for fun, the client decided to take a small drink of the plant/root-soaked water. Several hours after this, I was surprised that the client's contractions picked up substantially, and they delivered early the next morning.

<u>This is dried up</u>

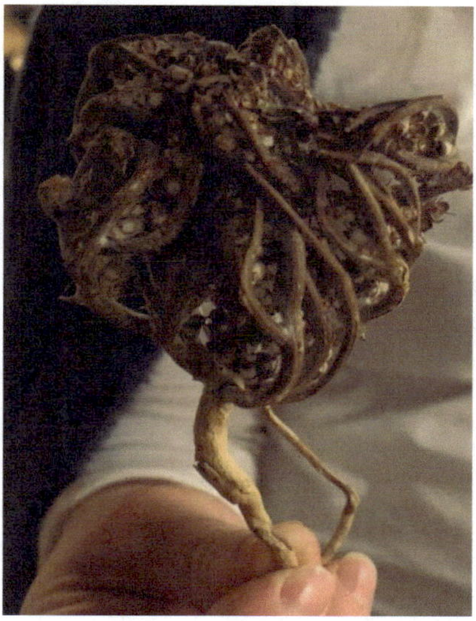

<u>This is watching it bloom in a container of water.</u>

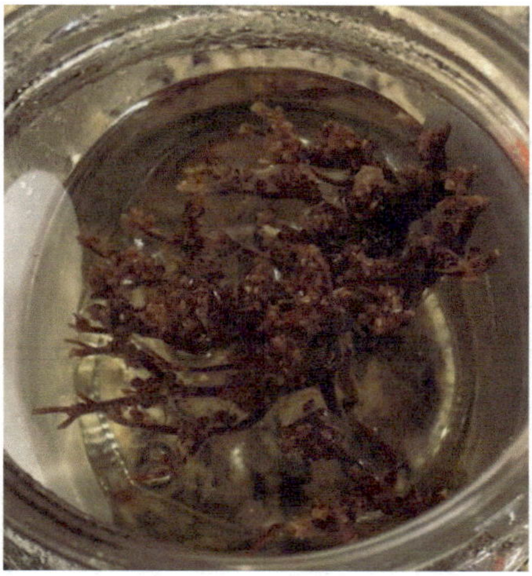

Author's Tip: *If you are not taking prenatal classes, talk to your care provider about procedures, pain management and alternative ways to deliver, for instance, Cesarean section, forceps or vacuum; this will help you make good decisions for your plan.*

Home Birth Wishes Plan: Start by discussing with your partner about any specific goals for labor. Who do you want on your birthing team? Midwife, doula, birth photographer, family members, special friends. What are your feelings about a natural delivery? Will you be using any specific birthing techniques? Birthing from within, hypnobirthing or others? Is there something you do not want? Think about what expectations you have and whether they are realistic. Birthing at home, you have the space to have family and/or friends, including your birthing team; there are no limits. You will be very familiar with your midwife by then, and your birth plan will be informal because you will have discussed most of the birth plan items already. But it is nice for the second midwife or other helpers, when they arrive at your home, to have a read.

When labor starts, have a list of names and contact numbers for the midwives or doulas and all other helpers and support team. Names of people in the home and who they are, i.e., grandparent helping and looking after other children, Sam, the dog walker.

A home birth is a different experience, gentle and not medicalized like the hospital, so there will not be any monitors to be hooked up to. The midwife will use a handheld doppler to listen to the baby's heart rate. But they will have all the necessary equipment needed for you and your baby. See the home birth list of items; most often, they have portable gas.

Home Birth with a Transfer to the Hospital: When planning a home birth, I would advise you to also make a hospital plan just in case you have to transfer to the hospital. This does not happen often, but as a precaution, have a bag packed with a hospital birth plan packed inside, along with your medical card. There will be no time to think about changes that might be occurring, and how you feel about interventions. For example, having an assisted delivery in the operating room. Do you want an epidural as soon as you get to the hospital? Put some thought into the 'what ifs' of going to the hospital.

If labor changes because you or the baby is showing signs of distress or they are not tolerating labor, the midwife will advise you to transfer to a hospital. The decision to go to the hospital will most likely be a rushed transfer via ambulance or car. When arriving at the hospital, the obstetrician will assess you and your progress and decide what you need for an expedited delivery. Your options may be a vacuum, forceps, or a Cesarean section. State your preference (if you have one); a Cesarean Section OR Forceps. Some people do not want forceps, and they have a definitive reason why.

If a Cesarean section is needed, ask to allow both your partner and the doula (for extra support and picture taking) to accompany you into the operating room. Your care provider will always come into the operating room with you.

Hospital Birth Wishes Plan: The hospital delivery suite is usually not very big, and there will be many more people than in a home birth. Your labor will include your care provider, a nurse and a doula (if you have one). Depending on how labor progresses, you will have extra people that come in for delivery. You may see two more nurses, paediatricians and obstetricians, in addition to your team. The hospital staff usually provides the following for you; gowns to wear, sanitary pads, diapers for baby, a towel to wrap baby in, a bassinet for baby to sleep in, a single bed and linens for you and foamy mattress on the floor or a bench for the partner. If you think you are going to spend time in the tub, wear a hospital gown. You do not want to have a hard time taking a wet bathing suit off when you are ready to push.

If you are chestfeeding, there will be a lot of advice and encouragement from the staff. If baby needs a 'top up' in the first 24-36 hours, they usually have a formula in small bottles.

Birth Wishes plan should be in *point form and one or two pages only.* I call it wishes because nothing in labor and delivery will happen the way we think it will; *expect change.* If you have said "no to any drugs during labor," you may change your mind at any time and have pain relief, set out what coping methods you want to use, possibly a tub or shower, or in the form of gas (nitrous oxide) or an epidural. Who do you want at the delivery? Ask how many people are allowed in the delivery suite, OR is there someone that you do not want in the room? The nursing staff and people in the delivery suite will help escort anyone that should not be there.

Care providers will be watching you and the baby constantly during labor. If they see signs that you or the baby is not tolerating labor, they will decide if you need to deliver with some help. Help may be forceps or vacuum in your delivery suite, or if they feel it best to go to the operating room, where they can do a trial of vacuum or forceps and if not successful, they can change to a Cesarean section.

If this happens, you most likely will have been laboring a long time, and you will be exhausted; making decisions about your delivery then will be difficult. It is important to talk about this topic before labor with your care provider.

The doctor will only suggest the procedure that they believe is best for you and the baby. I have seen people that have a definitive preference for their alternative delivery. So if you have a specific reason, explain briefly why you choose; no forceps - no vacuum - prefer to go straight to a Cesarean section. Ask for both the partner and doula to have admittance to the operating room for support and picture taking of you both and the baby.

A simpler option for making a Birth Wishes plan is the ease of making a one-page birth plan by downloading specific images that you choose from:
MamaNatural.com
https://www.mamanatural.com/visual-birth-plan/

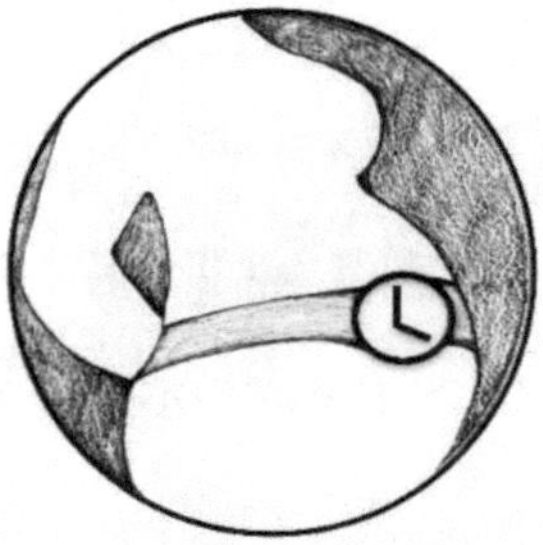

CONTINUOUS MONITORING

Many clients find it very helpful, and in addition, you can spend time looking at their fun baby information on this site.

Be open-minded and have fun making a flexible birth plan.

Make your plan reflect what is *Most Important for YOU!*

Start this document with the first and second lines being a statement of specific goals for labor that are very important to you. For some items, your partner may have a list and can verbalize to everyone your wishes.

My Name My Partner's Name, Contact number

Any other helpers at your birth - family, friend, doula (give names)

Dr Grant or Midwife Michelle Doula Kim

Due Date: January 1 Multip - 2nd baby

List the prescription drugs you are taking

List any Allergies, i.e., Shellfish

GBS +/- Yes/No for Erythromycin

Yes/No for Vitamin KYes/No for Oxytocin at delivery

Partner is queasy around blood and/or fluids and will faint

I want to try nitrous oxide 'Gas.'

I want an Epidural.

Limit Vaginal Exam - unless necessary.

Prefer auscultation by doppler for as long as possible

Prefer no IV unless needed for antibiotics, dehydration or epidural.

Gas & Air/Nitrous Oxide/the Laughing Gas

No Episiotomy, prefer to tear (seek advice regarding the difference for recovery).

I am open to all medications or procedures.

Please do not offer pain medications.

Wait till I ask for pain medications.

I want to use a tub or shower in labor OR use gas while you are in the tub.

I would like to have a water birth.

We are open to all changes/everything.

TENS machine & pads

No residents or students or interns attend me.

Prefer SROM (spontaneous rupture of membranes)

Okay with AROM (artificial) if needed to augment labor or signs of fetal distress

Guidance to breathing during contractions

Guidance to change breathing, to hold breath for pushing

Guidance for breathing at delivery

Guidance to stop pushing as baby's head is crowing - to avoid tear

Guidance for when to start and how to push

Guidance with all different positions for pushing

Use of relaxation and meditation techniques to stay calm.

Want a natural birth - *explain what that looks like to you.*

Try walking, stairs, stand and shake or sway hips, squats.

With an IV and pole, try to move around.

Use of birthing ball to bounce on – squats.

Peanut ball if you have a posterior-facing baby.

Lots of movement, position changes for labor and pushing.

Nipple stimulation, by hand or breast pump etc., before starting Pitocin.

Use meditation techniques.

Use HypnoBirthing techniques and will put a poster on the clock and door.

Use birthing from within or other techniques.

Please do not remind me of the time.

Music to play from our playlist and speaker.

I want dim lighting, a quiet environment and minimal interruptions.

Gentle, hushed talking in the delivery suite.

Alternative pain management, acupressure, position changes, Tahitian hip shakes.

Massage, if it works, is awesome; but people sometimes do not want any touch.

Partner/Doula will do a massage or acupressure.

Partner to talk through my strong contractions to distract me.

I want a mirror so I can see the delivery and encourage myself.

Try as many suggestions for position changes while pushing.

Put a warm compress on the perineum for pushing when close to delivery.

Delayed cord clamping/stop pulsing before cutting (at least 2 minutes)

Partner or myself to cut cord

Partner brings and uses a sterile knife to cut the cord.

Partner would like to help catch baby, with care providers permission IF it is safe to do so (the CP will guide the partner at the moment at delivery to bring baby up to the chest area).

I want to reach down and have the baby put into my hands, to bring the baby up to me

Want the baby placed skin-to-skin for cuddles for the first hour after delivery.

Would like 'baby to find nipple' for feeding.

Leave Vernix on the baby to be absorbed in naturally.

I am keeping my placenta to take home; I have everything to store it in.

Your partner will take time to go and pray

Ceremonial Traditions at delivery; put honey put on the baby's tongue for 'their first taste.'

Doula or birth photographer has our permission and will take birth pictures or videos of the birth - excluding care providers or procedures.

Partner involvement - what are they not wanting to do or see? Are they excited to help and do anything asked of them?

What are you willing to let them see? For instance, clients have said ONLY above the waist or everything?

Ahead of labor, talk to your care provider about your birth control plans. At delivery in the delivery suite or the OR, your care provider may agree to placing an IUD.

At the one-hour baby check:

I want my partner to be involved and put the first diaper on the baby.

If I need to be separated from my baby, I want my partner with the baby at all times.

We have brought our own receiving blankets and prefer to use them on the baby.

If the baby has to go to NICU (newborn intensive care unit), my partner to stay with the baby.

In NICU, I do not want bottles given to the baby.

Allow and encourage the partner to touch and talk to the baby in NICU (if possible).

I understand there may be changes and exceptions in the moment - I trust my care providers to do what is best for the baby and myself.

Chapter 10: Doulas for Labor and Post Partum

A 'Doula' is a professional birth coach for birth and postpartum. They are excellent help at home or hospital births and later for postpartum. They give continuous physical, emotional and informational support to the birthing person before, during and after birth. You may be able to hire the same doula for your delivery and postpartum.

Labor and delivery can bring up anxiety from your past, or you may be listening to other people talk about their labor and birth or watching on the internet. It can be emotionally draining, and many people may have unnecessary worry, wondering how they will navigate their labor. Doulas can make your labor easier for you and your partner.

Statistics have shown that when you have one-on-one doula support, your labor is shorter, there are fewer complications, like forceps or cesarean sections, less drugs used, fewer epidurals, and more interaction with your partner. I have seen many partners not able to cope with some of the procedures and/or become stressed while watching the person in labor, and not knowing how to help them

Statistics are:

25% shorter labors

60% reduction in epidural requests

50% reduction in the caesarean rate

40% reduction in forceps delivery

40% reduction in oxytocin use

30% reduction in analgesia use

Continuous labor support offers huge benefits to birthing people and babies with no known downsides.

Start to look around weeks 25-34 to set up interviews for your Doula for birth and/or postpartum. My book called ***'What Does a Doula Do?'*** has a list of questions to ask at an interview, questions like; where did you have your training? Are you certified? Some Doulas have a set price point, or they may negotiate a fee or use a sliding scale. They are professionals, and this is their chosen career. Other doulas are new, or they do this part-time, so there are many options open for you.

A short list of things your Doula may offer (so ask them questions):

- Help you make a birth wishes plan.
- Offer private prenatal education.
- Ask how many prenatal visits there would be and for how long they would be.
- They use natural ways and techniques to keep you calm.
- One-on-one continuous support for labor and delivery.
- They support you if you do not have a partner.
- Tricks to lessen stress and anxiety for you and/or your partner during labor and delivery.
- Support and guidance for your partner to participate to their fullest.
- They will advocate for you and your birth wishes.
- Will never judge you and will always support any change in labor.
- Distract you by doing massage or acupressure points.
- They have many tricks to make labor shorter and more comfortable for you.
- Will support you when your partner needs a break or a nap.
- Never take over a partner's duties - unless asked.

- Bring peace of mind to your delivery and later in your home, postpartum.
- Supportive where or how you wish to deliver - at the hospital, home, planned C-Section OR as organically and naturally as possible, i.e., outside.
- Have a TENS machine you can use during labor.
- May document your labor and delivery by taking pictures or taking notes.
- They are a sounding board for you in early labor.
- Will guide you as to when to call the hospital to go in.
- They come to you in early labor as you transition into active labor.
- They will stay with you after the birth for approximately one to two hours.
- Do they have professional chestfeeding training?
- How many clients do they take in a month?

Doulas Do Not:

- Deliver babies.
- Are not medically trained and should never give medical advice.
- They will not or should not make decisions for you.

POSTPARTUM doulas are lovely when you want extra help in your home. It may be your first baby, and you have never held a baby, or you have one or more at home. I have had clients that have moved to my city and have no family or friends that can help.

When you hire a postpartum doula, you will discuss your needs; a price that you are comfortable with; specific times that work best for you, which could be; overnight 8 hr shifts or 4 hr shifts 3 days a week; they are paid hourly.

Short List of things Post Partum Doulas do:

- Give education and support for the first baby or other children.
- Help with learning how to hold and change a baby.
- Organize the baby station; make sure the changing table is in a good place and stocked properly.
- Feeding baby, bottles sterilizing and cleaning bottles; or chest feeding and pumping and storage; burping, comforting and settling the baby.
- Give tips for changing diapers and bathing.
- Help take other children to their activities or school.
- Help with the homework and play with the other children.
- Help cooking meals, cleaning dishes, loading and emptying the dishwasher, light housework, laundry, tidying, and encouraging other children to pick up toys.
- A doula can give you peace of mind to have a nap, shower or tub; while they watch over the baby, feed them, change a diaper and settle your baby.
- They may run an errand to pick up something from a store for you.
- You may need some help getting to a baby's appointment at the doctor's.

How to find the perfect doula for you: Find someone with whom, when talking to them, you *feel comfortable.* Before you interview a doula, read about their philosophy, how many clients they have helped, where they trained, and what they offer for their fee. Try to interview at least three people, then make your decision.

You can expect an initial complimentary interview that is approximately 30 minutes maximum (since Covid, interviews are conducted virtually). You should interview 3 doulas (or more) to find the best person for your labor or postpartum help.

My doula training was through 'Doulas of North America' *dona.org*. There are many different organizations that train birth and postpartum Doulas. Some Doulas are certified, others not. To help you find a birth doula or postpartum doula in Canada or USA (only), a colleague owns the amazing website, ***www.doulamatch.net*****.**

On this site, you can read where they trained, what their fee is and what their services include. You can learn about the person's philosophy, qualifications, training and experience, how many clients they take in a month, and how many clients they have helped in their career. Some have testimonials, their availability, and where they trained. This list will help you find three people to interview for a doula.

Sample wish list for a postpartum doula: If you hire an overnight doula, there are many different scenarios. Here is an example; think about what your needs are and ask the doula what you might expect, and what they charge.

A couple of scenarios might be:

The client wants to sleep through the night; they do not want you asking questions. The first night, I was given a tour of the kitchen, where the baby sleeps, where the baby is given bottles with formula (so shown where the supplies are), where I should be staying in the home and a list of the baby and their needs, much like the sample at the end of this document. So after they let you in the home, they go to bed and sleep until their alarm goes off.

The client wants you to come into the bedroom, pick up the baby and give the baby to the person for feeding, take the baby for a diaper change, settle them, and put them down to sleep. Then, you are to leave to another room until the baby's next feeding.

Night Shift Visit

Jack & Jill Parents
604 222-3333
1122 Main st
Vancouver

Start: August 18, 2022. Every Monday and Wednesday night. Start 7:30 pm - 6:15 am.

Baby:	**Sam**
Birth Date:	**August 1, 2022**
Birth Weight:	**6 lb**
Current Weight:	**6 lb 4 oz**
Amount of feed:	**80 ml.**

Breast milk 25%. Formula 75%. Brand formula from a can.

What equipment is used to mix formula and heat bottles? **None**

Heat up if not room temperature

Time of last feed ____________________

Wake baby to feed? **No**

Maximum hours to let baby sleep: **4 hours**

Soothing techniques, baby's likes: Shushing and swaddling, bouncing on a ball.

Can the baby have a soother? **Yes**

Do you use a white noise machine? **No**

Is there a communication book? **No**

Parent: C-section? **No**

Chest Feeding? **Yes**

Pumping? **Yes.**

Wake to pump: **Wakes on own**

If nursing, what drink/snack would you like brought into you? **None**

If pumping, how do you want the milk stored? **In fridge**

Is there milk in the freezer? **No**

Things to do when the baby sleeps:

If sterilizing, what type of sterilizer: **None; everything goes in the dishwasher.**

Laundry? **Fold only and leave on the dryer**

Empty dishwasher? **Not tonight**

Where to find:

In Nursery/Study	In Kitchen
Diapers	formula
Wipes	equipment to mix
Rash Cream	can opener
Change of Clothes	saran wrap
Burp Clothes	bottle warmer/mug
Swaddle Blanket	paper towel
Bibs	pump & accessories
Receiving Blankets	bottles
Crib Sheets	tongs
Soothers	soothers
White Noise Machine	laundry basket

Other: Is there anyone else in the house or anyone who will arrive during the night? **No**

What to do if siblings wake up? **Nothing**

Note from Parent:

____

____

____

____

We wake up at 6:00 am

Park on the street in front of the building

Testimonials from Past Clients

#1. Testimonials from both parents:

Nice to hear from you. I think I can say for both of us that what we appreciated most about what you did was responding, in the moment, with a clear head and stepping in to help the midwife in a medical capacity because the nurses weren't there. We really believe that your quick reflexes and clear head turned what could have been a negative outcome for the birth into a positive experience, and we will be forever grateful for that.

Thank you for your positive energy

All the best, Jinko (having the baby)

From Jinko's partner Brad

For background: You were the doula for our third child. The baby was born with the umbilical cord wrapped around her neck twice. Jinko labored mostly on her knees, but the midwife had to turn her to get the umbilical cord cut off. The equipment in the room in the hospital was not functioning properly, and in particular, one machine kept screaming at us and wouldn't stop. The nursing staff was not as attentive as we would have liked.

- Into all this, you injected a steady hand and helped navigate some very stressful moments.

- The midwife handled it all beautifully, but she needed help at certain points and needed it quickly, and it was you who was able to step in when the nursing staff was unavailable, and I was too stunned.

- You were the one who helped turn Jinko when the baby's head was showing, and you were able to deal with the malfunctioning equipment.

- I had been through a stalled labor and C-section for our first child and a normal vaginal birth for our second, but nothing prepared me for seeing our third child emerge with a purple head from lack of oxygen.

- Your expertise and reassurances were very comforting.

There is no substitute for experience, and a Dad just doesn't have it, no matter how many children they've had before.

Thanks again

#2. Hello, I would like to give feedback as your doula services were a blessing for our labor and delivery. Firstly my mom and Ian loved the ‘app’ that you used to time my contractions.

Ian’s points:

- Ian really liked reading and applying information, but the progression of labor was not as straightforward as our prenatal class or readings led him to believe. (He thought it was time to go to the hospital based on the timing, but it wasn’t).

My sense of smell was extra heightened in labor.

I loved the bathtub, but it did not help progress the labor since gravity was decreased.

We are trying for our second and will definitely be requesting your doula services again when the time comes.

Author's Note: Melissa and Ian did add to their family, and I was with them :)

#3. We were pregnant with our first baby when we had Esther. Then for my second baby, we hired another doula (they had moved out of province). The second baby was a much longer and harder natural birth. I compared both doulas' experiences; the things that were especially helpful were your 'positive affirmations' and generally having you around and helping us try different things. It was very helpful for my husband Mikael that you were there to guide him to try to help me through labor. I appreciated that you were both very active. I also **really** appreciated that you came over after the birth when I was having trouble with breastfeeding.

I have the pictures you took, but I think I look pretty bad after the birth.

Author's Note: She looked beautifully *in love* with their baby.

All the very best, Chloe.

#4. Birthing person points: Feeding help with the baby postpartum was really helpful.

The chance to revisit the birth story with you at the postpartum visit was invaluable. We could have gone through the photos at the same time, but it was all vivid in my memory at the time, so I didn't really need a reminder (although I love those photos).

Getting me to move to a better pushing position was helpful.

The best birthing help was that you explained to me that I had to hold my breath to push longer. I was just hyperventilating so much that it was interfering with the pushing.

I learned for myself to be more specific about the type of help that I like, even though sometimes it's hard to think ahead enough to ask for the type of help you need. For me, it was that I don't like people cooking at my house (because then things aren't clean as I like, plus there is more noise, plus them asking where things are). So I like mom, etc., to bring COOKED meals, even if they're cold. Actually, the second time around, anytime anyone asked what they could do, I said they should bring a cold cooked meal over or even a frozen one.

I've dealt with baby + food sensitivities twice. The first kid was full-on colic, starting at 2 weeks. I tried removing dairy and chocolate, and it didn't do anything. Colic is beyond draining and difficult. When baby #2 started the same, I eliminated everything except rice and chicken from my diet for 3 days. Colic went away. So then I slowly reintroduced foods to find culprits; dairy AND wheat. Just eliminating dairy would not have been enough. It's so hard to think through things like that when postpartum with lack of sleep, etc. Talking about these kinds of "breastfeeding complications" ahead of time would be great.

About colic - Mom needs to make a list of people who can come over and hold the baby. People she can call for "in a day or two or later today". See the previous point.

If people insist on buying you stuff and you don't want anything, ask for gift cards for places that deliver food.

Partner's points: He ALWAYS tells "pregnant" dads to "GET A DOULA! #1 thing to help Dad with birth; he really appreciates you telling him to take a minute and go outside "for a glass of water". Everything happened so fast, he was so overwhelmed, and the breather helped.

Jump in and take care of the baby - change diapers, offer to soothe for a few minutes. (Mom adds: Creates a great bond. I think that's been his "secret" to having a great relationship with the baby).

Love you Kim! Johanna

#5. Question to the client: What are the most effective techniques for the person in labor?

My wife will attest to this, that the best relief she felt during her labor was when you came in and immediately applied pressure to the tops of her bum and lower back. She was in on all fours at the time, and I can still remember the sigh she made when you applied pressure to that area.

Tips for the partner while pregnant or in labor and the 1st month home with the baby?

In general, I think you have to relinquish control around pregnancy and birth. You have to be able to go with the flow and do your best with the circumstances you are given. I don't think anything can really prepare you. You have your baby, and it's the expectations that can prevent you from being in the moment.

Find someone that you trust and whom you can ask for advice during the pregnancy. It can be overwhelming because everyone wants to give you advice, and I found it easier to have just a couple of people that I could go to, one being our midwife, who we trusted wholeheartedly.

When you bring your baby home, enjoy it if you can. When my wife and the baby, and I were all snuggled up in our room, it felt like a big sleepover! It’s rare that you ever get a chance to focus on one thing, so if you get paternity leave, relish every minute.

I appreciated having someone (the Doula) navigate the medical bureaucracy for me because it allowed me to focus on my wife and baby. It was great to have someone with us that could talk to the medical professionals and could translate it for us.

"Having a doula was such a great reassuring and calming presence at the birth of our son. Within seconds of walking in the door of our house, she changed the mood from one of fear and apprehension, to one of focus and determination. Obviously, childbirth can be scary, so having someone in your corner with such vast experience, for us anyway, was essential. For me, she gave me the ability to be an active participant, the knowledge to support my wife when she needed it most, and the confidence to be an involved father right from my son's first seconds. For my wife, she physically took away some of her pain, and she emotionally comforted us both in a way in which I knew I would be alright as long as I followed her instructions and listened to her reassurance."

What the care providers should have told us about labor?

We attended a series of prenatal classes as part of our birth program, so we felt pretty informed before the birth. I felt unprepared for the hospital experience and what nurses or doctors might ask you or do while at the hospital, such as cream on the baby's eyes, hearing tests, blood tests etc.

From Andrew

#6 A couple having their second baby, they delivered without a doula and in a different country for the first time. "It was nice to have doulas this time (I was mentoring a new doula). "Last time no one took the time to spend on us, it was such a nice change."

Anna and Ihor

Chapter 11: Vision – Birth Notes & Affirmations

People tell me that they have heard many horrible labor/birthing stories, and they wonder how they will get through their labor. So I came up with some tools for people to stay positive in pregnancy and labor whether at home or hospital. I have also included what clients have brought into the hospital (I include them with permission).

Some of the questions I have heard from clients:

- What if it is too long and too hard?
- How will I cope?
- How will I push my baby out?
- Can I love this small person?
- What if I can not stand the pain?
- Can I love a 2nd baby as much as the first?
- How long can I last without getting too tired?
- Will my partner be okay and fully supported?
- What does a safe or special birthplace be/look like?

MUSIC is a very important way to relax when you have concerns during pregnancy, especially during labor and later on when you put the baby to sleep. Many people choose a playlist that they would like to hear when they are trying to relax; or they want to get up and dance; to get the contractions happening; or when they need some incentive to get to 10 cm and push that baby out! Also, music will be beneficial when you are trying to sleep in the middle of the night and need to drown out the rest of the hospital noise, or maybe you are overwhelmed with the last 24 hours and need some calming - meditative music.

Visualize what your birth will look like.

Visualization and music are very comforting during labor.

Visualize a picture or drawing of something or someone that reminds you of a special time, place, or event; maybe special words which can encourage you. i.e., *I am birthing this baby with ease.*

How can I release fear around birth?

Nurture yourself and nurture each other.

Positive Intention: Is there something specific that you must have at your birth, or something or someone that you do not want at the delivery?

Music can motivate and transform us at any time, especially during labor. I suggest several playlists, one that is motivating or inspiring or gentle or exciting. The mood of labor will make many changes and different music at different times can help. Music you can dance around the room with or gently slow dance with your arms around someone; when you want to relax and rest, when you are about to start pushing.

Inspiration Cards: At the hospital, my client, Natalie, brought pre-made cards, similar in size to a recipe card but bigger. Each card had a single name of someone that they felt was strong and courageous, and special to them in some way; names included the partner, the baby, and Natalie. At the start of each contraction, the client started by reading the name and thinking about that person. Then, as they got more focused on breathing, one of us (in the Birthing Suite) randomly chose the card and read the name to my client. They concentrated on that one name for the entire contraction. There were approximately 30 cards, and as they went through the whole pile, I would shuffle them so they were not in the same order. The intention was to concentrate solely on that person for the entire contraction. They pulled strength and confidence to breathe through. It effectively gave them a burst of energy for every contraction. After the delivery, Natalie gave me, the nurse and our care provider the card with our name on it and said *Thank You*, for giving them the strength for each contraction. It was very touching.

Thank you Natalie, for including me in the cards. They were having their second baby, and this time wanted to feel especially connected to the labor, with no epidural. It worked, and *It was a fabulous birth!*

Count Down your Contractions: A client thought of how many contractions they might have in their labor. With that number in mind, when in labor, they concentrated through each contraction to count down from the 'chosen number'. Each contraction was one less than the last one. It was a huge distraction to my client to remember the last number, but it worked very effectively.

This is for after the baby is born. A **visitor's book;** my brother and sister-in-law had a visitor's book at the hospital. When a visitor came to see the new baby, they signed their name and gave their first impressions of the baby. Then they brought the book home for other guests coming to see the new baby, to write down their impressions and sign. It made for a lovely memory.

Positive Affirmations and Vision Notes: I have made this list to encourage clients at home, in labor and postpartum. Make notes on recipe cards with positive thoughts and special memories. Decorate the cards with pictures and/or something you treasure, a picture of the baby's ultrasound, favorite travel spot, pets, family, anything that always puts a smile on your face, possibly something that makes you laugh or gives you encouragement. Post these all over your home, mirrors, fridge door, or your workplace, on a desk, so that you can see them daily. Take your favorite pictures and make it your screenshot on your cell phone, iPad or tablet, or put together a collection of pictures and let them scroll on your device any time in labor and have your partner or other helpers read them to you often.

<u>My list of Suggestions might be:</u>

I am the Perfect Parent for my baby.

I Believe - I am stronger than I realize.

My body will 'know' how to navigate pregnancy, labor and birth.

I 'know' I can raise this person.

Baby and I are calm.

I speak to them Gently with Love.

Even when Contractions pick up, I am Safe!

We will see each other soon.

I Can Do This.

I Am Doing This.

My Body and my Mind are Open.

My Cervix/Body Opens, just like my favorite flower i.e. Rose.

Every Contraction brings my baby closer to me.

The stronger the Contraction, the more empowered I feel.

I embrace every Contraction.

I look forward to cuddling my baby.

I am surrounded by supportive people, that encourage me.

I feel Safe, I am supported and loved.

I relax in between every Contraction.

I relax during my Contraction and let my body do all the work.

Breathe in deep and slow, then Breathe out all tension.

Big LONG Breathe in - Big EXHALE.

I Breathe one Contraction at a time.

I am Strong with every Contraction.

I release all tension as I exhale.

I Breathe deeply, allowing my lungs to fill and give me and my baby lots of oxygen, then I blow the breath to the floor.

I know labor is long, hard, and complicated - BUT I am stronger.

I allow my body and baby to do everything they can with my help of movement.

I allow my body to gently push the baby down, closer to me, with each Contraction.

I trust my Body and my Contractions will bring my baby down closer to me.

I am strong and feel my strong body pushing my baby closer to me.

The more I relax, and allow my body to work efficiently, the closer my baby comes to me.

I often see people that look up at the clock in the birthing room and release a heavy sigh. They are visibly concerned and ask, 'When will this baby be born? This simple connection to time can draw out the whole birth experience. A trick for the clock in the birthing room would be to bring with you to the hospital a piece of paper and tape, then cover the clock on the wall.

This is a Sample of what a sign for the hospital delivery suite door might look like, and feel free to decorate it. (Names used are from my Clients, who made the poster.)

NATURAL BIRTH IN PROGRESS

YOU ARE ENTERING SACRED SPACE

PLEASE SPEAK IN SOFT TONES

BIRTHING PERSON IS ROBYN
PARTNER IS DAN

PIPER IS EXCITED TO MEET A BROTHER TODAY

NO DRUGS NECESSARY

WE ARE NOT CONCERNED ABOUT TIME IN THIS ROOM

THANK YOU!

Chapter 12: Cervix & Vaginal Exams – Baby Positions

Cervix and Vaginal Exams: Before labor, the Cervix is closed, firm, facing Posterior (toward your tailbone) and approximately 3 to 4 cm Long. Before you can start to push, your Cervix will become 100% Effaced and 10 centimeters open.

Effacement is when the Cervix shortens to nothing and thins out - to paper thin, so it can continue to stretch over the baby's head and body as they descend down the birth canal and are born.

Before labor **100% Effaced** **Fully Dilated**

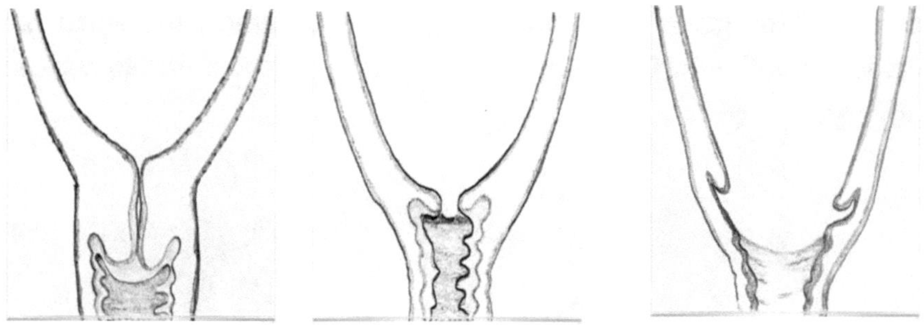

Dilation: The Cervix starts out closed and tight, and must open to 10 centimeters before you can start the pushing stage.

Soften: The Cervix is normally firm, like the tip of your nose. Care providers, when doing a vaginal exam, will describe the cervix as 'melted away' or 'butter soft'.

Station: It means how far down into your pelvis the baby's head is. The measuring system is + 4 to - 4. If the head is above 0, it means your baby's head is Floating or Not Engaged. At 0 and further down, the baby's head is engaged, and the higher into the plus, the closer the head is to the Perineum. So at + 4, we would say the head is on the Perineum and is very close to delivery.

To put this into perspective, if each station as a centimeter, - 4 to + 4 equals 8 centimeters or approximately 3 inches.

The station is very important to the care providers because it tells them how well you are or aren't pushing your baby down the birth canal. They may be able to estimate how much more time you may need for pushing. They watch the baby on the monitors, and it tells them if the baby is tolerating the pushing stage based on how much the baby's heart rate fluctuates. If the baby is getting tired from a long labor and long pushes at this stage, they may wonder if the baby is too big to come through your pelvis or if the baby is not in a favorable position. This gives them much-needed information for when they decide, if and when, to go to the operating room for an assisted delivery.

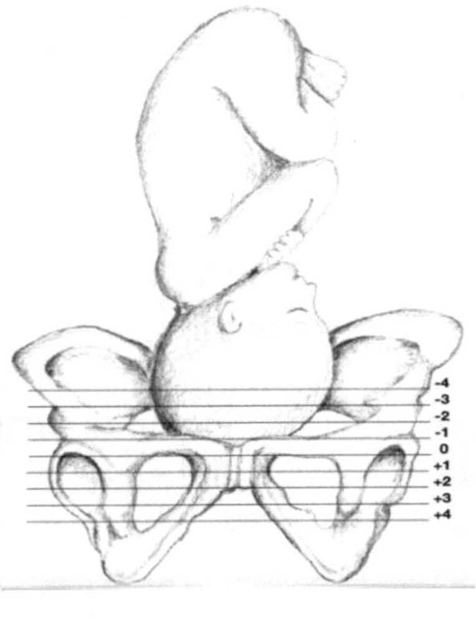

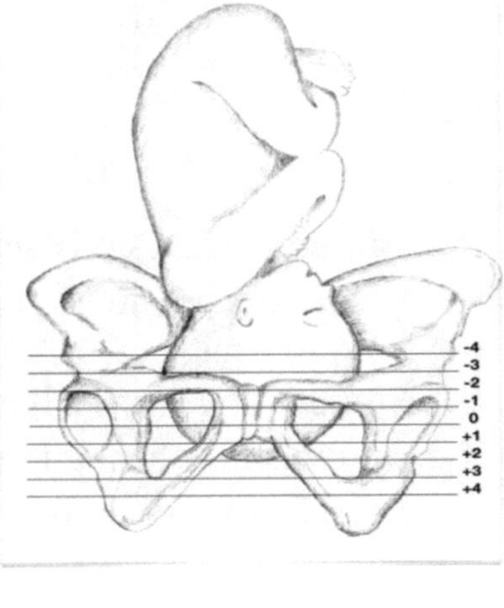

Head Position: During a vaginal exam in labor, the care provider, by touching the baby's head, can find out if the baby is in an OA or OP position. They feel for the cranial sutures (joints made of strong fibrous tissue) and fontanels (the soft spots that have not yet fused), and the baby's ears, making delivery easier by folding over and making a smaller head circumference to allow a bit easier descent through the birth canal. The Care Provider can tell which way the baby is facing.

OA means Occiput anterior position, Occiput means the 'back of baby's head' is against your belly button. It is the most ideal place for a baby to be in. They can make their way down and through the birth canal easier by tucking in their chin to chest, and the fontanels will mold to make a smaller fit. Baby is lying to one side of your belly facing, your tail bone and you can feel the all the wiggles and kicks on the other side from their back.

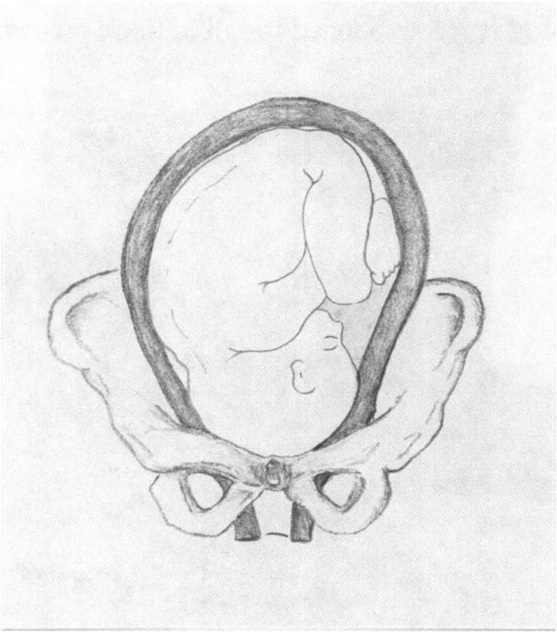

OP means Occipital Posterior position. In this position, the baby's back and spine is lying against your spine, and the baby is facing your belly button. People often complain about the discomfort in their back before they are in labor. When in labor, it is like having two different and distinct contraction 'pains' at once. This can make the last few weeks of pregnancy very uncomfortable, and harder to cope during labor. This also makes a longer and harder time during labor to come through the birth canal, as the baby's head will be flexed and not tucked down to their chest (chin to chin), making the baby's head circumference larger in the pelvis. I have seen OP babies looking up at us as they deliver, but this is only after a very long pushing stage or if the baby's head is not too big for the size of the pelvis. If the care provider believes it is safe to try a rotation (it involves putting a hand into the vagina and manually rotating the baby). The rotation often works, but sometimes baby has a cord around their body or neck, and they do not rotate. Or labor can slow down, making for complications that lead to having a forceps or cesarean delivery in the operating room. An epidural is recommended for all of these procedures.

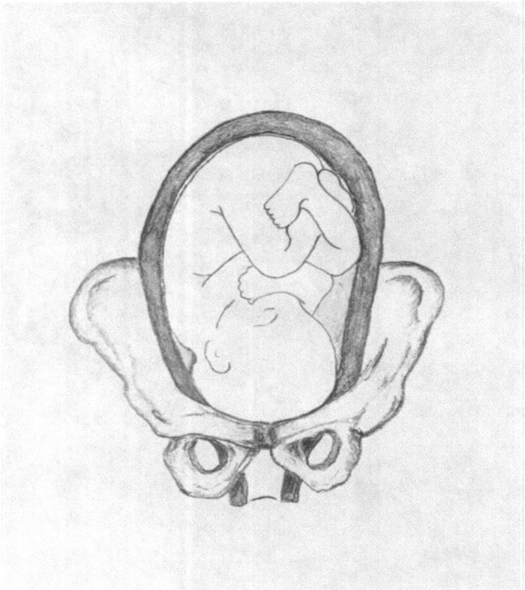

Author's Note: I have seen OP babies deliver face up and looking at the ceiling, but the push is very hard and is longer. You may be successful because you are extra strong in your pushing, or the baby's head and your pelvis are perfectly sized to pass their head through; this does not happen often. Many times we go to the operating room for help in getting the baby out, with forceps or cesarean section. Sometimes a baby has a big head that will never fit through your pelvis.

LOA means Left Occiput Anterior (opposite ROA is Right Occiput Anterior). The back of the baby is off-center in the pelvis and resting more on the left side than forward, and the head is facing towards your right thigh. Baby's kicks will be on the opposite side as *their* back. Ask your care provider when you are unsure where the baby is lying.

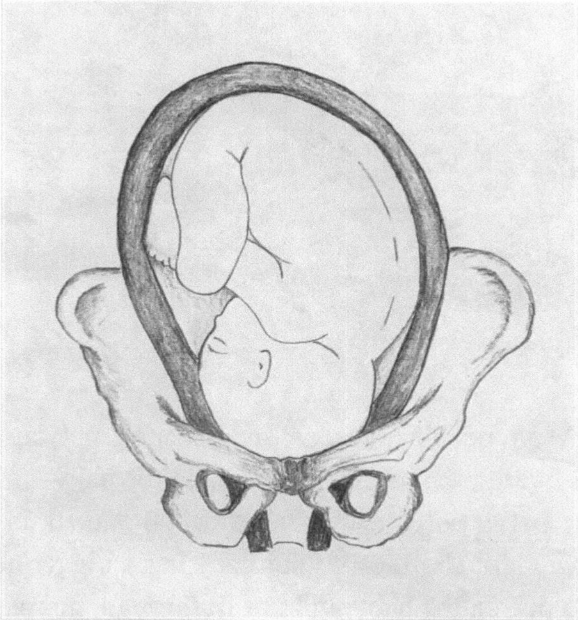

A transverse lie is when the baby is horizontally lying in the uterus. The baby's head is at one side of your tummy, and their bum is at the other side, and the head is nowhere near the pelvis. Once the baby is bigger, it is difficult for them to move lower, so the head does not get close to your pelvis for the descent. It is almost like they are suspended, with their limbs dangling downwards, or the baby can be lying facing upwards, looking towards the sky.

This makes for a very long labor, and it is hard for the baby to move on their own at 40 weeks because of their size. They simply can not place their head into the pelvis. These deliveries have a much greater possibility of a cesarean delivery. The sooner you know this position, the faster you can try to help the baby to move, head down. Your labor may not start because the head is not putting pressure down into the pelvis.

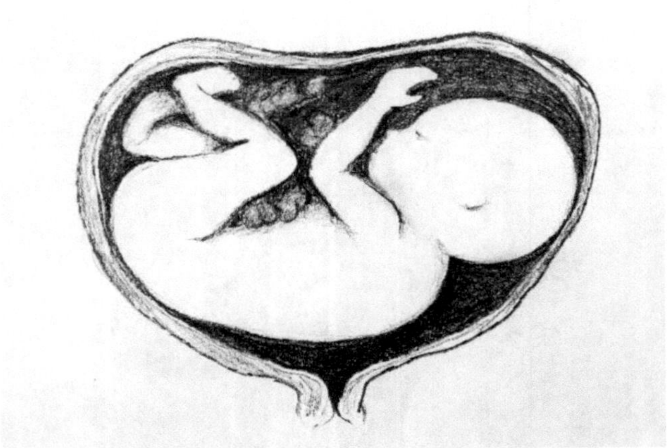

Pelvic Shape: Most people have an oval-shaped pelvis, and the baby's head will fit after the head 'moulds,' and the baby is in an OA position. If your pelvis is a heart shape, called "Australopithecus afarensis" or "Lucy" for short, or if your baby has a bigger head than your oval-shaped pelvis, the baby will not fit through, no matter how hard you try, and unfortunately, this is not something we can determine before labor.

Only until you go to the operating room for a cesarean section will some care providers tell you that the baby did not have a chance, your pelvis is small or heart-shaped, and your baby's head would not fit through your pelvis. During a vaginal exam and an extensive feel, if your care provider believes the baby's head is bigger than the pelvis and will not fit, then a Cesarean Section is advised.

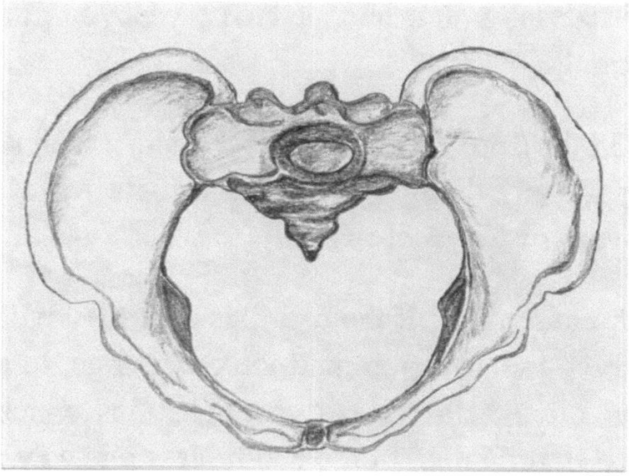

Oval shaped

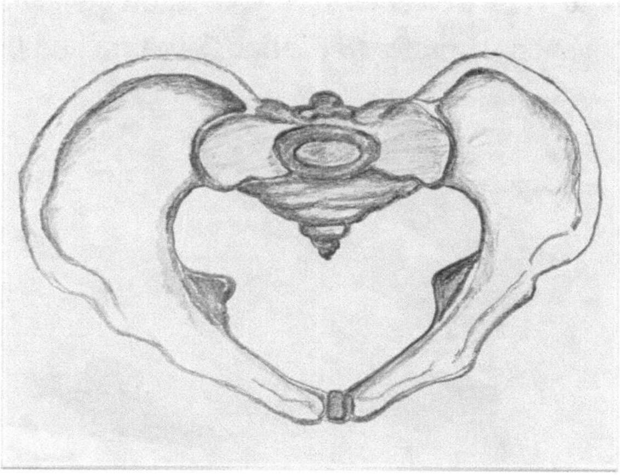

Lucy (Australopithecus afarensis)

Vaginal Exams: You may have a Vaginal Exam while having a pap smear, in early pregnancy. Unless there is any indication to specifically do another exam during pregnancy, you will not have another exam until you are about week 38. Vaginal exams are not comfortable and some people can not tolerate them.

One reason for a vaginal exam is to offer you a cervical sweep to possibly help start labor. It is intended to prevent you from going over your due dates.

At week 38 the Care Provider will ask to do a vaginal exam, they are checking for any dilation of the cervix, they may offer you a *Membrane sweep or Cervical sweep*

With your consent and if the cervix is soft, they will put a finger inside the cervix and sweep around the outer edge, to stimulate the cervix. It can often help release prostaglandins which start some contractions to start dilation of the cervix. It is one way of hopefully, preventing you from going over your EDD (estimate due date).

Ask your Care Provider, why they are helpful or necessary, when you get closer to your due date. It is your choice whether you want this or not, some people prefer to decline the exam and the sweep.

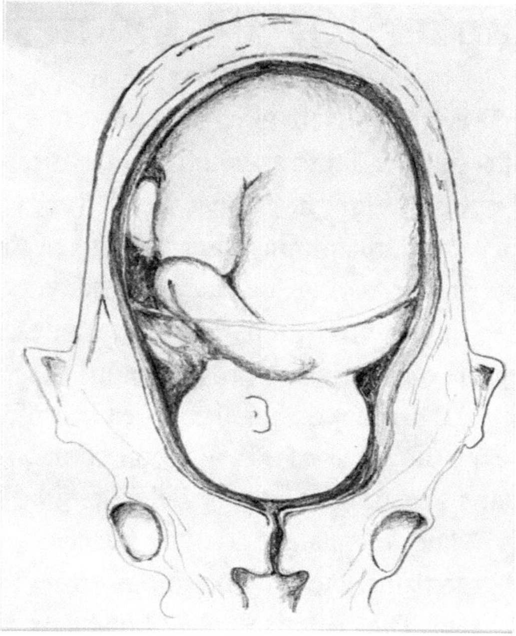

Most babies are surrounded by amniotic fluid and move about until they are too big, and movement slows down. The amniotic fluid consists of water from the pregnant person's body, the baby swallows this fluid and then the baby urinates. It contains nutrients, hormones and antibodies. Being in the sack of fluids is safe, and it helps to protect the baby from bumps and injury.

Chapter 13: 3rd Trimester

3rd Trimester Week 28 – Delivery: These last few months will be the busiest but the most exciting as your due date is fast approaching. Your baby will put on weight in the last 4 or 5 weeks and fill up any and all space in your uterus/tummy, and because of that, you should be slowing down and preparing for labor and delivery. I am amazed that so many people are busy preparing their homes. Many will be packing to move or renovating to provide more space for the baby. The farther along and bigger you get, the more uncomfortable you will be; you do not need the stress of all the preparations. I might suggest either doing things sooner than later or delegating by having friends and family help. Many clients get stressed because they are buying baby items and organising and moving things around in the home in the last month or two. They often tell me, "I just have to get this done before the baby is here," assuming that others can not help. Then it is very conceivable that the baby will come early with all the extra lifting and stress. Too many people go into labor and then come home from the hospital to a place not finished, which can cause more stress.

Your weeks will go by quickly, and you will have increased doctor appointments closer to your due date. They are monitoring the baby's health and growth by having several more tests and ultrasounds. They are also watching you closely to make sure nothing creeps up. There are so many different things that can change, from you needing to be put on a diet (for gestational diabetes) or complications and your baby coming earlier than their due date. Try to eat well and not over-exert or stress yourself, practice your breathing, and stick to a routine of fresh air, gentle exercising, and making sure the baby is in the ideal birthing position.

Take time to enjoy the last few months! Your life will get very busy when the baby arrives.

Celebrating the baby and the impending birth. Friends and family tend to get very excited when a new baby is coming, and often they will give you a surprise baby shower (party), or they may want to help with planning the baby's space in the home. There are many birth welcoming traditions to celebrate you and your baby, and they can involve a wide variety of themes. At the celebration, you can hire Artists that specialize in decorating with henna tattoos on hands, face, and belly, or on your belly, a variety of themes or pictures to be painted on your tummy. I have seen a picture of the baby in the position they are lying or should be lying, or of nature in a forest or water. They will usually last for a while and are quite stunning.

Belly casting is a beautiful way of preserving your 'belly'. The process consists of buying a belly plaster package which contains all materials and instructions. You would be wrapped naked, upper torso (tummy and possibly breasts included). You lay down and have someone that will attach the plaster to the belly, get comfortable, and have a tea party while you wait for the product to set. When it is set and dried, you can decorate the belly with paint in your favorite colors with designs or something abstract; possibly an artist can help. Personalize with special items, flowers, jewels (real or not), and ribbons; there are so many themes and ideas. This is a chance to have fun and express yourself, and have a memory of what your baby belly looked like. I have seen them displayed in people's homes, and they truly are a piece of ART. Ask your family and friends if they want to share in decorating.

My favorite thing is to hire a photographer to take pictures while you are still pregnant, go somewhere in nature possibly, a favorite or special place or into nature, or to one of your special spot. Photographers are creative and will go pretty much anywhere. There are birth photographers that go into the delivery suite and take birth pictures of your delivery, and then they send you a portfolio of amazing pictures. Afterwards, they will come back to your home to take pictures of the baby with you and the family. Or if your doula could take some pictures, although not professional ones. I offer to take pictures, and I ask my client what they prefer 'above' the waist pictures or 'below', meaning ALL birth and delivery pictures. Note there is usually a protocol in hospitals that as long as you do not take pictures of care providers or of the procedures, you are okay. Ask about the policies at the hospital you are going to attend.

Author's Tip for the Partner: You may have felt some anxiety that is settling into your home. As the birthing person gets bigger and more uncomfortable, they may seem to be cranky, but for really good reasons. They can not eat much at any meal because their tummy is squished from a growing baby, and they may have more indigestion or are feeling it for the first time in their pregnancy. They are definitely not comfortable in their bed, and there is no comfortable place. They pee *many* times every night, so there is no continuous sleep. They are counting down the weeks and days until they have to push this baby out! Which they have been told is hard and long.

As the due date gets closer, the more reassuring you should be by complimenting your partner and being positive in all conversations, and by being more helpful around the home. Encourage them to use all the tools from the Vision/Birth Notes and Affirmations document; you can maybe help them by saying some of the affirmations to them daily. You can start to learn all the acupressure techniques to help give the pregnant person some relief, and it will be good practice for you and the delivery suite. Start by doing more household chores or find help, maybe a family member or friend that can come to your home and help with baby preparations. Get to know routines for keeping the home clean or taking care of the pets or other children and their schedules. All of this will help. Surprise your partner by bringing 'take out' from restaurants or ordering in meals. Suggest that they have a massage, a manicure or pedicure, or take them out to dinner and a movie, anything that makes the pregnant person relax and feel pampered.

Your partner does not intentionally want to be cranky with you; it is because they have been watching their body grow and change, and experiencing fewer things they can do; they have been feeling all this 24/7 for months.

Learn the subtle luxury of Napping /Resting: You may laugh and say, 'I know how to rest'. From experience with my clients and many other people that have stress, they do not know how to take time in the middle of the day, to stop, reflect, be quiet and nap, or just rest. This subtle but effective time out for you will help when your baby is home and seems demanding (I am lovingly laughing at my comment, people often think this about their baby.); however, your reality can and will overwhelm you at times. The baby often seems demanding, but if they could speak, they would. Know that you will learn and understand all their habits faster when you can think straight, not when you are at your wits end from sleep deprivation. I have seen too many clients in their homes postpartum that *can not* sleep for fear of not hearing the baby or many other similar reasons while they sleep. It is imperative now to learn to relax, breathe and snooze, because the baby will rest every couple of hours, and you must also learn to take your break.

Sleeping comfortably can be a challenge. Pillows, blankets, and towels rolled up can make great props for the growing weight of the baby. Some support while lying down, for between your legs, from your knee to your ankles, and then your back. To relieve hip pain when lying on your side, you can put a small rolled-up hand towel under your ankle (of the foot that is resting on the bed sheet). Prop blankets behind your back to keep you from falling onto your back. Prop between the tummy and the mattress to help relieve some baby weight. I have heard some people sleep in a lounge chair, upright, for some relief, but I do not think that is very sustainable. From now until you deliver, try to sleep on both your left side and then your right side when in bed. Move to both sides frequently; this can help the baby as they descend into the pelvis as you get closer to delivery.

Positioning Baby: Always sit straight on a couch with your feet on the floor, or you could sit with your legs apart and heels together. Sitting forward on a chair with a straight back and legs spread wide apart. Be aware of sitting sideways on a couch with your feet tucked up under your hip; this can help babies get their heads stuck sideways in your pelvis. This is called Asynclitic and means the baby's head is sideways and tilted upwards. The chance of a baby delivering without help is slim to none because the head circumference is not ideal to fit through any person's pelvis. This will make for a very long labor, and only when you reach 10 centimetres of dilation, the care provider can feel for the baby's head position. If confirmed, they may recommend that you have an epidural for pain control because they will want to try to do a manual rotation of the head. If the baby is truly stuck and can not move, you will have to go for a Cesarean Section.

Week 34 Birth Tricks for Pre-labor until Baby Delivers: This document is a very important part of your birth preparation! Become very familiar with all of the content and start doing the 'tricks' and then increase weekly. These tricks help your baby to move into a more optimal position for labor and birth before they put on their last bit of weight. Their head moves sideways and then lower, they twist their body through the pelvis, which puts more pressure on the cervix, and in labor, the uterus will more efficiently push the baby lower into the pelvis, the result is a shortened and easier labor. Follow through with all exercises, *in labor and until you deliver*.

As I am writing this book, in the past two days, I attended two Multip's births; both babies were bigger this time, not in an ideal position, both were stuck, both clients went to the OR for Cesarean Sections, and neither client knew the second baby was going to be bigger. Not exactly sure if they did any birth tricks or worried about positioning the baby with their second.

It can be hard for you to judge where the baby is lying; ask your care provider the position; they can usually get a good sense of where the baby is lying by touching your tummy, then look at the diagrams of the baby in OA, OP, LOA, positions, in ***Cervix & Vaginal Exams*** document. It is ideal when their back is laying on one side of your tummy (it can be left or right). They must be head down and looking towards your spine, called '*OA*'. These tricks help you to put the baby into *the* most ideal position for delivery, to descend into the pelvis to make your labor shorter and easier.

Family Members are usually excited to help you during your postpartum time. Many cultures support the new parent and the baby for several weeks postpartum. The family will come and stay at your home, or you go to their home and stay for the first few weeks; if this is possible, it can make adjusting to parenthood easier. What I like about family helping is that it is a safe environment, and the knowledge that your parents have is sound advice regarding how to take care of the baby's needs. Family can help you adjust to your baby's demanding schedule until you can learn the baby's routine. They will help by doing the cooking, tidying, and watching the baby while you rest and recover from your labor and delivery. It's quite a unique environment. My mum came to help me with all of my children, and I found it very comforting to have her with me.

If the family is not available and you can afford the higher-priced postpartum nanny, they will live in your home for up to six weeks or how every you want. They cook and tidy and look after the baby and allow you the chance to sleep at night while they bottle feed the baby during the night feedings. You should be considering hiring someone sooner than later, they are very busy, and they book in advance.

Prenatal Classes should be starting soon. If you have been unsure about taking classes, you may still have time to find a place that has space. Meeting other people in your community that are also having babies around the same time as you will give you an advantage of resources from the class and will help make the journey into parenthood easier. If you have missed all available classes, go to 'YouTube' to find online classes for many pregnancy-related topics. For example, prenatal yoga instruction is brilliant, and it helps to keep you fit in a gentle way and position the baby. Clients rave about being connected to other parents and other support groups. Once you're a member and you know they are safe, you can set up text, email, and online support circles with other new parents, some in your neighbourhood, or many that are virtual, on social media, in any part of the world. While you are at home with your new baby, you can ask for and get help in the middle of the night when you have a question about the baby.

Weight Gain: It is easy to think that we can eat what we want because of our cravings, or you think no one will know. It is very important to stay with a healthy diet, not sneaking foods that will cause you and your baby to gain more weight, like starchy foods, or sugar, greasy or high calories, it will be especially difficult to lose after the baby is born. With an unhealthy diet, you run the risk of getting gestational diabetes, anaemia, high or low birth weight (which might put you in the operating room for an assisted delivery) and more. Then after the baby is born, you will have many things to do, like taking care of the baby, and there will be no or little time for exercise, and dieting is not recommended for the first few months. You still need to eat a healthy diet to grow a healthy baby while chestfeeding. Most importantly, the first few months are all about sleep deprivation.

GBS +/-: A swab test will be done in your care provider's office around this time. The results come back within a few days. If the results are positive, they will recommend that when you are in labor, you have an IV and start antibiotics. If you go into labor before they get your results, you may have to stick with GBS+ protocols and have the IV and antibiotics as a precaution.

Body Changes: During pregnancy, extra fluid retention in the body and the pressure from a growing uterus can cause swelling (called Edema) in the ankles and feet, hands and fingers. This is very common in the third trimester and can be very uncomfortable, and it always seems to get worse as you get closer to your due dates. Swelling can put a strain on your body, which makes regular chores, work, and exercise more of a challenge. You may have leg cramps that are uncomfortable or give a prickling feeling.

Carpal Tunnel Syndrome is from swelling that pushes on the nerves and causes numbness and pain in the hand. (This may make pushing complicated and more difficult, in that you can not hold on to your legs while pushing.) If the swelling is sudden, it may be a sign of pre-eclampsia, which should be monitored by your care provider as soon as possible. Hormones relax all of your ligaments and joints in preparation for delivery. There can be a greater risk of strain in parts of our body, hips and knees. Your breasts and tummy are slowly getting bigger, and this can have an effect on your back and shoulders. You will find that your balance is off, which can cause you to fall. Take special care of what you are doing, and try not to over-exert yourself. If your natural routine of a vigorous exercise routine, like biking, hiking, running and more, you might start to slow things down as your tummy grows. On occasion, your care provider will ask you to stop, especially in the last trimester.

Consult with your care provider about how much and how long you can keep up your routine before delivery, and then when you feel good after birth, you should not have any problem getting back to your regular exercises.

Baby movements should be happening a lot more now.

Your baby will have definite awake times and sleep times, but they do change.

Wearing jewellery, rings, and bracelets might be difficult, and you might decide to just take them off until your body comes back to pre-pregnancy, or at least until the baby is delivered. Try not to stand too long or stretch often when sitting for long periods; gently do all the birth exercises regularly. Take extra time to rest with your feet up, have someone give you a massage or have acupuncture treatments and most definitely talk to your care provider for advice.

Exercise Ball: I recommend buying a ball now for birth tricks and then for your labor and postpartum; it is the most important item to have in your home. This inexpensive item will help with positioning the baby in the pelvis before labor, progressing labor and then postpartum. You should be using the ball daily, from week 35, in labor and until you deliver. Make this your favorite place to sit, and while sitting, spread your legs apart wide to stretch. This will help the pelvis relax. You can be gentle or vigorously bounce on the ball, move your hips in a 'figure 8' or sideways on the ball that gets the baby moving lower. This is ideal for the babies to help them get into a better position AND puts pressure on the cervix. During labor, it can help with dilation or to pop the bag of waters.

After delivery, it is a very effective way to settle and help calm the baby and have them fall asleep. If you do not have access to an exercise ball, find a corner of a bed or couch that is soft enough to bounce on.

Your center of gravity is off, and it is important that when you are bouncing, you are in a secure place where you can not fall off the ball and injure yourself or your baby. Sit on the ball between other chairs or a couch and wall.

Decorating and stocking a nursery can be fun and filled with anxiety at the same time. It may be financially impractical to outfit your nursery with everything the baby needs right away. I have seen so many sweet little themed nurseries, for instance, 'baby animals'. There are many ideas on the internet, a fresh coat of paint, mobiles and books. Decorating with mobiles that hang from the ceiling, stuffies and teddy bears and toys, and many books to read to them even when they are still in your tummy, and then afterwards.

The most important thing is, where will your baby sleep? It is recommended that the baby is in the same room where you sleep, in a bassinet is ideal. They are too young and small to be in a crib; wait to set that up for a few months. If your partner works and needs rest, then you may need to have a separate space that you can go to and be with the baby as needed.

Bassinets/Cribs: I believe a baby does not need to be in a crib until they are older and bigger, and their brain has developed and when they feel a sense of security, and especially when they are starting to roll over. This is when they can transition from a bassinet to a crib. It does not mean you have to buy a specific bassinet for several months and then move the baby into a new crib. This expense should be thought out, a cost that fits your bank account. A newborn needs 'something' big enough that has a firm and not hard and plastic-covered mattress (2 inches) plastic for the wet diapers. I know of baby stores that sell newborn boxes for this transitional time. It has to have strong and deep sides, so they do not roll over. When the baby is bigger and rolling over, a crib is ideal, and there are many choices. The baby will need a sheet that covers the mattress and can be secured under the mattress. Babies grow so fast in the first few months that they will outgrow their bassinet and then need to go into a crib anyway.

Start with the basics, some blankets or receiving blankets, a thinner version of a warm blanket to wrap the baby. Clothing might be an undershirt that snaps under the diaper, sleepers, a pyjama-type clothing that has feet and a zipper or snaps that starts from under the diaper up to the neck for easy access to change diapers. They are designed this way because you will go through many diaper changes and spit-ups during one 24-hour period.

The baby at home can regulate their body temperature, and there are many ‘sleeping bag’ type sleeper/blankets that will keep them warm enough. This type of blanket prevents them from getting wrapped up in regular blankets. There are many on the internet and in stores to choose from.

Note: If the crib you want to use is older and for sentimental reasons you want the baby to sleep there, it may not be recommended for health and safety reasons, possibly because it has lead-based paint or the space between the ‘bars’ are too wide, and you want to put a bumper guard (a short 12 - 14 cm padded cloth), so baby does not get their head stuck. These are definitely not recommended to keep baby safe. You should consider a new crib or something that is transitional for the time being.

SIDS, Sudden Infant Death Syndrome fact sheet, see the document after the PPD Post Partum depression chapter in this book or go straight to www.Canada.ca for more information.

Chair for YOU to feed Baby: Whether you want the baby in your bedroom for the first weeks or a couple of months, or you want the baby in their own space, you will need a place to feed the baby. You can buy a new chair, or if you are able to borrow from family or friends, a chair that was once used for another baby. It has to be comfortable for you and must have a sturdy back for your back support, one that rocks is especially nice for soothing the baby back to sleep in the middle of the night. A footstool for leg support and a feeding pillow for propping/supporting the baby. This should be in a quiet area to ensure you can cuddle and burp the baby back to sleep.

You will benefit from having a small table beside your chair that has all essentials needed for you; water, snack, tissue for you or baby as needed; baby wipes and a diaper; a tv or music wand to watch tv or listen to music, and your cell phone (on silent).

There are many parent and baby groups online that you can exchange or buy and sell baby clothes and baby items for very reasonable prices in your neighbourhood. Social media is a popular way to find a group that is not necessarily close to you, that can support virtually or can be helpful in finding things for your baby or giving good advice and recommendations.

Author's Tip: When buying clothes or diapers, I often tell people to wait until the baby is born and know what the birth weight is. They may be bigger or smaller than expected, and you can often buy the wrong size. You could buy the size of diaper that you *think* your baby is going to be at delivery, then the next size bigger, they will grow out of their diapers and clothes quickly. If your baby comes early, they will be a 'preemie' born early, weighing around 3 kg or less, or 'post dates' over their due dates, which are heavy babies around 4+ kg. They will not fit into most clothes or diapers that an average 40-week baby does. Then you scramble to buy these items after the baby is born.

If your baby happens to out grow their clothes, and this is your last baby or you end up having extra disposable diapers, you can donate everything to your local thrift stores.

Diaper changing table is going to be used for a good year or more. Find the space where you want to change the baby's diaper and often dress and change their clothes (this will most likely be used many times daily). A small dresser or bookshelf next to the table or close by for your easy access to reach for something and space to stock (many) diapers and disposable wipes or cleaning cloth and diaper cream for their bottom, then separately clean cloth for wiping their face and body, and many options for their clothing, for sleep and for being up during the day. All other supplies needed, low light in the room, garbage for soiled wipes and/or disposable diapers, and separately a place for dirty clothes.

Infant car seats are mandatory in my country for babies, it is the safest way to transport an infant, baby or young child. They come in different sizes for the smaller baby and until they grow bigger into toddlers. These specially made seats are also good for many other types of transportation like taxis, planes and some that fit into a special stroller. The stroller may hold an infant, and then as they grow, they will need a bigger style stroller or have space for the bigger baby; options are plentiful.

Baby Wearing: A favorite thing of mine is to put the baby in a sling. There are many different styles, and they are easy to use for both infants and bigger babies. They are bundled in to keep the baby close to your bodice, for snuggling and keeping them warm, and to hold them when you are puttering around your home or when you go for a walk. Babies get fresh air and are so close to you that they hear your heartbeat, and they can sleep in them. Babies do not last too long in these because they grow fast and get heavy, and that can put a strain on your back, but it is a nice option as an infant that you do not want to put in a stroller yet. After several months when they are more alert, they will want to look at everything as you stroll them around. There is a huge assortment to choose from.

Feeding the baby, chest or bottles: In my career, I have seen many people who, for a variety of reasons, can not chestfeed their baby; clients that physiologically can not produce enough *or any* milk for their baby to thrive. More commonly, if you have had a chest augment or reduction surgery, you may have challenges feeding the baby.

You need space for the plethora of feeding items to choose from, bottles, short or tall; bottle liners; angled or fast flow nipples or the size of the nipple. Your baby may not like the nipple you have chosen, but a new different one may also not be correct enough to entice the baby. It may be trial and error to find the best one. Bottle and nipple sterilizers, as opposed to the 'old fashion way' of boiling water in a pot to clean everything. Babies under three months are still in the process of building their immune systems, and it is recommended to sterilize bottles, so you may want a machine to sterilize everything that way. If you need a pump for extra milk to store and/or to encourage more flow, there are many brands for you to choose from. Deciding on a brand of machine for electric pumps or simpler but not as efficient manual hand expression pump, can be daunting. There are different types of machines with different price points. They can be expensive so this item may be a good suggestion as a gift.

Author's Tip: Ask your family and friends; some may have recently had a baby or know of products, or have recommendations on brands that have good reviews. I have seen many clients purchase a huge supply of 'feeding paraphernalia' that they can not use or do not need because they successfully chest feed.

Consult with your care provider for their advice about preferred brands of formula if you know that you will be feeding your baby this way. There are many brands of formula, and each different brand of formula boasts that they have A+, are Fortified with iron, and are better and enriched. My personal concern is, 'does the baby need that?' Many clients over the years have asked me why their baby is having stomach aches and throwing up, so I ask if they use regular formula or fortified formula. They always say 'fortified with extra' stuff, so I ask them to try the regular formula and see what happens. Then they usually go ahead and switch to the formula *without* all the 'Extras'. It seems to settle the baby's tummy straight away; no more discomfort. *This is not scientifically proven, it's just an observation on my part. I do not recommend or endorse any formulas for feeding the baby. I prefer to have them at the chest exclusively, but I understand it is not always the case.*

Tip from clients: "Bring your breast pump to the hospital with you and ask the nurse/lactation consultant if they can show you how to use it properly." This is great! Because the pump and all of the paraphernalia can be hard to figure out in our fuzzy baby brain that we seem to acquire after delivery.

I encourage you to read the full chapter, **Feeding Baby by Dr Jack Newman.** This chapter was exclusively written for this book, and this is my favorite feeding GURU, Dr Newman. This chapter is filled with expert advice and many tips, their clinic is in Toronto, Canada, and they have been in the exclusive business of chest-feeding babies for MANY years. *Please excuse me, but I have chosen not to change the language (pronouns) that they use or any of the content in their chapter.*

High chairs and so much more are not necessary for the first several months, but they do have many options that look more like a car seat with lots of support. Newborns have small lounge-type chairs with a slight incline and are strapped around their waist and under the diaper. As they grow, their options explode, then after many months and when your baby is able to sit up on their own, they will go into a high chair.

There are many lounging chairs for a baby; they are very popular. I call them entertaining seats, for a lack of another word to call them. They look like an 'entertainment center' that are very sophisticated for your new baby and offer to stimulate the baby. These chairs can rock or vibrate or swing, both sideways and back and forth, many now that you plug into an electrical socket, meaning you do not have to wind up the swinging chair, as I did with my first baby. They are padded for the baby's comfort, along with a variety of music, toys, mirrors and lights that can flash or blink. Parents use these for the baby's sleep time (not so good to do this) or to go into the bathroom for a quick pee, or a secure place to put the baby when making dinner and the seat can be in eye-sight view.

The expense of a baby now is overwhelming! Doing all of this in the hopes that you have everything the baby might need and you are totally prepared, ask for help! Make a list for any family member that would like to gift you any of these or other baby accessories.

Cell Phone Apps: *There are many uses,* and they all have different advantages. This is a personal choice, but I happen to believe it is necessary in streamlining your new life with a baby. Once in labor and until your baby is approximately one year, is when you will come out of the baby fog, so until then, have all the help you can get.

Firstly, this is a fabulous way to count contractions when in labor; then the first few months, when the baby eats and when they pee or poo, your baby's Doctor will ask you these questions regarding how often and what the 'business' looked like. Take some time now to research and download one of the many apps to choose from, all about labor and pregnancy and then postpartum. Most are free and easy to use. They will make the first few months postpartum easier to navigate. If you do not have access to cell phone apps, then you can make your own list with a piece of paper and write everything down.

Count Your Contractions: This will help you keep track of your contractions and is very easy to use. When you are having regular and stronger contractions, push the button to start timing and then push the button again to stop timing. It will record the length of your contraction and how far apart they are. There are usually many other features, like a baby movement/kick counter and how strong, out of ten, your contraction was. When you call the care provider, the first thing they ask you is, "How long are the contractions - how often are the contractions - how long has this been going on?" The formula for

511 or 411 is what they go by to determine whether you should come to the hospital. These are all very easy to use, even if you are alone when you start contractions.

Pee, Poo & Feeding: Yes, this is a great way to keep track of the baby's business. It is important in the first weeks and in the first couple of months to keep track of how often and how long the baby feeds, if chestfeeding, which side, left or right, did they start on, and how long the feed was. This is especially helpful for the middle of the night feeds because you are very sleepy and *you will forget!* Another question for a formula feeding is how much did they eat per feeding, 2 ounces? How often do they void or have a bowel movement, and what color is the stool, if different from the normal? How often does the baby sleep, and for how long?

Your baby's doctor wants you to keep track of what goes in and comes out, and wants you to report back to them at the baby's next regular visit. They have to watch that baby gains the proper amount of weight and does not have any issues. Your mind is already on overdrive, wondering if the baby is sleeping okay, eating enough, wondering if you have time for a bath, or to make yourself a meal or anything else that you want to do. It is impossible to remember any of these statistics about your baby. Your sleep pattern will be at the utmost minimum for the first several months until your baby finds a good sleep routine. These first few months for all new parents can be an anxious time, so make it easier for yourself.

Post Partum Support Groups: Search for groups that you can converse with (globally) via texting. Other new parents or experts that you can ask questions to, get advice or have a chit-chat with while feeding the baby in the middle of the night.

WEEK 36 **Drink Teas**: There are many herbal teas you can buy in the stores that state they help to ripen the cervix, for example, Raspberry leaf tea which has been around for many years and is still being used. Other teas go by the name 'Last Trimester or Third Trimester' teas. You can find these in the natural foods section of your grocery stores, health food or organic stores that sell tea. I have encouraged clients to try them.

When you are in the store, take the time to look for **Witch Hazel** (my preference is Thayers, and it is actually a facial toner, so it can be used on the face, it is alcohol-free); this is for after birth. This product is clear and does not sting when you put it on damaged skin. It helps heal soft tissue damage, cuts and bruises quicker than any other product I have used. I have used it on myself and my children. It can be used on the perineum to heal stitches and a week after a cesarean section on the incision. Put some of the product on a pad, and put the pad onto the damaged tissue inside your panties to hold it in place. In addition, this is a very gentle product that can also be used on anyone else in your family that has a cut or bruise. It has been used on my kids to heal road rash from skateboarding arms and legs many times.

Be Prepared for labor: Get all preparations finished and ready for the baby, as they may arrive early, anytime from week 36 through week 40. Have your bag for the hospital, postpartum calendars, your kitchen filled with food and diapers, and your car seat bought and installed in the car! Being prepared takes away all the worry and pressure if your baby decides to come earlier than week 40.

Week 36 or 37: Refer to the '**Birth Wishes Plan home/hospital**' to start writing your birth plan, be prepared in case your baby surprises you by coming early. This is best done when you include your partner and or primary support people, as they will be very involved when labor starts. If you are planning for a home birth, you should also have a hospital plan on the rare occasion you have to go to the hospital because if you have to go, it will be in a hurry, or if you are having a hospital delivery.

Ask your care providers questions because they know all your medical issues regarding changes or how your labor might be, for instance, an induction or possible early cesarean section, there are many reasons. Do some research to get all the essential information that you need to know all your options for if/or when labor changes and you need a different way to deliver the baby. This document tells your team important information for both your labor and delivery in case you can not make a decision at the moment.

Labor can change at any time for many different reasons. When you or your baby are not tolerating labor, and you may be offered an assisted birth, forceps or vacuum or Cesarean Section, it will be difficult and stressful to make decisions at the moment, so consider all your options. What would your preference be for a variety of changes and scenarios?

Ask for some help from your care provider if you are not clear about what procedures might entail. Then have your birth wishes plan ready for anyone that is coming to help you at home, in the off chance they have not read it yet. And when arriving at the hospital, and getting settled in a delivery suite, have your partner give the birth wishes to your nurse. They will put it in your chart, along with your medical history and test results.

Some things to consider before you start making your birth wishes plan if you have animals or other children in your home. Dogs but mostly cats, are very sensitive and protective over you; they know something is not right and become anxious and fussy. You may be able to put them in another room, but they may scratch at the door or make crying noises, especially when you go to the hospital, they may be left for quite a while, and that is not good.

A pet sitter can come by and take them elsewhere, but if that is not possible, take your dog for a walk while you are laboring. *Both pets and children can be a huge distraction for you.* Your children can be distracting; they may come to you for hugs and attention while you are laboring, and when you ignore them (because you are so focused), it may make them sad or confused. Have a plan for family or friends either take your children to their home for a sleepover, or if they are staying in your home, have someone to look after them. It would also be nice to ask people to bring or make meals or snacks for everyone, tidy, make sure children are taken to school, play dates, or naps and bedtime, or entertain them while you are in labor. Calling helpers early in labor to take and look after other children or furry friends, the sooner you can relax, and focus on your contractions. If you want children present during the birth, have someone that can be with them if they get tired or to have their needs met, eating, napping, and school, as they can be demanding of your attention.

At a home birth, doulas or midwives will take turns keeping you hydrated, but they are there for *you and your labor*, and in active labor there is simply no time to be away from you. You want your partner with you as much as possible and not tending to others. ***Birth Wishes Plans are in a separate document.***

Prepare a PostPartum Scheduling Calendar: If your baby surprises you and delivers before their due date, I highly suggest you have a plan in place *earlier* than their due date. Once the baby is at home during those first few weeks, there is no time to do anything other than take care of the baby; you will be very busy and exhausted. This is a conservative estimate of the time it will take to feed your baby, burp, diaper change, then cuddle time and put to bed, which is approximately 2 - 3 hours. Your baby will want to feed every 3 hours, every day and night. Find time for you to eat, go to the washroom, dress yourself, my goodness take a nap! Your memory is compromised because of lack of sleep, so preparing yourself now, will make your life much easier.

Take a current calendar or make one or print a copy from your computer and customize it for all your needs. Write a list of everyone's name and contact information. You may need to make changes in case your baby is sleeping or is fussy. Ask friends and family if they are able to help with meals, cleaning, taking you and the baby to care provider postpartum appointments, or taking your other children to school or activities. Make sure ahead of time you give your permission to teachers, and any other activities or sports, for your helpers to ensure an easy drop-off or pick-up. On the calendar, have times for pick up and drop off and addresses for events and activities.

Make specific lists of all things that you want your friends and family to help with; tidy your home; do laundry; do dishes; watch the baby while you have a break or a tub or a nap; run errands or buy fresh food for you; take you and or baby or *other* family members to appointments.

Set up a meal train and be specific; who will buy and prepare food to be made in your home or dropped off, or restaurant-bought food, have take-out menus handy and how you will pay for the meals. You may have special requests, for example, if you are vegetarian and how you prefer your food prepared or if you have allergies. I suggest you try to finish general household shopping, including extra diapers, several weeks in advance of the due date. Make some meals that you can freeze and eat in the last couple weeks of pregnancy and for the first week of the baby's birth because you will feel too tired to cook.

***I highly suggest you schedule some special 'timeout' for yourself on the list.*

Pack your Hospital Bag: Many people are caught off guard when they go into labor early. I have a *long* list of suggestions for what you might want to take to the hospital. Your partner can always go home to get things. Bring the essentials, whatever you might want, a camera for pictures of the baby, a cell phone and wall chargers. Most important, in my city, all babies are required to be in a baby car seat when leaving the hospital. Check out: ***Pack Your Hospital Bag in a separate document.***

Take the time to drive past the hospital and know where to park and which door you go into. Some hospitals close most of their doors at night except the birth and delivery suites entrance. This is especially helpful if you are having a home birth in case there is an emergency. The birthing partner will likely follow the ambulance to the hospital; it will be helpful to know exactly where you can park and get inside the correct door quickly.

Signs for your front door: Make these in advance, the time when you get home will be busy with the baby. It will be nice to inform people that come to your door that you have a sleeping baby or you are both sleeping; suggestions might be;

Sleeping Baby

Do not ring the buzzer - do not knock hard. - Knock Gently Please

New Baby in the House

For *Delivery People* - We are sleeping, please leave the package in the box container next to the front door. Thank You. OR, quiet, please leave us a message on the notepad, and we will check it when we are up from our nap (then have a pen/pencil and notepad handy).

Put a sign over the doorbell that says 'Out of order - New Baby.'

Put the 'silent' mode on the cell phone, so no one can text or call you while you and your baby rest.

~ Then ~

Advise all your family and friends that the ringer on your phone may be off.

Perineal Massage Diagram: During birth, the tissues in your perineal area will be stretched to allow your baby to be born, which often results in a tear. Here are a few tips for stretching and loosening the tissues and reducing damage during delivery. Find a place that is safe, so you do not fall, and that is comfortable, possibly lying on your bed, or while sitting on a toilet, or in a warm tub, which will naturally help soften the tissues. I will leave this to your imagination.

With clean hands and the use of some lubrication, an organic or natural oil, or massage gel to help relax the tissues, you, or if your partner is interested and wants to help, can help with stretching *very gently.* It can be hard for you to reach around your baby bump. This is a very tender area, so use fingers to gently pull and stretch sideways and downward towards your anus. Do the massage for approximately 5 minutes at a time daily, every few days until delivery. This may not be for you; some clients say it is uncomfortable and/or hurts, or they are not comfortable doing this massage. Separately, another suggestion would be to put this in your birth wishes plan. Ask your care provider to apply a warm compress on your perineum while the baby is crowning (being born).

Please do not do this massage if it is uncomfortable.

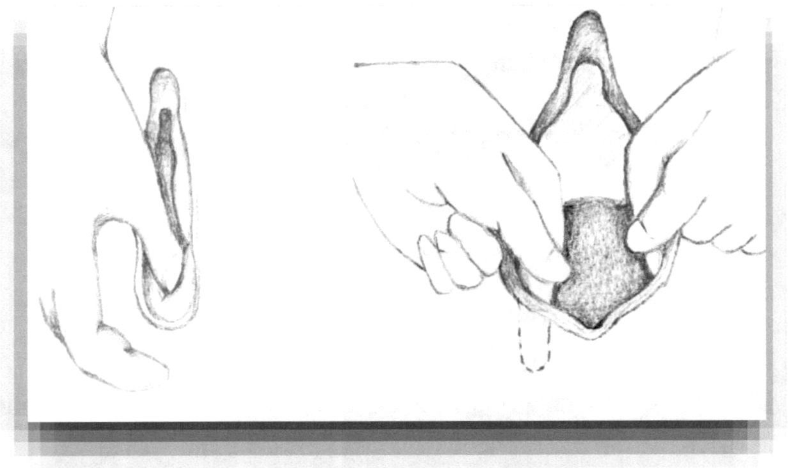

If the baby is breech, it means they are 'bum' down, near but not in the pelvis. Ideally, the head should be downwards to go through the pelvis first. If a care provider feels your tummy and suspects you have a breech-positioned baby, they will send you to confirm the exact position of the baby at an ultrasound appointment.

Do not do any birth tricks until your baby moves; they will only get stuck!

There are several different breech presentations. The baby's head is at the top of your tummy, making it difficult or impossible for a vaginal delivery. Most people find out that the baby is Breech during a belly check, and then it is confirmed by ultrasound.

Breech is bum down in the pelvis.

Frank Breech is when the baby's legs are positioned straight upwards towards their chin.

Complete Breech is the baby sitting with crossed legged with feet near their bottom.

Footling Breech is when a foot or both feet are below their bottom, and the foot or both will come through the vaginal canal first.

If the OB doctor believes they will be successful in trying an ECV, an External Cephalic Version, they will try this at the hospital. This procedure is a bit intense to watch and worse for the person having it done; it is very uncomfortable for them. The doctor will confirm the baby's position by using an ultrasound. This will help them to decide exactly the best way (turning left or right and down) to help the baby to move. The procedure will be done while listening to the baby's heart rate, which is monitored the whole time and using ultrasound imaging.

The doctor using their hands externally, presses gently on the tummy to help rotate the bum out of the pelvis, then gently touches your tummy and baby, encouraging them to move. If successful, you can start the exercises and wait until you are in labor and then deliver the baby. Most often, they will move, but when they show signs of not tolerating the procedure or do not move, the doctor will stop. You will be offered a scheduled Cesarean section for delivery, and they will set a time and date. There are not many obstetricians, doctors, or midwives that deliver breech babies, and waiting for a provider that has the experience to be on call to deliver a breech baby is not practical; there can be many complications involved.

If you happen to be at the hospital, in labor, and it was discovered you have a breech baby, and there is a provider that has experience in delivering breech, you may get lucky enough to have them deliver your baby. You will need to have an epidural for this type of delivery. It is extremely painful, as the baby's bottom comes first, and it can be a longer push. This delivery is very tricky and can have many complications. Often around week 35, a baby will rotate on their own and go into a head-down position, which is ideal for delivery. If the baby does not naturally turn and gets stuck, you will be scheduled for a C-Section, as many care providers do not have the experience to safely deliver a breech baby.

There are several ways you might help baby to move their position naturally. In water, a lake, an ocean, or a swimming pool, you can do a handstand, with support from someone standing beside you to guide you or help if needed. It may be hard to hold your breath, but you can give it a try. The water will make you buoyant and wiggling in the upside-down position, and you can help the baby to move with no pressure points. This can be very effective in encouraging the baby to move. Try only at your comfort level; it may not be easy to go upside down.

Another way to get into an upside-down position is to lie on your back on a secure and flat surface. For example, a big piece of plywood at least the same length as you, as long as your head is near the floor resting on a pillow and the wood is supported on the side of a couch and elevated at a 40-degree angle. You should have someone to help you to get into this position of laying on the wood - laying on your back, then stay with you while you are on your back for several minutes or until it is uncomfortable. Then they can help you get up from this position. Mind that you might feel light-headed.

You must have at least two people to help support you for this next position. Have them help to place your head onto a pillow on the floor, with you facing the back of the couch. Start with your knees on the couch, then with someone supporting your legs, lift your legs up straight; this would look like doing a handstand, BUT with someone fully supporting your legs. Then you help to support yourself with your arms on the floor. Stay as long as it is comfortable, and you can do this several times.

ALWAYS have a support person in place whenever you're doing an upside-down exercise. When you are doing any of these 'upside-down' activities, your equilibrium is unstable, and you should not be allowed to fall. Especially if you feel light-headed, stop and possibly try again later. It may take several times, but do this only as long as you can be in that position. The baby will try to turn themselves into an ideal position, which is head down. Many times babies will move on their own around week 35. Be proactive because the other option for delivery is a Cesarean section.

Baby Positions are shown in Cervix & Vaginal Exams document.

Author's Story: *I remember with my first baby, I was at dinner in a restaurant, and I had the most uncomfortable 5 to 10 minutes of the baby moving. I must have looked really silly with my back arched,* *leaning way back in my chair. It did not hurt, but the sensation of the baby moving was a very weird experience. I actually did not know what had happened and was a bit worried. I called the doctor the next day. I did not know that my baby had been breech.*

Author's Story: *I have seen approximately 20 breech births. One time during a routine vaginal Hospital delivery, I looked down and saw a foot coming out of the vagina. In utter surprise, I looked to the care provider that was going to catch; they had been looking at someone else, answering a question. I leaned into the person and quietly said, "There is a foot!" What a surprise, no one suspected. We got lucky that day; the care provider happened to be very experienced at catching breech babies. They turned to the staff in the room, and gently asked for everyone to help set up for a breech delivery quickly, and for the paediatrician to be present in the room for delivery. There were a few directions to inform everyone in the room. Our client delivered their baby within a few more pushes. It was very amazing to be there for that birth!*

Acupuncture and Acupressure at Week 37: The use of these pressure points should be in full use daily. I would highly advise going for a treatment at the acupuncturist. You go and lay on their bed/table for approximately half an hour or longer, the treatment is very relaxing, and you can remember exactly where different pressure points are used (to do them at home). ***All Acupressure points and Double Hip Squeeze in a separate document***

Author's Tip: There is a fabulous documentary that my sister recommended; it is 1 hour of fascinating information about how a baby grows in the womb during pregnancy - how twins are made? Triplets and Quads.

http://topdocumentaryfilms.com/the-nine-months-that-made-you/

Week 38 Vaginal/Pelvic exam, Membrane Sweep: Your care provider has many reasons to do an exam. It gives them a reference point of your cervix; and helps them find out whether it has started to soften, thin, or open. This can indicate that labor might start on its own soon in the next few days. If there is no indication that the cervix is starting a change, they may suggest ways to help prepare the cervix. There are many reasons why you should be delivering at 40 weeks or earlier. For instance, if you have gestational diabetes, we do not want a baby to grow too big, but each person is very different. This is a very good precautionary way of having a successful vaginal delivery and a healthy baby, and a functioning placenta.

Vaginal exams should only be done by a primary care provider, a doctor, a nurse, or a midwife. Sometimes, vaginal exams are necessary at a clinic appointment or at the hospital. The exam is done (with sterile gloves) by putting the index and middle fingers into the vagina; the person can feel for any dilatation and effacement of the cervix and can get an idea of where the baby's head is in the pelvis, is it high and not 'engaged' in the pelvis, or is it lower, and if so, how low.

While doing the VE (vaginal exam), if there is a slight opening of the cervix, the person may offer to do a sweep of the membranes. This is when they put a finger into the cervix and wipe all around the inside of the cervical wall. The exam and the sweep may be very uncomfortable. The outcome is that it aggravates the cervix and should give you some contractions, in the hopes that labor will start. It is not 100% efficient in achieving this, *but* on the other hand, it can be very efficient in putting you into labor. It has more to do with whether your cervix responds well to the sweep.

Last few weeks: Until the baby arrives, you may be asked to do many things to ensure that the baby arrives at their due date or close to 40 weeks. Foods that 'might' help ripen and/or soften the cervix and to stimulate and/or irritate the gut to start contractions, try any and all. Try dates - pineapple – extra strong garlic, extra onions, SPICEY on all your food, *only enough that you can still eat it*. Liquorice, not the sugar-filled candy, but the natural black liquorice, is a stimulant that can start cramping in the bowels, similar to a laxative, which in turn will produce some uterine cramping, *it is recommended to eat only very small amounts*.

Sex: The release of sperm on the cervix has a high amount of prostaglandin and is a natural way to ripen the cervix and help start labor. At this point, you may be saying NO to all of that. However, it has the natural ingredients that are synthesized in the products that may be used for an induction of labor. Kissing and nipple stimulation means 'rolling the nipples' releases oxytocin in your body. Double up all the birth tricks and acupressure points that are possible. Other options might be to make appointments for moxibustion, acupuncture, and the Webster technique done by a chiropractor.

Aromatherapy is not allowed in many hospitals; there are restrictions, so it is best to inquire before taking a scent into the hospital. If you are allowed to take it to the hospital, a good way to transport it is to put your chosen scent onto some tissues or a facecloth and into a secured (zip-locked) plastic bag. When in the birthing suite, ask the staff if it is alright to take out and use. People working in the birthing suites may have an allergy to different scents, for instance, lavender, and many people in labor can be *very* sensitive to scents. For example, if your partner comes into the room with food or a coffee, you may demand they get it out of the room! This can also be the same for any essential oils - aromatherapy that you HAD wanted; you may not want any scent in the room during labor.

MUSIC can motivate and transform us at any time, especially during labor. I suggest several playlists for different times, one that makes you want to dance and giggle your hips, gentle music for a slow dance with your partner or when taking a rest break, calm meditative sounds when you are having a nap (when you have an epidural) or after baby delivers. Then something vibrant when you are 10 cm and need the incentive to push your baby out! (I once had someone play the Star Wars theme). Music will be beneficial when you are trying to sleep in the middle of the night and need to drown out the rest of the hospital noise, or if you are overwhelmed with the last 24 hours' events. Visualization might be favorite pictures or drawings of something or someone that reminds you of a special time, place, or event. Special words and sayings that encourage you, i.e., *I am birthing this baby with love and ease.*

Signs that your body is getting ready to start Labor:

Diarrhoea is common at this time. Prostaglandin, a hormone, is released in the body, which can hyper stimulate the bowels, but it can help the uterus to start contracting and help soften and dilate the cervix.

Back pain: If you have any back pain, do all the *birth tricks for* an OP baby, and the back pain will go away; the baby has not moved if you still have pain. You may have a baby that is not in an ideal position and is lying on or near your spine. Ask your care provider for clarification on their position.

Sleep is your biggest barrier to the longevity of labor progressing. Nothing is comfortable for you now, and you are both excited and anxious that things should be starting. Sleep is one of the biggest factors in how you will cope during labor, so try to take breaks and rest.

Mucus Plug seals the opening of the uterus. It usually comes out either before labor starts or during labor. It can dislodge and fall into the toilet in the middle of the night when you void, and you may not notice it. If you do see it, it looks like a small ‘blob' of milky white jellyfish, around the size of a walnut. It may have some stringy red blood attached to it. The slimy mucus can come out randomly any time up to a few weeks before or a couple of days just before labor starts. It is an indication that the cervix is starting to change for labor.

Bloody Show is different from the mucus plug, and it indicates the cervix is changing/starting to dilate. There may be small amounts of blood or a blob of mucus and blood, most times dark brown, pink, or red in color discharge, which is called bloody show. After having a vaginal exam at a prenatal visit, you may have a tiny bit of bloody show on your pad or panties.

NOTE: If you have a substantial amount of blood, approximately 2 - 3 cm in size or more, then contact your care provider; they may want you to take a picture on your phone of the amount of blood that lands in the toilet or on a pad, to show them. They may also ask you to come into the hospital or their office.

SROM, Spontaneous Rupture of Membranes: Your baby lives in the uterine sac that is filled with a 'bag of waters' called the amniotic fluid, and most often, it will let go or break on its own. Water breaking can happen any time of the day or night, but unlike in the movies, where they show a large amount of fluid spilling down your leg and flowing all over the floor and down the hall, the amount is seldom more than a 1/2 cup of water.

If you are having contractions, the pressure of the contraction and the baby's head being well applied to the cervix can put enough pressure to break the bag. With the release of the waters, often baby's head may slide a bit further into the pelvis, and that helps to put more pressure on the cervix. You should notice the contractions become more intense. It is common to leak small amounts of fluid with every contraction, so you may want to wear a pad in your panties. If you do not have contractions when the sac breaks, it should start contractions, but it does not always.

When your waters break or a rupture of membranes happens, it is very significant information, and you will need to tell your care provider to explain *when* your water broke. Be prepared to tell them the amount of fluid (i.e., 1/4 cup of water) that came out and explain the color the fluid was. The color of the waters has different meanings of importance. If it was clear with possibly a small amount of pink/reddish blood or brownish blood, OR was it a slight brown, green, or yellow. When the water is brown or green, it is called meconium, which means the baby has had their first bowel movement inside (not all babies do this until delivery). There will be different protocols for your delivery with meconium in the waters. One important change will be having a paediatrician in the room when you deliver. If you are past your due dates, many babies will often have a bowel movement, especially if your baby has been under stress, possibly because of the labor OR many other reasons.

When waters break, and if you are GBS+, you will need antibiotics at least four hours before you deliver (unless you have declined having this). Your care provider will want to have an intravenous put into your arm or hand for the antibiotics when you come in for an assessment and usually before you go to the delivery suite.

Author's story: Only twice have I seen what the movies portray, the pregnant person walking down a hallway and their waters break, and the amount was literally a bucket of water, slowly flowing down their leg and all the way to the end of the hall. One time I was with a client, and they were given an artificial rupture (AROM); they were on the bed, but the fluid kept coming like a small river that continued for approximately five minutes. It ran right off the end of the bed.

AROM, Artificial Rupture of Membranes, is explained in the labor chapter. This is a procedure that is done during labor to 'augment' or bring on more contractions or help with the progression of labor by dilating the cervix.

It is normal to feel depressed or cry at any moment of the day or have mood swings. You are getting bigger, and you are not sleeping because you can not get relief from the weight of the baby, and you are uncomfortable. Many people are concerned that they will not know how to take care of their baby. Emotions can swing from low to high several times a day. The future of this baby becomes *of most importance.* You wonder, 'Can I deliver this big baby in my tummy?'

Primip is your first baby. It can be described as the first baby that opens the pathway inside your body. This birth can be challenging because they are usually a very long labor and then a tough and long push. There can be many complications, and often but not always, you may have help with the delivery. Your subsequent labor should be shorter in duration and have less complications.

Multip: You have your second or more baby. Second babies tend to come faster and be shorter in duration, but not always. However, a third baby can be a 'hodgy podgy' type of a labor, meaning it can be almost as long as your first, or maybe as fast as the second; you never can tell. Babies that tend to come faster, do it with more intense pain, but then the pain is gone much quicker because they deliver faster.

I explain to my clients that with a multip baby, once labor starts, you can dilate faster, then deliver quickly, even the push is faster, so it can feel like being on a 'roller coaster' ride, but with all births, when you have pushed your baby out, and placenta is delivered, there is no pain! Well, except for the repair, but then the care provider will give some freezing for that.

Prodromal is the early labor that seems to start and stop randomly, over days or a couple of weeks. You may or may not have experienced prodromal labor from your first, but I have seen people with second or third babies have this. It can be very difficult, because people expect labor to progress into active labor, but it does not; it just becomes very tiring and hard to cope with the sleepless nights and uncertainty of when labor will progress.

Week 40 What if I *don't* go into labor: There are times that the baby does not fit into the pelvis, the size of their head is big, or your pelvis is shaped in a heart shape; it is called 'Lucy' or '*Australopithecus afarensis*', our babies head *does not* fit, even if their head is a bit smaller. The problem is that we do not know that 'you' might have this type of a pelvis until you have gone to a Cesarean section and the surgeon takes a moment and notices the size and shape of the pelvis. I have seen doctors tell clients in the operating room that it might be best not to try for another vaginal delivery. (Take a look in **Cervix & Vaginal Exams** for a picture of Lucy)

Why you have not gone into labor is a difficult question, so the care providers will be asking you to go in for non-stress testing to make sure the baby is responding as expected, then to an ultrasound to measure the amount of amniotic fluids and check the baby's body and head circumference. Is the baby in a good position and in the off chance baby is breech, if you and the baby pass all of the testing, you will be given a bit more time to wait for the baby and your body to start the birth process.

This is the **Time to Double up *all* Doula Tricks**, they should be done as often as possible and daily with as much vigour as possible! Stay hydrated and continue eating small meals or healthy snacks. Go see an acupuncturist for several visits. Do ALL of the acupressure points and often. Shake hips! Stomp downstairs! MOVE! Then at the end of your day, eat spicy foods, take time to relax, have a tub or shower, and get some sleep or rest. Your care providers will make an appointment for you to have a sweep of membranes and/or an induction of labor.

Author's Tips: Stay Positive - Focused, and Breathe - You will fall in love with your baby! I can definitely say that our heart grows whether you are having your 2nd or 6th baby. I also believe that we innately know what to do with our babies and how to raise them.

For the pregnant person, the last few weeks can be the slowest of the entire pregnancy. You should be reserving time to do things with your partner that will be hard to do after the baby is home, like going on a date, meals out at restaurants, movies, and other forms of entertainment. It is time to pamper yourself with a massage or pedicure, or manicure before the baby comes, so enjoy this free time.

My motto in life and especially in labor:

Breathe and Believe ~

Birth Knows NO Date or Time - Expect Anything - Be Prepared for Everything and DO NOT get fixated on having a Labor and Birth *Your Way*.

Chapter 14: Birth Tricks - Pre-Labor Until Baby Delivers

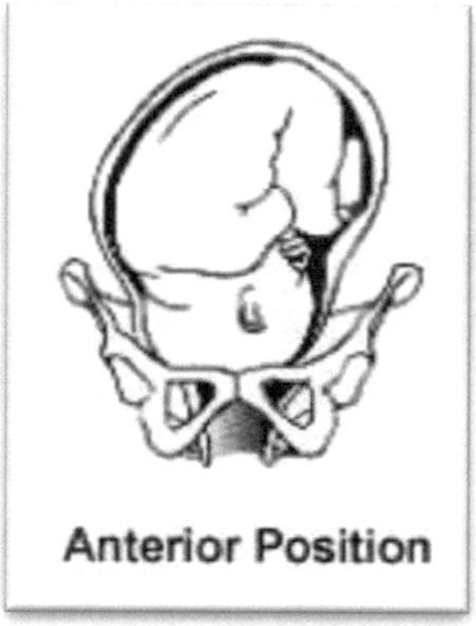

Baby in OA Position

Birth Tricks and 'Exercises' I use the word 'exercise' loosely, but when you faithfully start these tricks and do them several times a week or preferably daily, it results in an easier labor. These tricks help your baby to get into the most ideal birthing position OA, Occipital Anterior. When they tuck their chin into their chest, the fontanels on the head gently fold slightly over themselves, making the circumference of the baby's head smaller, so the head comes down, through the pelvic area easier. This is an ideal position for a baby to be in for a shortened labor with fewer complications. This puts more pressure on the cervix as the baby gets lower into the pelvis resulting in a shorter and easier labor. *You will be able to continue all acupressure points in labor.*

Author's Tip: If you have more than one baby growing in your tummy, ***do not*** do these tricks without asking your care provider what they feel is best practice for you, OR if you are physically uncomfortable doing any of these, then stop.

If you find out your baby is Breech, no more exercises until baby turns to a head down position. You do not want the baby's bottom stuck in your pelvis. Your care provider should be able to tell you where your baby is lying.

Start at Week 34: Start all tricks and gently increase exercises, with each next week, until you deliver.

Hands and Knees in this position, cushion your knees on a small pillow or a folded towel as needed. Then as if you are 'cleaning the floor', swing your hips back and forth and side to side for 20 minutes every day. It may help to break it up into shorter times but more frequently. Other places that you can do this is on a couch or leaning against a tall countertop; you will lean forward and wiggle the hips, changing it so you can do both slow and vigorous hip shakes.

Lay on your back, lift your pelvis up high, and stay in this position for a few minutes or as long as it is comfortable. Do this three times a day.

Sleep on BOTH sides. Try sleeping on the side you do NOT favor, the uncomfortable side. Use a rolled-up blanket or towel behind your back to prevent you from rolling back over to your favorite side, also another blanket or towel between your legs, from the knees to ankles. You are trying to get the baby's back centerd in the front of your tummy, looking at your spine. If you have hip pressure, put a small hand towel, folded under your ankle, of the foot that rests on the bed.

Squatting when you are brushing your teeth, or anywhere else you can squat, try this many times during the day. If this is uncomfortable, you can use a yoga block under your bottom to support yourself. Then with your elbows, push your knees outward for a wider squat. Squat any place, and often, if it is uncomfortable, sit on a chair and spread your legs as far apart as possible and for as long as you can.

Check with your care provider before doing the squat position in labor.

Sit or Bounce on an Exercise Ball: If you can comfortably sit on the ball, it is a great way to be upright and take the pressure off your legs. This is also helpful to open and relax the pelvis and to put the baby deeper into the pelvis. On the ball, ensure that you support yourself from falling sideways and rolling off. For example, position the ball beside a couch and wall. On the ball, you can do figure '8' with your hips and then bounce *both* slowly and vigorously up and down, do this often and every day, for at least 15 to 20 minutes at a time; it may help you to stay longer, by listening to music or watching tv.

If you do not have room for a ball, sit on the corner front of a couch and bounce, or when you are at the dinner table, spread your legs wide. The ball can be used after the baby comes back home from the hospital after delivery. To comfort the baby, you will hold them in your arms while bouncing on the ball when they cry in the evening, and it helps soothe them to sleep. These balls are easy to find and very inexpensive.

Climb Stairs and Lunge: At the bottom of a flight of stairs, lift your leg up 2 steps and lean into a deep lunge (do left leg then right leg) support yourself by holding both sides of wall or railings, then walk to top of the stairs. When coming down the stairs, let your leg and foot **drop heavily**, to the stair below. Do this daily as many sets of stairs as you can, *especially* when you are in labor. Clients tell me that a Lunge helps stretch and relax the legs, they like the feeling of stretching.

Chair and Lunge: This can be done on a chair or at the bottom of the stairs. Put your foot on the chair (a chair that is stable against a wall and will not move) and support yourself by holding on to the wall, a railing or your birth partner; do a slow lunge with the left leg, then the right leg, repeat this several times every day.

No sitting sideways on the couch with your legs tucked up and beside you with feet curled under your bottom. Your baby will settle into the side you favor and most likely will get stuck in the wrong position. Ideally, you need to sit straight and upright, with your legs spread apart (opening the pelvis).

Walk for 30 minutes, 3 times a week. At week 35, increase walking to 45 minutes. At week 36, increase walking to 1 - 1.5 hours per week. Before you go walking, do some Tahitian hip shakes for at least 45 seconds and more. Then do intermittent shakes (see next paragraph), then walk 100 metres, and repeat, repeat as much as possible.

Tahitian hip shakes are fun and the best exercise to do **daily.** Stand with your feet 6” - 12” apart (so you are comfortable), knees bent, back straight, shoulders square, and start to Sway your hips quickly back and forth, shaking hips to Tahitian or Indian music or your favorite fast music. The *Hawaiian shake* is a slower version for when you need an easier ‘shake’. Then as you get better at the shake, start to *shake* and walk around the room, clench your fist and with arms at your side, with bent elbows, around the room swinging your arms. Then for fun, you stomp around the room! Start this for 30 seconds, then increase the duration and length of time, every day and as often as possible. Do the Tahitian hip shake from each room you go in and out of daily. During the day, shake your hips as usual, then walk as much as possible. What does a Tahitian hip shake look like? Envision a Hawaiian dancer, with a green leaf skirt, shaking their hips from side to side. You can find a visual if you look on the internet to find out how to swing and shake your hips. Choose your favorite dance music.

Some of the tricks were created by a colleague Doula Noriko Ishibashi and a website that has similar techniques is the Miles Circuit **www.milescircuit.com**

The above exercises help ensure a well-positioned baby. All these tricks should be done before labor starts, AND *especially in labor.*

Variations might be to slow dance, wiggle, jiggle, Salsa, fast crazy dance, shake your hips, stomp around to put baby deeper into the pelvis, and especially in early and active labor, and try to swing your hips WIDE. These are all about helping baby wiggle down deeper, the key is to find a great playlist filled with FAST and SLOW music - all your favorite choices. (Then use these songs in labor).

OP/Posterior If you suspect the baby is OP because you feel their 'kicks' and movement of knees, arms, and feet in the front of your tummy, you can help them move. With the pregnant person on hands and knees, resting their arms on an exercise ball, OR leaning against a countertop, sway or wiggle your hips, side to side, until you are tired or it is not comfortable anymore. Put some ice into a bag, and place the ice on the side of your tummy for up to 15 minutes, where the baby's bottom is. They will feel the cold and will try to move their back and bottom, which will naturally move towards the center of your tummy. Also, you can place the palm of your hand on their bottom and with gentle massaging and moving their bottom towards the *center* of your belly; you can help them move.

If the baby is not moving from the OP position, they may be stuck; you can try this *before and IN labor*. It is called ***Shake the Apple Tree,*** and visuals of this technique are on the internet. Get down on your hands and knees; you need to relax your glutes, the muscles in your bottom. I help people relax by gently giggling their hips and butt and by doing a few acupressure points on the back and bottom while they are standing.

On hands and knees, have someone standing up, and behind you, they can use hands on your hips OR can use a rebozo wrapped around and below the belly, holding the ends high up above your back. *Vigorously* giggle your glutes and hips for a good 2 minutes break and repeat (and repeat again) until you feel the baby has moved. This technique can be done in LABOR if you find the baby is in a posterior position. You will know you have moved your baby because you no longer have back pain.

Peanut ball is another kind of exercise ball; this is specific for moving a posterior baby. It looks like a peanut; many hospitals have these, but buying one for at home because you know the baby is OP will shorten labor. If you have to wait until you are in the hospital, ask for one straight away when you get there. The birthing person lays on their side, and the ball goes between their legs at the knees. The bottom leg can be straight or gently bent. The leg that goes over the top of the ball rests around the top indent of the ball, with the hip jutted forward. Laying there for as long as you are comfortable. If you need a break, take one. If you do not feel the baby has changed, repeat the position on the ball, and have someone do the **Pressure Point BL67** on both of your baby toes for a minute or two at a time, and for at least 10 - 15 minutes, then repeat after a short break (do not lay on the side that baby's back is - lay on your side with baby's back at the top side of your hip)

Author's Tip: Randomly, during every labor, I feel the client's glutes, to see if they are tensing their bottom. I gently jiggle the bottom and do pressure points until I feel them relax. Mostly, every person clenches, and this can hold the baby up in the pelvis, so I do the 'bottom check' often during labor. The other pressure point is on the top of the shoulders, 'Gall Bladder 21' shown in the acupressure points document. Anyone can do this often.

TENS machine, 'Transcutaneous Electrical Nerve Stimulation', is a small hand-held machine, battery-operated with wires that are connected to 4 small sticky pads that adhere to the skin on parts of your back, shoulder, besides the spine, and legs. One set has two pads that have black, and the other two pads have red. They are separately controlled, giving more or less intensity from the pulsing. Pads on the back can be placed on either side of the spine (black on the left and red on the right side of the back), and the bottom part of the pad can start at BL32 and move upward to the panty line. The other two can be placed approximately 5 - 6 inches higher directly above, or to encourage the shoulders to relax, use both GB21 and then SP6. Try all positions so you can 'feel' which pressure points give you the most relief, both before labor and during labor.

You regulate the machine with a handheld controller that you can turn up for more intensity when you have a contraction, and down for less intense pulsing when the contraction is over. The pads release a gentle pulsing feeling that floods the nervous system, then reduce the pain signals to your brain, helping you relax.

Your Doula may have one to borrow or you can rent one or you can buy one online. If you purchase one for yourself, you can use it before you are in labor and all during your labor, then they come in handy when you or your family member have muscle pain or strain. The other two pads can be placed approximately 5 - 6 inches higher directly above, or to encourage the shoulders to relax, use GB21 and then SP6. Try all position to 'feel' which pressure points gives you the most relief, both before and during labor.

There are several spots on the body where the pads can be used on. Of course, the internet can show you, but the most effective spot for labor is on the back.

Yoga poses are great for Pregnancy! Practicing yoga for the ideal positioning of the baby for labor is also a lovely way to de-stress and relax tired muscles. As there are many beneficial poses, it would be easier for you to watch on the internet or read a book for exact positioning of the poses. There are specific positions for an OP baby.

Week 36 You can start drinking any of the '9 month' or '3rd Trimester teas'. They are made specifically and have different names, and some have red raspberry leaves known to ripen the cervix, but have many more ingredients. Find them at health food stores or in the organic section at grocery stores, **and** while at the store, purchase Witch Hazel (my personal brand preference is Thayers) for after birth. This product helps heal soft tissue damage quicker, around the perineum, or if a c-section then on the incision. You should put some Witch Hazel on a regular pad and apply directly to the perineum or, if a c-section, on top of the bandage already on your incision, BUT I would advise waiting until you are at home and the incision is at least a week old.

Acupressure Points: Practice acupressure points and become experts now until the baby has delivered; these will help to release stress from your mind, strain from overused muscles, and baby weight, and can help the baby to move into an ideal position for delivery and prepares your body for delivery. Start to practice now for up to an hour daily on all points so you and your partner know the correct placement and strength of pressure. These points will be especially comforting during labor, giving you relief from the pain of the contractions. Try them on each other for fun.

Spleen 6, there is an exception - start at Week 38. This pressure point can start contractions, and if you go into labor earlier, it may be too early to deliver the baby. If you are told that you need to have the baby sooner, for instance, around week 36, then you can start Spleen 6 earlier. Do this pressure point for 20 - 30 seconds, then break for 20 seconds, and repeat for at least 10 to 15 minutes, several times per day, until labor starts.

*Stay Hydrated once in active labor. *This is probably the most important thing that your birth partner needs to make sure you do. Drink plenty of fluids. A large container that you can put a straw in is the most comfortable to have handy. You will not remember to drink as you transition into each different stage of your labor. There can be many complications that come up during this time that can affect how the baby reacts to the labor and how your performance and endurance are tested.* Look for ***Labor Aid Drink recipe***

Author's Tip: If labor starts gently in the late afternoon, I would advise you to eat a spicy dinner (to aggravate the gut and give stronger contractions), then have a tub or shower to take a relaxation break, then Tylenol and Gravol (recommended by Care Providers) get comfortable in your bed, and rest in between contractions; getting some rest is better than being up all night. You will be tired the next day; we would expect you to be getting more active in your labor; it helps when you *stop thinking and let your body go.*

There are many reasons that the body does not go into labor naturally; we can only try and help to encourage labor. You most likely will understand after the baby is born.

BY Week 38: These Tricks will help start labor if you are doing all acupressure points, eating spicy food to aggravate the gut; Nipple stimulating (rolling them) as often as you can, hugging, kissing, cuddling, oxytocin is released in our body, the hormone can stimulate contractions in the uterus. Sex, if you think you can…

During the day, walk as much as possible, and shake your hips by doing all dance moves. Do lunges and climb 'many' sets of stairs. This should start or bring on more contractions. These should be done daily and often; the more, the merrier!

Get aggressive on all Tricks!

Chapter 15: Pack Your Hospital Bag

Pack your Hospital Bag at week 36; there is a chance you may go into labor early. Ask your care provider what you can expect during your hospital stay. Suggestions to include might be:

Your medical care card (cash or debit or credit card as needed in your hospital).

Birth Wishes Plan.

Prescription drugs that you regularly take (This may be different in other countries).

Insulin and tester if you have Gestational Diabetes.

Medication or Tylenol for your partner (hospitals do not usually give anyone else medication).

Food in hospitals is not spectacular, and some hospitals do not feed the partner.

Have snacks and beverages for your partner while in labor; they will get hungry.

During labor, you can order in from restaurants or have someone bring you food.

After delivery, I see many people have family bring in meals, or they order into the room from outside restaurants or the hospital cafeteria. Hospitals hours for serving food are usually 7:00 am to 6:00 pm.

What is available in your birthing room or on the ward? Possibly a tiny fridge in your room Or a fridge, coffee maker, kettle, toaster or microwave that is shared with other patients?

Hospitals should have water and ice machines.

A pregnant person in active labor usually refuses food and prefers fluids. The hospital will allow people to eat small and easy-to-digest snacks. If there is an indication that labor may end in the operating room, it will be suggested to stick to clear fluids, such as:

Labor Aid, to put into water or make into popsicles (see the recipe in the book).

Clear Juice, Water, and Coconut water with ice.

Popsicles can be made from fresh fruit at home or bought from a store.

Frozen fruit, for instance, grapes.

Jello cups, buy them from the store.

Instant chicken broth - I have seen many people who like this.

Bring in your own drink container, make sure it has a bendy straw, so you can sip from it in bed or a bathtub.

You may deliver in the middle of the night, and no food is available for you. Bring your favorite snacks, granola bars, cut-up fruit, dried fruit, whatever you like, that does not need a fridge to be stored in. (Most hospitals have a fridge but may have restrictions on who can put food in the communal fridge). They may or may not have a microwave.

Music from a cell phone or laptop computer, with a portable speaker and headphones if you decide at any time you want to listen to music and blank out the sounds of the delivery suite, and for listening afterwards. During labor, music is very encouraging and soothing, depending on your playlist. Download your playlist in advance; hospitals usually do not have good wi fi.

Camera, cell phone, batteries and/or chargers for all devices. Playlist downloaded; hospitals usually do not have good wi-fi.

Throat lozenges, just in case you make lots of noise during the pushing stage, you may strain your vocal cords.

At our hospitals, after delivery, I make the person toast with peanut butter and/or jam and freshwater or juice or tea. Bring your favorite tea with you, or instant coffee packs, and organic or homemade condiments.

If you have a c-section, you will be put on a light menu.

TENS Machine and Pads (extra batteries).

Witch Hazel - to put on pads - for the perineum, to help heal.

Pillow & sleeping bag - extra for the partner.

Birth Cards with All the strong people you know on the cards.

Visuals - Pictures of Favorite people, places or things, possibly pets.

Ear Plugs: Listen to music while in labor or after the baby is delivered it can be noisy, possibly with other babies crying.

Sleep eye cover if you want to nap with an Epidural or to help you sleep after the baby delivers because there may not be a way to darken a hospital room.

Personal items for the short stay at the hospital; brush or comb; toothbrush & paste, soap, cream for hands & face, lip balm; vitamins; glasses; contact eye solution and container.

Hospitals usually have pads for You and the bleeding and Diapers for the baby.

Bathrobe and slippers, change of clothes for both you and partner to come home.

Clothes for baby, and blanket to cover them - depending on how cold it is when you leave, warm jacket and hat. In my country, a car seat is essential when taking a baby home.

When in the hospital, you can use hospital gowns, even when you are laboring in the tub or shower. I do not recommend you take a bathing suit to go into a tub; they are not comfortable to labor in and are very difficult to take off when you are wet. I have seen people wear an oversize summer dress or a big floppy t-shirt. Most often, laboring people do not like to wear constricting clothing or anything at all.

Chapter 16: Colostrum Collection by Nadia Hawkins

Collection of colostrum before labor and storing is ideal for giving to the baby at delivery and in the first few days, especially if anyone wants to chest feed. The expression of colostrum can take a bit of time to practice, to do it correctly, but when the baby is born, they will be able to taste and ingest it. I see the baby go to the nipple with a bit more excitement when there is colostrum at the nipple. If you do not want to store and take to the hospital, then the act of being able to squeeze at the moment truly is ideal for them.

People can have sensitivity at the nipple, so it may be uncomfortable, so you may prefer not to do this.

Try massaging the breast and pushing the colostrum down towards the nipple. You should be able to squeeze a tiny bit of sticky, yellow drops from the nipple. This concentrated first milk is all baby needs in the first few days born. I explain to clients that the baby's tummy is still so small - the size of a cherry pit, that they really do not need much colostrum. I equate the few drops of colostrum as being the same as astronaut food; we see them in space, squeeze a caloric package of energy food in their mouth, which is packed with a high amount of calories. Similar to what toddlers are being given when the parents are on the go, a meal in a pouch.

Hand expression in pregnancy can assist you in having an easier time starting and continuing feeding the baby. It may also help your body be ready for labor. It is normal to not collect any colostrum while hand expressing. Keep expressing! This act of doing hand expression that helps you to have More Milk Sooner.

When can I start expressing? Before starting, discuss with your OB, doctor or midwife; there may be special considerations prior to starting if:

Your baby is measuring small for gestational age.

A previous or multiple previous Cesarean sections.

Any number of other obstetrical or medical issues.

If you are pregnant with more than one baby.

Do Not Express in pregnancy if you:

Have threatened or actual preterm labor.

Have a short cervix, cervical incompetence or a cervical cerclage.

Have had bleeding during your pregnancy.

Have a low-lying Placenta or Placenta Previa.

Do not worry if you cannot express in pregnancy. Focus on hand expression in the first hour and 24 hours after birth will get your milk production off to a great start.

Bring your frozen colostrum to the hospital.

Collecting and Storing your Colostrum.

In the first week, you might consider practicing in the shower or tub to help you learn; it is a place that is warm and comfortable. Once your colostrum starts dripping easily, often in the second week, start collecting! Families say using a syringe to suck up the bead of colostrum right off of the nipple works best. Using a breast pump may stimulate the breast too much and can bring on labor, *which is a trick to start labor.*

When going to the hospital to deliver, bring only three syringes unless you are delivering far away from home and would not be able to get someone to bring your frozen colostrum.

If you do not have access to refrigeration, do not worry about collecting and storing the colostrum but still do the hand expression for practice.

Birth Tip: Parents often say the partner is able to collect more colostrum when they do hand expression while the person relaxes.

For visual explanations and instructions, learn how to Hand Express for the Colostrum collection. Please go to YouTube, at 'More Milk Sooner' or MoreMilkSooner.com with Nadia Hawkins, BScN RN IBCLC.

Chapter 17: Labor Aid drink and Cookies recipes

Labor Aid Drink Recipe:

In a blender, mix

1/3 cup fresh lemon, cranberry, grape, or your preferred flavor of clear juice

1/3 cup honey (to taste)

1/4 tsp salt

2 calcium/magnesium tablets, crushed or liquid equivalent

Water to make 4 cups

Honey is for calories, to fuel your body

Salt keeps electrolytes balanced through the hard work of labor

Calcium/magnesium feeds hard-working muscles - 'Labor Aid.'

Water - Hydrates

Make the drink to your taste, with more or less sweetness or salt

Mix well and freeze in ice cubes trays or popsicle containers

Puree fresh fruit, then freeze it into a popsicle container

Frozen fruit, grapes, for instance, has a bit of sugar for energy

Mix up a batch ahead of time just before the due date. When frozen, put in a zip-lock freezer bag, ready for home or hospital births. Frozen cubes are easier to take than a jug of liquid. The cubes can be put into a glass of water to dilute.

Use when the laboring person no longer wants to eat, to keep their energy up, while still giving nutritious fluids. Hydration is essential, especially as they go into active labor, and up until delivery, they can have sips.

A container with a straw is also *encouraged*, as they may be laboring in a tub or laying on a bed, and the straw is very convenient for them.

Flavors can seem stronger in labor, so put the cubes into a glass of water to dilute.

Coconut Water and Emergen - C mixed into a glass of water are other ideas for hydration.

Labor Cookies:

There are a variety of cookies that you can find on the internet. If eating cookies can help to start your labor, it is worth trying. I am using *Mrs Dillon's recipe* from the internet, for example. I imagine some of the spices, especially cayenne pepper is the culprit in aggravating the gut, which is good for starting some contractions. Also, you can change a few ingredients if you have allergies or intolerances example, the flour. If you are really clever, this may give you ideas about other types of food that you already love that you can *Spice* up.

2 1/2 c. flour

1 1/2 tsp. baking soda

3/4 tsp. cinnamon

1 tsp. ground ginger

1/2 tsp. ground cloves

1/2 tsp. salt

1/2 tsp. cayenne pepper

8 Tbsp. butter

1/2 cup sugar

1 cup brown sugar

1/3 cup molasses

1/4 cup egg whites

Preheat oven to 350 degrees. Combine flour, baking soda and spices and set aside. Cream the butter and sugars together. Add the molasses to the creamed butter, then add the egg whites until combined. Add the dry ingredients slowly. Chill 1 hour (up to overnight).

Drop spoonfuls of chilled dough onto a baking sheet. Bake for 8-10 minutes. Sprinkle with coarse sugar if desired.

Once cool, eat as many as you can possibly stomach, lie down for a nap and wait for labor to begin. Mrs. Dillon recommends eating at least 5 cookies. (Makes 30-40 cookies)

Chapter 18: Massage for Labor by Paula Jaspar

Basic Swedish massage techniques for early and active labor. These relaxing massage techniques can be done on the laboring person, hand to skin, or with clothes on.

There are four basic principles of massage:

General to specific to general - is in regards to the body part and hand surface.

Superficial to deep to superficial - is in regards to depth.

Proximal to distal to proximal - is in regards to opening up blood flow to the heart first..

Periphery to center to the periphery - is in regards to pain

Massage Applications:

Biomechanics is the study of the most effective use of your body during a massage. This is imperative to the prevention of injury. By using your whole body as an instrument, not just your hands, it becomes an integral part of the treatment. Your awareness of the center of gravity is vital. The more stable your base, the more effective your massage techniques. Often, you will be reminded to move through the center of gravity.

Compressions can be used as a palliative technique when applied lightly. When deeper pressure is applied, it stretches muscle tissue and increases blood flow when pressure is released.

Effleurage is a gliding motion applied in the direction of venous flow using the entire hand surface, molding to the contours of the structure. It is applied in a smooth, continuous fashion with pressure on the upstroke and a light return pressure.

Effleurage can be used as an introductory stroke to accustom the person to your touch. It is also used to apply the oil. Increases circulation and warms the tissues when applied progressively deeper (Superficial to deep to superficial).

Palmar Stroking is applied with the entire hand surface moving over the body part. If minimal pressure is used, it can be applied in any direction as long as that direction is maintained. If moderate or heavier pressure is used, the direction should support venous return as in effleurage. It can be applied with a single hand, one hand on top of the other reinforcing the stroke, or alternately hand over hand.

Stroking can also be applied with the fingertips and thumbs. Stroking can be used to clear the tissue of exudates after deeper techniques have been used. When applied lightly, it can reflexly affect the nervous system.

Petrissage is a movement applied with one or both hands, which uses alternate pressure and release of soft tissue. Pressure is applied by lifting soft tissue up from underlying structures (i.e., wringing) or by compressing down toward underlying structures (i.e., kneading or rolling the structure)

Wringing is performed facing the body. Hands are placed on the opposite sides of the structure being massaged. Hands should be relaxed and molded to the body part. Pressure is applied to the area by the palmar surface (full, molded hand contact) with equal pressure from both hands. Tissue is lifted up and away from the underlying structure.

This technique stretches tight and hyper-toned muscles, thus affecting pliability, circulation, and tone.

Palmar Kneading is applied in a rhythmical, circular motion with alternate pressure and release. The pressure is applied on the upward stroke of the circle and released on the return. Full hand contact at all times. Movement is directed away from the midline of the body.

Due to the alternate pressure and release, veins are alternately drained and refilled. As a result, there is increased capillary blood and lymph flow, more nutrients are supplied to the tissue, and metabolic waste is more readily filtered. Kneading will stretch and elongate tight muscles.

Fingertip/Thumb Kneading: This is similar to Palmar Kneading, but the pressure is applied through the pads of the middle three fingers in fingertip kneading and the pads and outside length of the thumb in thumb kneading. The circles are much smaller, and the remainder of the hand rests on the body.

In both types of kneading, a single hand can be used or it can be reinforced with the other hand on top, or both hands can be used at the same time simultaneously or alternatively.

Basic Principles of Application:

General to Specific to General: This refers to the area of the body, massage techniques used, and the part of the therapist's hand.

A rhythmical flow of massage is best achieved by treating a larger or broader area of the body (general), then proceeding to smaller areas (specific), then gradually back to the larger area.

General to specific to general also pertains to the choice of techniques. The therapist should commence application with broader strokes, progress to more specific techniques, and then finish with the broader strokes.

This principle also pertains to the part of the therapist's hands. For example, with palmar kneading, the whole hand contact accustoms the client to your touch and allows them to relax. With digits and thumbs, more specific work can be done to affect more specific tissues. Return to general with full palmar contact to ease off, ensure sufficient venous and lymphatic return (clearing), and soothe the area that was specifically treated.

Superficial to Deep to Superficial: Begin the movement with relatively superficial light strokes, progress to deeper and/or firmer strokes once the soft tissues have relaxed and circulation increases, then gradually go back to superficial contact.

Proximal to Distal to Proximal: When discussing the treatment of the limbs, the heart is the most proximal. Begin at the most proximal part of the limb, which is closer to the heart. Progress distally, farther from the heart, and then return proximal. As well as intermittently incorporate general strokes to the proximal area to maintain relaxation and circulation so that the circulatory pathway to the heart remains open.

Periphery to Center: A well-trained massage therapist knows to avoid treating the specific area or pain or source of dysfunction first, even though it will be the main focus of treatment. If this is approached too deeply too soon, it will only exacerbate the client's discomfort, and a protective mechanism will prevent any massage from being effective.

Components of Application of Massage: These components are always viewed with respect to; a person's health history, stage of the dysfunction, and what the person wants to accomplish.

Pressure: Deeper pressure is usually applied toward the heart to support venous flow. There is more pressure on the upward stroke on the limb and less on the return stroke. Pressure is adjusted according to the constitution/condition of the client.

Rate is dependent on the effect you wish to achieve. Generally, faster rates stimulate the nervous system, and slower rates soothe and relax the nervous system.

Rhythm is even, smooth, flowing, consistent, fluid, and continuous. Constant contact is important during a massage. If the connection is broken, re-establishing contact must be done gently and carefully. The transitions between two different massage techniques need to be smooth.

Duration: Generally, the length of the treatment is dependent upon the client's needs and reaction to the treatment.

General Massage Routine: Skin on skin or through sheet/clothing.

1. BACK

Place one hand gently on the sacrum and the other hand at the top of the spine.

Have the person take a few deep breaths

Undrape the back

Effleurage - bilateral - both sides at the same time - apply oil

Wringing - bilateral

Alternate Palmar Stroking - unilateral

Palmar Kneading - unilateral, start at shoulders to low back

Effleurage or Wringing - to link to the other side

Repeat the sequence as on the other side, starting with:

Alternate Palmar Stroking (unilateral)

Reinforced Palmar Kneading (unilateral)

Wringing to link to the other side

Effleurage to finish

2. LEG

Massage one leg and then the other. The following can be adapted for the arms and hands.

Effleurage - entire leg starting at the ankle

UPPER LEG

Lymphatic pump 4-6 gentle compressions over the femoral lymph chains. Located at the hip crease

Wringing proximal to distal to proximal

Alternate Palmar Stroking

Effleurage to link to lower knee

KNEE

Simultaneous Fingertip or Thumb kneading or Open C kneading

Effleurage to clear and link to the lower leg

LOWER LEG

Alternate Palmar Stroking - make a V between the thumb and index finger

Effleurage - to link to the lower ankle

ANKLE

Alternate Thumb or Fingertip Kneading - all around the ankle bones

FOOT

Alternate thumb Kneading - top of foot

Light Stroking - between the bones

Compression - to toes and slight traction

Thumb Compressions - bottom of the feet

Alternate Thumb Kneading - bottom of the feet

Knuckle Stroking - bottom of the feet

Range of motion - of the ankle, foot and toes

Effleurage - entire leg. The intention with the pressure on the up stroke and light return stroke

3. ARM

Effleurage the whole arm starting at hand to shoulder

Shoulder

Alternate Palmar Stroking

Effleurage to link to the forearm

Forearm

Alternate Palmar Stroking - make a V between the thumb and index finger

Effleurage - to link to the wrist

WRIST

Alternate Thumb or Fingertip Kneading - all around the anklebones

HAND

Alternate Thumb Kneading - back of hand

Light Stoking - between the bones

Compression - to fingers and slight traction

Thumb Compressions - over the palm, follow the long bones or over the thicker tight areas

Alternate Thumb Kneading - over the palm of the hand

Knuckle Stroking - over the palm of the hand

Range of motion - for the wrist, palm and fingers

Effleurage - the entire area. The intention with the pressure on the up stroke and light return stroke

4. HEAD

Simultaneous Fingertip/ Thumb Kneading - on the scalp. Scalp massage can be done lightly (moving the hair) or deeply (moving the skin). Alternate the light and deep scalp work. Alternate between large and small circles. Alternate between circle and lines. Address the whole head.

Fingertip Compressions - over the midline of the scalp, where you could part the hairline and on hair line where the hair meets the face.

Light Fingertip Stroking - middle of face to sides working from chin, over cheeks, over the forehead

Light Finger Kneading **-** over muscles of the jaw

5. FULL BODY LIGHT STROKING - This technique focuses on rhythmical strokes from the top of the head to the tips of the toes. It can be performed with two hands simultaneously or one hand then the other. The intention is to be rhythmical and light. This creates a neurological response.

Special Techniques

Sacral Counter Pressure

Position 1

Birthing person Standing

Partner/Helper facing the birthing person's back

Hands in fist formation, positioned over sacrum

Apply pressure during contraction to stabilize sacrum

Position 2

Birthing person Side lying

Partner/Helper seated, facing the birthing person's back

Hands in fist formation, positioned over the sacrum

Apply pressure during contraction to stabilize the sacrum

Position 3

Birthing Person on hands and knees

Partner/Helper facing the birthing person's feet

Sitting and using ischial tuberosity or *sit bones* over the sacrum

Apply pressure during contractions to stabilize the sacrum

This is a useful technique to decrease the pain caused by ligament stretching and sacral movement due to the force of the baby's descent.

Double Hip Squeeze

Position yourself behind the birthing person, facing their back. With your hands in a 'fist', place your hands over the buttock muscles. One hand on each side. Press your hands together towards the person's sacrum. This will help separate the ischial spines. It will help to open up the pelvis and ease some pressure of the baby's descent.

Modified positions are standing, sitting, side lying and all-fours position.

Chapter 19: Acupressure Points & Double Hip Squeeze

Acupressure is beneficial in preparing your body to relax and help start labor, which can effectively result in shortening the labor and pushing stage. This practice uses the same spots on the body but without needles by applying pressure from a finger, thumb, or hand. The meridians or energy lines that flow through our body respond quickly when pressure is applied in the correct spot on the body. Universally this technique is very effective in relaxing muscles, reducing stress and anxiety, and coping better in life, especially for people in labor.

Ask your care provider for a recommendation to see a practitioner that offers Acupuncture, one that is in close proximity for you to visit. I highly endorse going and having a treatment(s) to feel revitalized, especially as your baby grows bigger. You should call by week 34 to discuss when you can start treatment and make a few appointments for future dates for Cervical Ripening and, if necessary, positioning of the baby. At the appointment and if you are unclear exactly where the pressure points are, ask and watch the practitioner placing the needles. They will be the same spots that you need to press on for your acupressure points at home.

Start practicing these acupressure points by week 35, so your partner can learn the correct placement of finger or hand on some of the points, so by labor, they will know the exact spots. Give feedback when they press, if you do not feel anything, they are not pressing hard enough or not in the correct spot. Then in labor with contractions, advise them if they are too strong or not enough pressure for the contractions; people can be more sensitive in labor.

I have come across many people that do not like to be touched during labor, if that is the case, do not try any touch.

Make this a daily practice by doing all pressure points, they will help you get through pregnancy, delivery and into the postpartum time.

Benefits: It will help with positioning the baby in the most ideal 'OA' position for labor and birth.

- Turn a Posterior baby
- Help baby to descend into the pelvis
- Reducing anxiety
- Shorten Labor
- Manage pain during contractions
- Relax the tightness or tension of muscles
- To relieve some pain that comes with contractions
- Reduce a Cervical Lip
- Increased Fetal Heart rate
- Relieve nausea
- Expel retained placenta
- Reduce Cesarean Sections

Author's Tip: *I use pressure points often, anytime and intermittently using a variety of pressure points and vacillate between them.* ***Where*** *I do pressure points depends if the person is on their back, standing or on hands and knees. These are my most important tricks during labor. In early labor, where ever you are, have your support people start doing pressure points until you deliver.*

The following pressure points are in no particular order. I use an asterisk * beside my favorite and most used pressure points.

SP 6 or Spleen **6 *** is the ONE ***exception*** I do not encourage using before Week 37. This will help start contractions. Baby is considered fully developed at week 36, and they will gain more weight in the weeks leading up to delivery. Then I wholeheartedly want you to do this as often and as long as you are comfortable with doing it. Do this on your own or have your partner help, and maybe have them give you a foot massage.

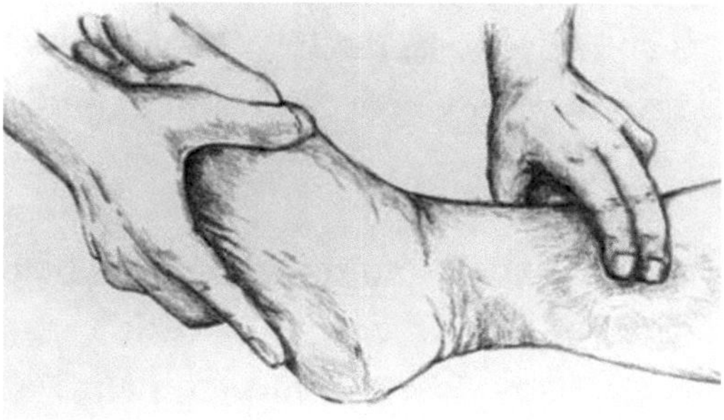

Start with the tibia bone, and on the inside of the leg, follow up four fingers from your ankle bone. Then just beside the bone, towards the muscle, is a sensitive spot. You should be able to feel the correct spot when pressure is applied, if not, move the fingers slightly up or down.

Author's tip: I use this pressure point to help dilate the cervix; to start and regulate contractions; to increase contractions that have slowed down, especially during the pushing stage.

When the care provider does a vaginal exam and says there is a cervical 'lip', it means there is still a tiny amount of cervix that is a bit swollen, and you are asked to refrain from starting your push. It may have been that you were involuntarily pushing before the cervix was fully dilated (10cm).

Use both Spleen 6 and BL 32 at the same time to help reduce a cervical 'lip'.

Use all three Spleen 6, BL 32 and LI4 to induce labor after waters have broken.

BL 32 * There are dimples on the buttocks, and if you run your fingers down the spine, then just towards the hips about an inch or two, on both sides of the spine until you feel the dimples (which is above the gluteal cleft - butt crack). Use your knuckles or fingers or thumbs in the dimples, straight on pressure, then stop and repeat. This releases and relaxes stress and tension in the lower back. The birthing person may push backward towards you at the beginning of contractions for relief.

This stimulates nerves that go into the uterus and help blood flow. It is relaxing during labor, but when the transition starts, it is MOST effective. It helps the baby descend into the pelvis and, at the same time, relieves the pain that is felt. This is used to help induce labor or augment labor, get rid of a cervical lip, and back pain.

Find all 4 (both BL 32 and BL 54) and press randomly or 20 seconds at a time, continuously before labor and during labor. This stimulates nerves that go into the uterus and helps blood flow.

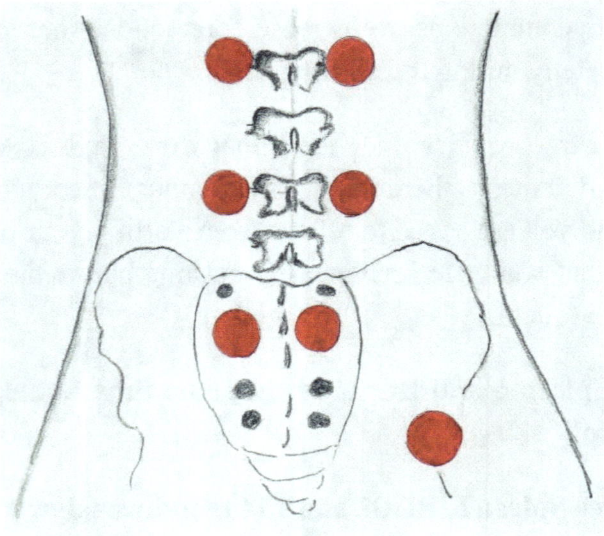

BL 54: This is in the middle of the buttocks, a few inches down from BL32. When you apply the heel of your hand, straight inward and

slightly upward, at the same time, it helps to relieve pressure from the baby's head, but also allows the baby's head to descend.

Separately, find the top of the butt cheeks, then a bit lower, toward the sacrum and the coccyx, put pressure with the heel of your hand, and press gently straight on and upwards at the same time, onto the back.

BL 60: This is right behind the ankle bone in the small depression. This can help with descent and the first stage of labor.

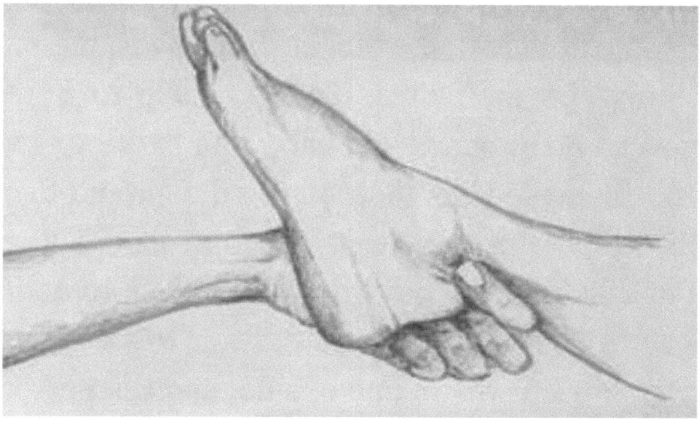

BL 60 and SP 6: To help the baby into a better position, OA is ideal. They can often be in any of the other positions LOA or ROA, (left occiput anterior or right occiput anterior) or LOP, ROP (left occiput posterior or right occiput posterior).

Using both of these points on all four spots (both ankles and both leg points) for up to two minutes at a time, OR ankles then leg points for two minutes each) for as long as the person will tolerate it or up to ten minutes, then break and do it again.

Double Hips Squeeze: At the end of massage for Labor by Paula Jaspar, they talk about the Double Hip Squeeze and using the hands and arms. An alternative way of doing this technique is to use a Rebozo. It is a long flat garment, similar to a shawl which has been worn by people for many years. It was worn over the head to shade the sun, and around the upper body to keep warm. It has been worn to carry babies in, and around the torso in many cultures. If you do not have a Rebozo you can roll up a bed sheet, and wrap it around either the hips and under the tummy of the birthing person, and it is also a great way to hold a cold or warm pad against the back of the laboring person.

The rebozo has been made popular for laboring people because it is useful not only on the hips for counter pressure when pushing *but* earlier when you need to help move the baby if they are in an unfavorable position in the tummy. They can get stuck in any number of positions, some not ideal, the bigger the baby is, the more difficult for them to move on their own. To help them to move, have the birthing person go on to hands and knees, on the floor (with padding for the knees), the person has their butt in the air and their head on a pillow, on the floor. Put the sheet/rebozo around the tummy, then stand above and behind the person. With NO Contraction, you can pull on the Rebozo or sheet, upwards and side to side simultaneously. Have them take big breaths in and exhale, and the person is literally shaking the belly sideways.

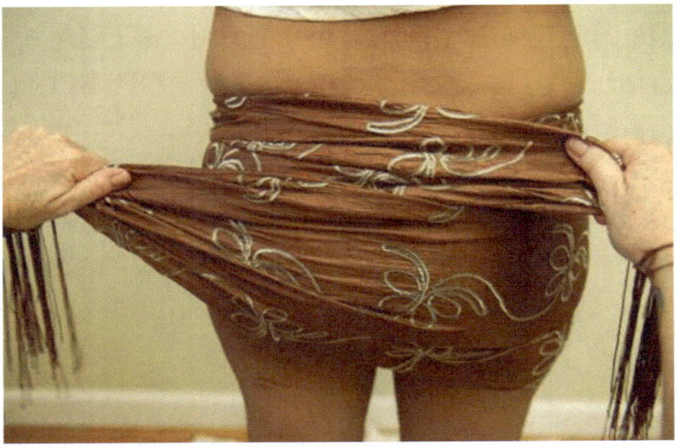

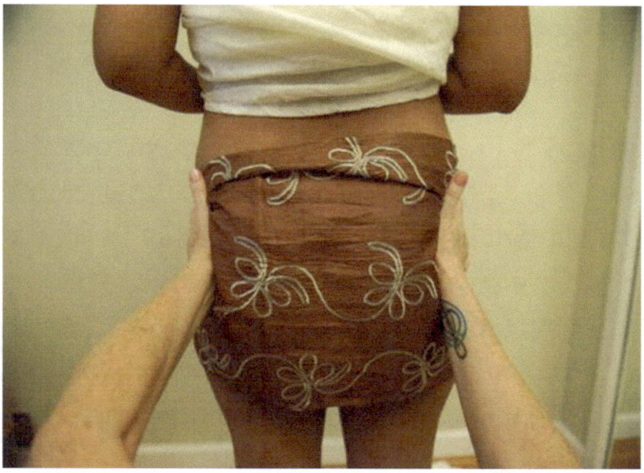

Similar motion is the 'Shake the Tree', where the pregnant person is in the same position, hands, and knees, the partner stands behind and above their hips, put their hands firmly on either hip, then shakes quiet vigorously, use this only when there is no contraction. The ‘shaker’ is literally shaking the hips sideways. Continue as needed, as the person is comfortable and the baby should move.

Double hip squeeze will help to relieve pressure for the person. During contractions, pull the rebozo up and cross your hands, while squeezing inward and tightening pressure on the hips. The birthing person will tell you which way to move your hands. Pressure on the sides of the hips with the palms of your hands. Pushing towards the center of the body.

Baby sometimes does not want to move, no matter what you try, if that is the case, an Obstetrician will come into the room, and if it is possible, do a manual rotation of the baby’s head with their hand, inside the vagina (you will definitely need to have an epidural for this procedure). Most times, it is very effective, putting the baby in a more ideal position and continuing pushing. If not successful, you can preserver and push much longer. However, if the baby gets tired, and we would know this by the monitors acting up, and the baby’s heart rate being high or low, it will be suggested to go for a Cesarean section.

BL 67: If the baby is in an OP position, they need to be the more ideal position OA, (OP is a posterior baby that faces your belly button, they need to be facing your spine). This helps them to turn and descend into the pelvis. On the corner of the outer edge of the baby toenail, with *your* fingernail or a blunt pen with a cap or similar, apply pressure for 30 seconds at a time, break, then repeat pressure for at least 5 minutes. Do this on both toes at a time if possible.

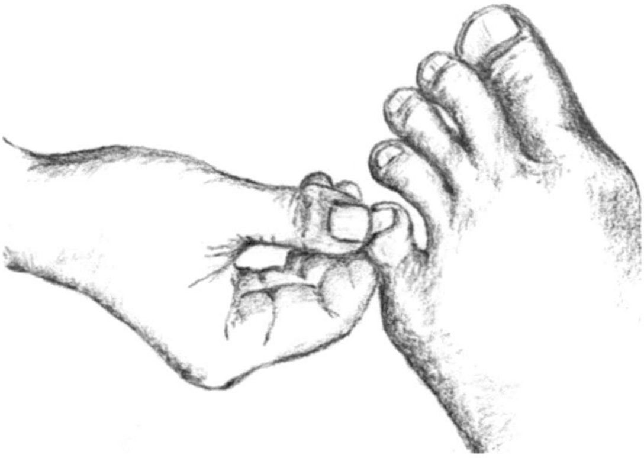

LI4: This spot is between the thumb and index finger. With your thumb, press firmly straight inward of the 'V' toward the middle of their hand. This helps in providing general pain relief (headache or contraction) in labor. It is very useful when people are starting a 'transition'. It is helpful when contractions do not need regular 'intensity' to even that out. It can help the baby move lower into the pelvis and helps the birthing person push more effectively.

LI4 and SP6: These two pressure points used in conjunction are good when the baby is in a good position but labor is not progressing; this will help for more efficient contractions and cervical dilation.

GB 21: At the top of the shoulder, between the neck to shoulder, feel the muscle (many people have a very tight muscle) with 4 fingers or knuckles, and press straight down towards the floor. This instantly releases tension in the shoulders and back, and the person will probably give a sigh of relief as everything releases. This helps the baby descend at the pushing stage, expel the retained placenta, helps to allow the 'let down reflex' for chestfeeding the baby.

Author's Tip: You can use this pressure point every day, it reminds you that we carry too much stress in our bodies.

LI4 and GB21: When a person is fully dilated, and you are pushing, but the baby is not descending very well, doing these two pressure points for 5 - 10 minutes can be used.

Hand Point: Wrap your fingers around a small comb in your palm, and press the teeth of the comb along the crease of your hand during a contraction. Press until you can feel the pressure but are not hurting yourself. This is the spot where endorphins are released into the body. Endorphins are a 'hormone' that your body produces to ease pain and make you feel calm and happy.

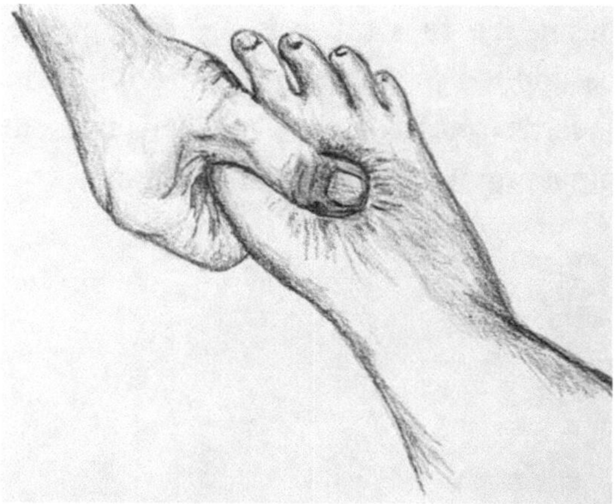

Liver 3: This helps to regulate contractions and relieves stress during labor.

Fun Fact: We release endorphins when we chest-feed a baby.

Pericardium 6: On the inside of the arm and proximately three fingers from the wrist and between the two tendons, press on that spot with two fingers. This can help with nausea and vomiting, which are common for many birthing people.

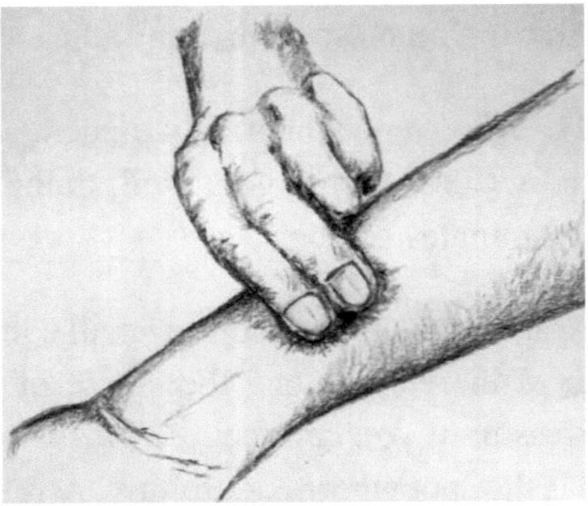

KID1 This point is in the top one-third of the sole of the foot. Easily located as a depression formed when the foot is placed in the planter flexion (by pulling the toes towards the sole of the foot). Strong pressure can be applied in the depression with a knuckle, pushing inwards and upwards towards the big toe. This is useful if feelings of panic occur from a previous birth or other trauma.

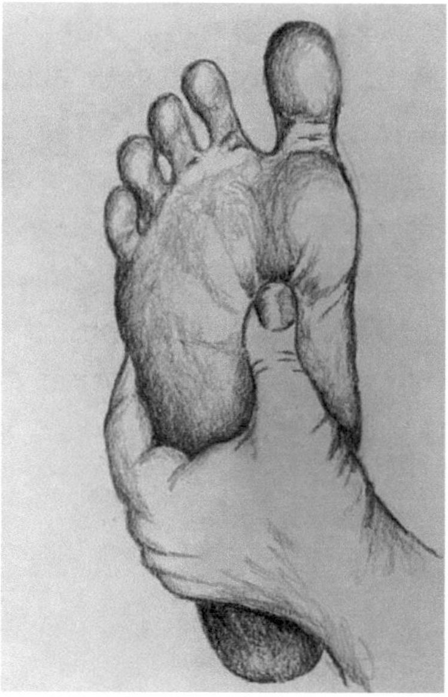

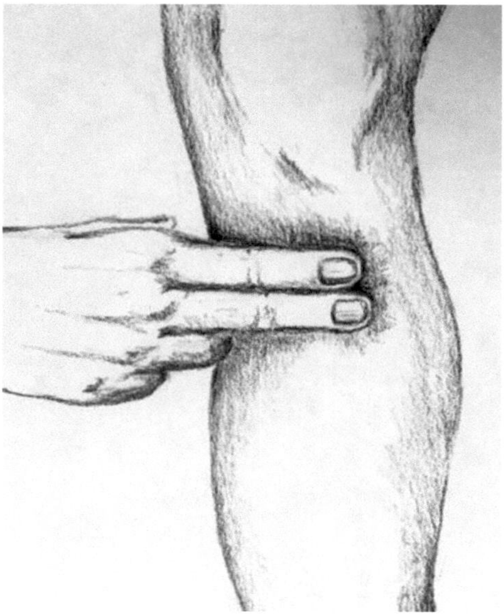

ST 35 (calf's nose) and **ST 36,** the pressure point, is just below the knee cap and on the bone. With two fingers, used at the same time on one leg, if manageable, use both your hands (one hand per knee). Give gentle but constant pressure during a contraction. This can be done until the person is calmer. This can help release muscle tension and reduce and manage pain from labor. This is only used when you have access to the knees. I use this pressure point if contractions become overwhelming or the client is anxious, anytime during labor.

Chapter 20: Procedures & Terminology Explained

Author's Note: The following document is from my perspective. From having watched hundreds of procedures, I offer a quick and simple explanation for some of the more common procedures that might be offered to you at the birthing clinic or the hospital. I live in Vancouver, Canada, and am aware the rest of the world may have very different procedures and protocols. Ask your care provider for current and exact explanations for any and all procedures for the benefit of you having a positive and healthy outcome for you and your baby(ies).

There are many reasons why you may need help to entice your body into starting the labor process that takes you through labor and delivery. If your cervix has not started labor to make the change that will start your labor, or if your labor stalls or your baby gets stuck on the way out, and you need help to deliver the baby, it can all be a bit of a mystery; a reason why you need the procedure or the procedure itself.

I feel for clients that think they have failed the birthing process. It may be as simple as your baby being too big or not well-positioned. There are ways to entice the cervix to ripen and dilate and then ways to deliver a baby in the operating room. If you have ended in a Cesarean section, you should find out why you had a section, and then with your next pregnancy, you may be able to try to have a VBAC (vaginal birth after cesarean).

When labor starts spontaneously, our body releases endorphins to help us cope with the increase in pain coming from labor contractions. Many times if labor does not start on its own, induction can work well to help start labor or to stimulate contractions to become more active, but the process does not give us that slow natural start. Induction can be difficult, and can give us the feeling of 'being out of control' it is common for people to ask for pain relief sooner.

Induction of Labor: Cervidil is similar to a tampon that has medicine on it. The medicine is similar to a hormone we naturally produce called prostaglandin. It helps to relax the muscles of the vagina to stimulate and dilate the cervix for inducing (starting) labor. This procedure is done in the hospital, and the care provider will do a vaginal exam. Then the Cervidil is inserted next to the cervix, and you are put on the monitors for an hour or two to see how the baby responds. You will be sent home in the hopes that your cervix will soften and open, and you will start having contractions over the next 24 hours. It can be a difficult time to manage at home, and many times is not successful in starting labor. When you are back at the hospital, you will have another cervical exam to see if there has been any change. If not, the staff will assess and determine if they can put a new Cervidil in for the next 24 hours or consider changing up the options for induction. This will all take into account many other factors of your pregnancy. If you find that the Cervidil has fallen out and plops in the toilet, it will mean that your cervix has dilated at least to 2 cm, you may or may not have contractions, but it can be encouraging that things are slowly starting. This is the time to be aggressive by doing all the Birth Tricks!

Membrane Sweep or stripping the membranes; this procedure can help induce labor when you are close to, at or past your due date, and can prevent or reduce other induction methods that are more invasive and are started with medication. This is usually done in your care provider's office. With a sterile glove on, they will put a finger into the vagina at the cervix. If it is closed, it may not be possible, and they will not do the procedure. If a bit soft, they will sweep inside the cervix in a circular motion, aiming to separate the amniotic sac and membranes from the uterine wall. This separation triggers the release of a natural chemical called prostaglandins, which will help soften the cervix and stimulate contractions that leads to labor starting.

The procedure can be uncomfortable while having it done, then later on, after you go home, many people will have mild and irregular contractions that carry on all throughout the night, or it will give you strong sensations that last for a long time, and it can be hard to rest or sleep, you can just go about your daily routine. This procedure does not always work the first time, and it may be repeated several times, still with no positive results in starting labor. On the other hand, it is often successful and starts contractions that progresses into labor.

Along with mild discomfort or irregular contractions, there may be some bleeding or bloody show. If there is any excessive bleeding or severe pain, you should call your care provider straight away. Not everyone will respond to this procedure the same way.

Foley Bulb Catheter is used for the induction of labor. It is a small soft silicone tube with a balloon near the tip. One side is deflated and inserted into your cervix. Once the catheter is placed inside, it is inflated with a saline solution. This puts pressure on the cervix to encourage the cervix to soften and dilate. The catheter will fall out when your cervix becomes 3 cm.

IF labor has stalled and you or your baby are having complications, i.e., high blood pressure, high heart rate, or a fever, there are many scenarios that may result in you having an expedited delivery. It may be an emergency, or if you have some time to ask, I have listed some questions to ask your care provider:

- What exactly is; Forceps, Vacuum or Cesarean Section?
- Are the care providers certain you do not have any more time to labor longer?
- What can you change or do to help encourage more active contractions?
- Are there any other alternatives, and what would that look like?
- What exactly are they planning on doing?

- What might you expect afterwards?
- Who will be doing the procedure?
- When do they want to start?
- How long is the procedure?

How is your postpartum recovery going to change?

Augment Labor: When your contractions have slowed down or stopped, and your cervix is not dilating at a rate that is needed to make a change to the cervix to fully dilate to 10 cm, one question the care provider might wonder is that is there enough pressure from the contractions on the cervix to make the change? How can they help strengthen the contractions so the baby descends into your pelvis? It can be hard to know the 'fit' of a baby's head and your pelvic size and shape. The obstetrician will come in to assess the cervix and feel for where the baby is laying, and then they will watch the tracing to see how often and how long the contractions are and determine if the baby is tolerating labor. Then they will decide if you need Oxytocin (also called Pitocin) medication to stimulate the uterus for stronger and increased amount of contractions. If that is their recommendation, medication will be given through an IV intravenous infusion placed on your hand or arm. The stronger contraction can be overwhelming, and you may want to try using nitrous oxide (gas) or decide it is time to have an epidural. You and the baby will be monitored throughout this time, and the nurse will check on you often.

Gas or Nitrous Oxide or Gas & Air: You wear a mask over your mouth and nose OR hold in your hand a mouthpiece. At the beginning of your contraction, you take the mouthpiece and breathe the Gas very deeply into your lungs, then with a *big* exhale back into the mouthpiece as you try to relax. You will take 3 deep breaths for each contraction. Having someone that can do some acupressure points as you exhale, especially pressure point GB21 at the top of your shoulders, and reminding you to relax. Sometimes the Gas can make you feel loopy or light-headed. If that happens, take the gas away and breathe several deep breaths of fresh air, it will dissipate quickly. Not everyone likes the gas, but on the other hand, it is very effective with many people through some or all of their labor.

GBS + or -: You would have had a test taken around week 36 to determine whether you have tested negative or positive for GBS, Group B Streptococcus. If you are 'GBS+' as a precautionary measure, you would be asked to go to the hospital to have antibiotics administered through an IV drip (care providers would like one dose to be administered into your body before the baby arrives). If this is your first baby, you will most likely have plenty of time. If you are a multip and in very active labor, there is a slight chance that they do not get an IV sited and/or have time for the antibiotic to be administered in time before the baby arrives. Your care provider can explain everything you need to know, IF you are tested positive and how this might change your labor slightly.

Ultra Sound, Fetal Monitoring, NST nonstress test to confirm where the baby is lying, check body movements, muscle tone, and amount of amniotic fluid to confirm the baby's health. When it is a high-risk pregnancy, for example, with more than one fetus, or you have high blood pressure or diabetes, they may want to monitor the baby weekly. With fetal monitors strapped around your abdomen, they measure the baby's heart rate as the baby moves in the amniotic sac; measure to see if there is enough or too much amniotic fluid. To ensure the baby is moving *more or less* than normal. If you are a high-risk pregnancy, you will be used to having an ultrasound and non-stress testing. Doctors always want to know how a baby responds to contractions when stimulated by oxytocin or nipple stimulation. (This is one way of knowing if you can stall having an Induction for a bit longer.)

EFM Electronic Fetal Monitoring in labor is when the care providers watch and listen to how the baby is tolerating labor. They listen to the heart rate and track your contractions for an extended period. There are two monitors that are round and flat, hard plastic discs, and they are placed onto your tummy and held in place with a wide elastic stretchy cloth strap around your back and tummy that stays for a period of time (usually for several hours). These on your tummy means you will need to stay very close, within 3 feet of the monitoring machine (hospitals may have wireless monitors, which gives you much more space to be mobile and move around).

The monitors are cumbersome and do not stay on a round belly very well, and you often have a nurse fussing with them, for a better pick up, as you or the baby moves. Of the 2 bands, one monitors the baby's heart rate, and the other counts when the contraction starts and ends, so they know how often and how long the contractions are. You may have the monitors on for hours, then be allowed off of the monitor to move around freely or to be in a tub or a shower. They do not necessarily hurt, but most people do not like them. They are constricting and attached tightly, but it is a very necessary tool for all of your team of nurses, doctors, and midwives to know if your baby is tolerating labor.

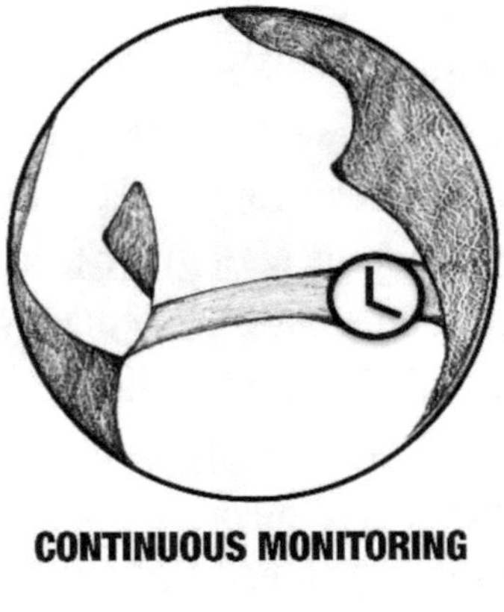

CONTINUOUS MONITORING

Intermittent Auscultation: This is when the nurse, holding a small wand that is attached to a handheld machine, is held against your tummy, and they can listen to your baby's heart rate. This is used during a routine exam at your care provider's office but also in labor.

This is usually done every 15 minutes or so and gives you access to move around the delivery suite more easily.

A **Paediatrician** is a specialized baby doctor. They are usually called to be in the delivery room at birth, especially when there is meconium in the waters, in case your baby swallows some of the waters at delivery or if the baby is giving us any indication that they are not tolerating the labor and their heart rate is dipping (there are many reasons why), the paediatrician can take the baby to the bassinette at the back of the delivery room immediately after delivery for assessment. The paediatrician is always in attendance in the operating room for cesarean section, forceps or vacuum delivery, especially when there are multiple babies.

Epidural procedure 'simplified': When you are not tolerating your increasing strength from contractions or have decided that you are ready for 'something more' and want total relief from the pain or want to rest from the longevity of your labor, you can have an epidural at any time. I have had clients get an epidural at 10 cm. However, when they are that far along, they usually do not have time, and the baby delivers. This procedure *usually* gives complete comfort from contractions, but on occasion, it does not.

The anesthetist is highly specialized in all care of providing anaesthesia and pain management to patients before, during and after operations and all surgical procedures.

They will go over all the risks and side effects and will describe the epidural procedure, they will also ask you to read an information sheet on epidurals. (Then afterwards, they ask you to sign a paper for your consent to allow the Doctor to administer the epidural).

You will be sitting on the hospital bed, with your legs dangling over to one side of the bed and your feet placed on your partner's legs, who will be sitting in front of you on a chair. You will sit still, with your shoulders curled forward and downward and put your chin to your chest, cuddling your arms around a pillow. Many people use nitrous oxide - gas for contractions while having this procedure. The procedure is done in a sterile environment; your back is cleaned with an antiseptic solution, and your back is draped with a plastic sheet.

A needle to freeze the area is given. Then there is a tiny catheter that is inserted into your lower back, into the epidural space. The tiny and flexible catheter will carry the drug that keeps you comfortable. The catheter is covered with a large and sterile tegaderm bandage that will keep the cathedar from dislodging.

The catheter is attached to another tube and a pump, where the drug is administered. The first injection of the drug is given and takes effect within 10 minutes. The procedure is usually done within 15 to 30 minutes; it can be harder to place the tube if you have scoliosis or an injury of the spine. Once the tiny tubbing is placed, they tape it to your back so it stays in place. I tell people that the needle to freeze the area where they are working is the worst part of this procedure.

The nurse will make sure that you have the EFM bands around your belly and that you will have many blood pressure reading on your arm. They monitor both you and your baby. They do an ice check to make sure the pain medications are working properly - that you do not have more on one side or the other of your body. Relief starts slowly, and you feel your contractions get shorter with each next one you have until you do not feel them, just the pain-free pressure. This is approximately 15 - 20 minutes. Then you start to relax, and your smile comes back.

Once the procedure is done, the goal is to be pain-free and still feel light pressure from your contractions. This lasts until after the baby is born and after the placenta is delivered and the repair is done. Then they will turn off the medication and take out the epidural. You should be able to get up to void your bladder approximately 1 - 1.5 hours after delivery. You will be given your baby at your chest for bonding and initiate feeding.

On occasion, for a variety of reasons, the epidural doesn't give enough coverage from pain, the doctor will access it, and they may re-site the epidural.

The anesthetist's job is very precise, and they are very accomplished at their jobs. Honestly, in the delivery suite, they get all the 'love' from the laboring person.

- With the epidural, you should be comfortable, pain-free and not able to 'feel' the contractions, and that will allow you to relax and get some sleep.
- A 'walking' epidural is not always achieved when your legs feel heavy and unstable, so you can not support yourself to stand or walk to the bathroom and void your bladder. It can be common that your mobility is compromised.
- Anytime in labor, it is hard to void; you may be offered a bedpan. I can say I have only seen a handful of people successfully void this way.
- You may not be able to stand near the bed or sit on an exercise ball, or squat while pushing.
- You may not feel pressure or the urge from the contractions when it is time to push. So pushing may be harder, but you will be guided on when to start pushing and how hard to push. Someone, usually the nurse, will touch your tummy so they know when a contraction starts and tells you when to start pushing.
- Epidurals can slow the contractions; if so, your care provider will talk to you about needing to 'augment' the labor by giving Oxytocin (intravenously) to increase the contractions.
- An epidural may make you itchy, mostly on your torso. I always joke with my client that if the itchiness is too much, we could ask for the epidural to be shut off; it makes them

laugh. I give them a cold, wet cloth to wipe on the itchy spots; it does not take away the itch but does make it feel more controllable.

- The epidural can make your blood pressure go down, which might affect the baby's heart rate, but care providers or the nurse will monitor the baby closely. They need to make sure the baby is responding well to contractions.
- If you have to go to the OR for a trial of forceps or a Cesarean section, having an epidural already in can make this an easier trip. The anesthetist would put a stronger medicine in your epidural called a 'top up'. Making it easier and faster to have your procedure started and done.

Morphine & Gravol is an option if you come to the hospital and are having contractions that are strong and frequent, but your cervix has not dilated past 1 or 2 cm. If you are offered this option, it is a way for you to go home and, over the next 4 to 6 hours, get some rest (many people can sleep), or if you are too uncomfortable, then you can at least have a break from feeling all of the strong contractions that your body will still be having.

The procedure is administered by a needle with morphine and Gravol that is placed into the outer side of your butt cheek. You will be asked to go straight home to rest, it will make you sleepy and/or groggy, and you may need help getting into your home and walking upstairs and getting to your bed. The drug allows you to rest while your body dilates.

NOTE: So you are aware when the drug wears off, you *should be* in a very active labor and more dilated. Most likely, you will want to be going back to the hospital. I have seen clients come back and being *3 or more* centimetres dilated.

General Anesthesia: If you have been laboring at the hospital and, for some reason, the care providers believe that the baby has to be born very quickly! You will be whisked into the operation room very fast (if you already have an epidural, they will top it up). If not, then you will be given a general anesthesia, meaning you will be put to sleep, and the baby will be delivered via Caesarean section. Usually when this happens, your partner will not be allowed with you in the operating room; anaesthetists, paediatricians, nurses and surgical staff are only allowed in. (I have been in the OR a few times with the partner at these types of deliveries, the atmosphere is very tense for all surgical staff, as they do their work.) I will try to calm and assure the partner that the baby is getting very good help from all staff and especially the paediatricians. Then you will go into the recovery area for 1 to 2 hours or more, usually after you have woken up. At my hospital, the partner can stay with the baby in the nursery or where you are resting, depending on how your baby is and if they need some special attention.

Why your **Labor might Stall or Fail to Progress…** there are many possibilities as to why:

- Asynclitic is when a baby's head is looking at *their* shoulder and tilting their face up to the sky. The care provider may have a difficult time rotating the baby, or the baby does not want to move or can not be moved, and the baby does not tolerate the manual rotation.
- The baby's head circumference is too big to descend into the pelvis.
- OP - Posterior positioned baby, they are facing your belly button, your care provider tries for a rotation of baby, and they do not move or do not tolerate a rotation.
- Failure to progress the uterus/contractions did not dilate the cervix to 10 cm, for unknown reasons, after a long labor.
- The umbilical cord prevents the baby from coming down the birth canal; they are wrapped in the cord and/or holding on to the cord.
- The baby is getting tired from a long labor.

- You are showing visible indications of not tolerating labor (you have a fever).
- Surprise Breech position (bum in the pelvis). Not many care providers can or want to do a Breech delivery unless they have experience and they happen to be in the hospital at the time you are in labor.
- You may have pushed for longer than 4-5 hours and are exhausted.
- At any time, if we see a visible indication and/or abnormalities with the baby's heart rate on the monitors, with the baby and with you becoming more tired and not coping with a long labor, it will be advised to expedite delivery - usually in the operating room.

Author's Note: The size of your hips, if you are petite or short, does NOT indicate whether your pelvis is too small to birth your baby. I have seen many small petite people easily and quickly birth their baby, *but* people can have a narrow or heart-shaped pelvis (this is not known until you have a cesarean section, the surgeon can see this and would tell you after the procedure a VBAC would not be recommended).

Does your partner have broad-shouldered and/or have a big head that might have been the reason for a failure to progress? That might happen, but many people can push a baby out with a partner that is a larger person.

Options for Delivery Vacuum, Forceps or Cesarean Section: There are so many reasons why your labor needs help; it usually is discovered 'why' after delivery. If you are not fully dilated or you or your baby need a quick delivery. You will be rushed to the operating room for a Cesarean section.

Vacuum: This procedure can be done in the delivery suite IF the doctor doing the procedure is confident it will work. The birthing person must have a very good epidural working already. The vacuum is a hard plastic (shallow) cup with a suction device on the end, which is placed on the baby's head. There is a plunger that puts some pressure to stay onto the head, so it does not slip off. During a contraction, you push, and the obstetrician will pull gently to help the baby's head come under the public bone. If successful, they take the vacuum off, and you will push the baby out on your own. You will only be offered this option if the baby is *very low* down into the pelvis, and they expect you will deliver successfully. If the baby shows any sign of distress (by having a high or low heart rate tracing), the care providers will not proceed, and you will be offered a Cesarean section.

The OB will only do a trial of forceps or vacuum IF they are very confident it will work.

Episiotomy: Where I practice, the care providers *do not* make a routine episiotomy; they let the skin tissue tear naturally. Some Care Providers believe it is easier for the patient's recovery to do the repair by putting the skin and tissues back together in their natural way. Some reasons for a tear would be when the head of the baby 'does not' fit or the tissues are very tight, or the baby is in distress, and the provider wants an imminent delivery. There are 1 - 2 - 3 - 4 degrees when describing the tear or cut on the perineum. Usually, the higher the degree means, the deeper and more severe, and sometimes the tear is close to or near the muscle around the anus. An obstetrician would come in to repair the most difficult tears or cuts. Afterwards, you may need to sit on a 'donut' shaped pillow until the incision heals. I have told many people to use witch hazel on a pad and to put it straight onto the perineum to help heal all repairs faster (when you get home).

The Decision for the following procedures is after the Obstetrician has been in the delivery suite and has assessed several things; where your baby is positioned in the pelvis (birth canal), their progress, the baby has had good tracings on the monitors (there have been several hours of baby 'looking' like they are tolerating labor contractions) how you are coping, does baby need expedited delivery, there are many reasons.

Forceps or Vacuum delivery can be done in the birthing suite when the obstetrician believes it will be a straightforward 'trial' of forceps and is confident that it will work. When the Obstetrician suggests that they will do the procedure in the operating room for a trial of forceps in the event that the forceps do not work, the staff can switch to a Cesarean section quickly. Making it an easier transition for operating room staff to achieve either delivery for you. You will need a very good epidural in place, and once in the operating room, it will be topped up for extra coverage. Forceps are metal and look like large and elongated salad spoons, they are gently placed into the vagina and placed on either side of the baby's head (if the forceps do not fit properly, the obstetrician will not proceed), and when a contraction comes, you push very hard, and the Doctor gently pulls baby downwards. They will try once or twice; if the baby does not move, they will quickly make a couple of changes, and you will have a Cesarean Section. If the baby moves (it is only a few centimetres for the baby to get under the pubic bone), then they take the forceps off, and you do the last couple of pushes and birth your baby.

Cesarean Sections can be urgent. If you or your baby have complications or the baby is not responding well to labor, you will need an immediate delivery, called an emergency Cesarean section. If you have a good working epidural, the anesthetist will top that up. If you do not have an epidural, they will give you a general anesthesia, and you will go to sleep. The partner will stay in another room until the surgery is over and the birthing person goes into the recovery room. If it is not an emergency, it is very civil; it feels like just another procedure done in the hospital operating room.

In the Operating Room, I have been in many Caesarean sections. I am amazed as I watch everyone there, they have a specific role to play, and every part works like a ballet, with ease and grace. There are many people in the operating room, there are bright lights, and it is very sterile. Often, someone puts music on, or clients ask if they can listen to the music they brought in with them on a cell phone. The birthing person lies on the operating table and is prepped for surgery. Once the medication has been administered, they are usually so exhausted from a long and hard labor, they rest their eyes.

My job is to wait with the partner, both of us in scrubs (the only thing allowed in the room is your cell phone to take pictures) until we get an escort to our place in the operation room. The partner is seated beside the birthing person that is on the operating table. There is a large blue drape in front of the surgeons, so we do not see any of the operations, they have usually just started the procedure as we sit down, and we expect the baby to be born soon.

The anesthetist is beside us, making sure the patient is well taken care of. When the baby is delivered, the surgeon will lift the baby high enough over the blue drape while they are screaming or crying for the new parent to take a few pictures. (I always get a few pictures of that and always get one picture of the time on the clock when the baby was born). Then a nurse wraps up the baby. If the baby is happy and crying, they are brought to the birthing person to have skin-to-skin and the first cuddle. I take lots of pictures of both parents with the baby as they meet their baby face-to-face for the first time.

A few minutes go by, and the paediatrician comes to get the baby, and I escort the partner to watch the assessment. The baby is weighed and measured, and pictures are taken. I ask if the parent can put the first diaper on their baby. Often, it is the first time they have done that, more pictures. Then baby can go back to the birthing parent.

If the baby does not cry or looks like they need some extra attention from the paediatrician, they will go straight to the baby bassinet for a full assessment and any assistance with breathing or suction; all of the baby's needs are taken care of. Most often baby comes back to the parent, but if the baby needs more help, they will go to the NICU (neonatal intensive care unit).

Sometimes when it is an emergency, especially having twins or more, it seems that it *should* be high levels of stress, but it is not. With the large group of people, many people from the NICU helping and assessing baby(ies) for any issues, all the while talking in whispers.

Thank the heavens, we have ways of getting our babies out when needed!

After the Birth, the birthing person has had the tummy repaired and is cleaned up and now has the baby to cuddle; they are taken to the PACU (post anesthesia career unit), where they are monitored for an hour or so. We usually get the baby to start suckling at the nipple. Then they go to their recovery suite, where all post-surgery people stay for up to three days.

Afterwards, and most often, we find out why the baby had a hard time coming down the birth canal, but sometimes we do not. Most often, they are perfectly fine, but many times they are not. If the pediatrician believes they need more attention, they will go to the NICU or neonatal intensive care unit for extra attention and stay there until they are healthy enough for them to go home. My hospital is beside the children's hospital and has space for many new babies at all levels of care.

Chapter 21: Pelvic Floor by Kim Vopni

Your pelvic floor is a group of muscles (3 layers) that run from the pubic bone (it is actually a joint called the pubic symphysis) to the tailbone, as well as the sitz bones. The pelvic floor is a highly vascular (a large blood supply), as well as a highly innervated (a lot of nerves) part of the body. The nerves, muscles and connective tissue work to keep you continent, provide support to the internal organs (the bladder, the uterus and the rectum), stabilize the spine and pelvis, and contribute to your sexual satisfaction. It also plays a major role in childbirth. Because it is not visible, the pelvic floor is rarely thought about until there is a problem, and then it becomes the only thing you think about because it plays such a central role in so much of what you do. Problems will often show up during pregnancy or after childbirth - problems such as incontinence, pelvic pain, organ prolapse, sexual challenges, back pain and/or hip pain. These problems, also known as pelvic floor dysfunction, can develop from a variety of reasons such as overuse (muscles that don't relax and that are tight and weak as a result), under-use (muscles that lack tone and are weak), injury (perineal injury or nerve injury from birth, sports, accidents, surgeries), or from poor posture and alignment. The pelvic floor is the foundation of your core and deserves a lot more attention than it gets!

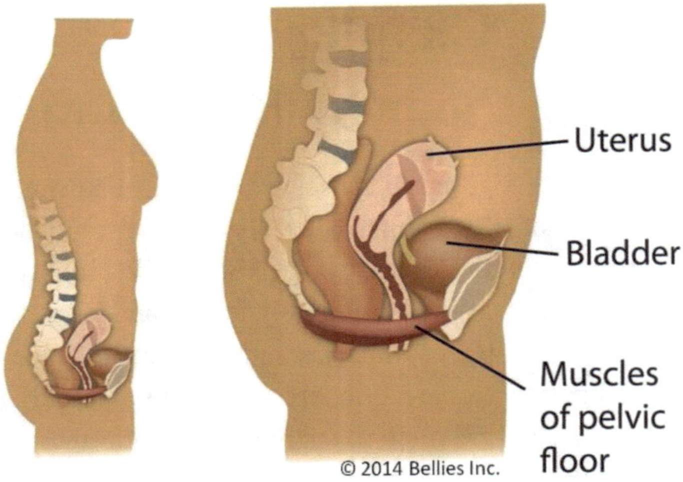

When functioning optimally, the pelvic floor helps support your spine and pelvis, holds your internal organs in place, helps keep you continent and contributes to sexual satisfaction. Unfortunately, as we have discussed, pregnancy and birth can impact the ideal function of the pelvic floor and can contribute to some common types of pelvic floor dysfunction. (Notice we said common, not normal).

Back pain, pelvic pain, tearing, incontinence, diastasis recti, organ prolapse and unsatisfying sex: these things are often thought of as 'normal' once you become pregnant or have a baby. The truth is, while they are common, they are not normal, and they don't have to be a part of your pregnancy or postpartum experience. Healthcare professionals might say, "These are just part of being pregnant." But that's not true. You have the power to do things differently and prepare your body for birth and recovery.

The pelvic floor is often never really thought about until a woman becomes pregnant, and even then, not so much. After the baby is born, when things don't feel right, it is the only thing a woman can think about because it plays a role in so many aspects of daily life. Women suffer in silence because they are embarrassed because they think their core is weak or that it is just 'normal' after having kids. They suffer in silence which in turn affects their relationships, their moods, their activity levels and their overall well-being.

Thoughts about the pelvic floor in pregnancy usually center around - '*how am I going to get this baby out and still be able to hold a tampon in*?" "*Will I still enjoy sex?*" "*Will my partner still enjoy it?*" "*Will I pee my pants when I exercise like my mom does?*" These are all valid concerns, and by thinking about them during pregnancy, you are more likely to take steps to prevent and maintain your pelvic floor wellness. The good news is that the body is designed to give birth, and with the information, awareness and preparation, you will gain from this program. You will support your body and set yourself up for a better birth and recovery that has you still enjoying sex, able to keep a tampon in and not leaking!

A deeper understanding of the pelvic floor and what it actually goes through in pregnancy and birth can help prepare you both mentally and physically for the big day! Seeing a pelvic floor physiotherapist during and after your pregnancy (and then once a year after that) is an ideal way to prevent and treat pelvic floor dysfunction.

Pregnancy and birth are miraculous, and often, our marvel of this miracle makes it easy to forget that it is a very physical event that can really take a toll on the body. With the right information and preparation, this toll is minimized.

Posture, hormones, number of babies, size of babies, number of pregnancies…these all affect your body, and many women wait until they are 'done having kids' to 'fix' their bodies. While it is never too late, waiting means you have a much bigger recovery hill to climb.

By being proactive, you will be able to prevent or minimize the issues that are commonly associated with pregnancy and birth and be in a better position to get back to the body you want.

Let's look at some of the more common aspects of pregnancy and birth that can contribute to core challenges.

Pregnancy:

The abdominal wall, pelvic floor and low back undergo increasing strain with the weight of the growing baby, the uterus and the additional fluid. Adding to this strain is the effect of the hormones affecting ligament laxity, making the joints less stable. These changes all contribute to alterations in your posture. The pelvis will often start to tip anteriorly, the shoulders round as the breasts grow, and the head juts forward. (Actually, the forward head, rounded shoulder posture is the one most people live in all day, every day, without being pregnant! All the driving, computer work, desk jobs, texting, etc., is creating core dysfunction everywhere! The difference, though, is in the pelvis. People who sit all day usually sit with a tucked or posteriorly tilted pelvis. Many women actually start their pregnancy with elements of core dysfunction - huh - who knew???

In pregnancy, the center of gravity is shifting. Women try to counteract the forward shift in body weight by leaning back, pushing the hips forward and clenching the butt muscles. The tailbone tucks and the hips thrust forward, and stability is then attempted by gripping in the butt, the obliques and the rib cage. This butt clenching and rib gripping are non-optimal strategies and are the body's way of trying to stabilize itself when the muscles that should be supporting the core are not working properly because of poor posture and alignment.

These non-optimal strategies are compensations and need to be prevented or changed. These poor core stability strategies overuse the posterior pelvic floor and move the pelvic floor into a less supported position. It also inhibits and weakens the glutes and creates an increase in intra-abdominal pressure, which is not good news for the abdomen or the pelvic floor. Add to this the extra weight from the growing uterus, and you have a pelvic floor that is overworked and out of position!

The good news is that even if you go into pregnancy with an element of core dysfunction, and even if you already have some aches and pains, you can take steps now to reverse them and prevent things from becoming a bigger problem!

Diastasis Recti

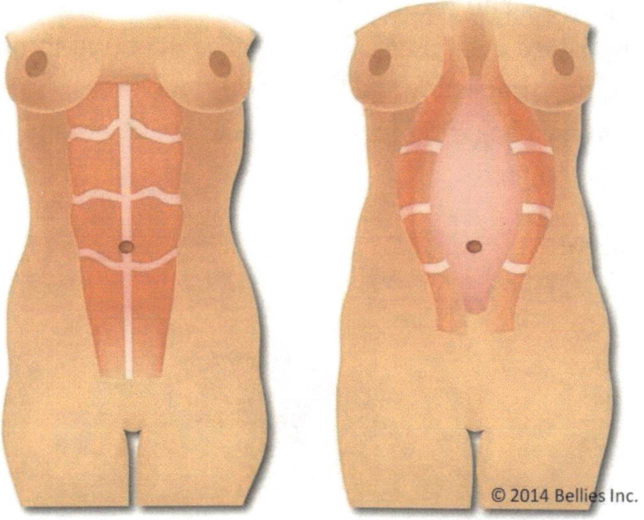

During pregnancy, the outermost abdominal muscles (the rectus abdominis) become stretched and weak and will start to move away from the midline as the linea alba (the connective tissue that holds them in place) thins and stretches. This means less support for the spine and pelvis under the increasing load of pregnancy. This stretching of the muscles and connective tissue is a normal part of pregnancy (to an extent) and is how your body adjusts to accommodate the growing uterus and baby, but it can certainly wreak some havoc on the function of the core. The other thing to consider is that with weakened connective tissue and muscles, as well as muscles that are not in optimal alignment, pushing can be less effective, which may mean a longer labor. The good news is that with the right posture and alignment and by choosing the right preventive exercise, this havoc can be minimized.

Breastfeeding:

Who knew that breastfeeding could have an impact on core function? Breasts become enlarged during pregnancy which can contribute to alterations in posture and alignment. Slouching has become a typical posture for us in our computer-driven world, even without pregnancy and birth, and once breastfeeding starts, you will live in that posture even more. Paying extra attention to posture and alignment during pregnancy and then as you start breastfeeding is key! This program will help you identify how to stand, sit and move with your core well aligned.

Childbirth:

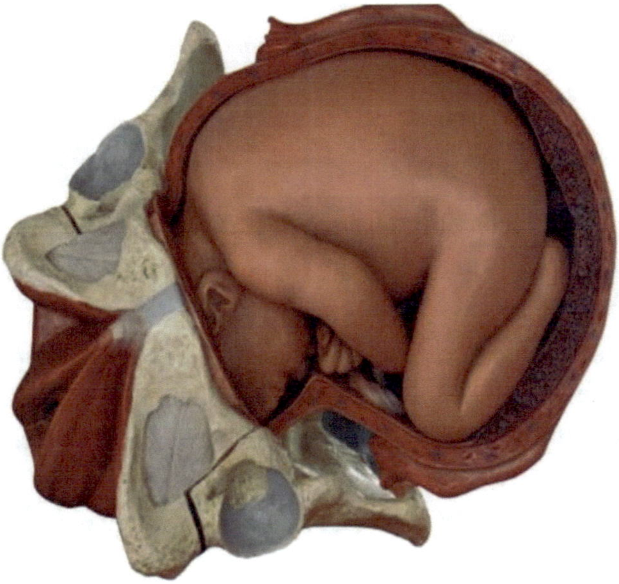

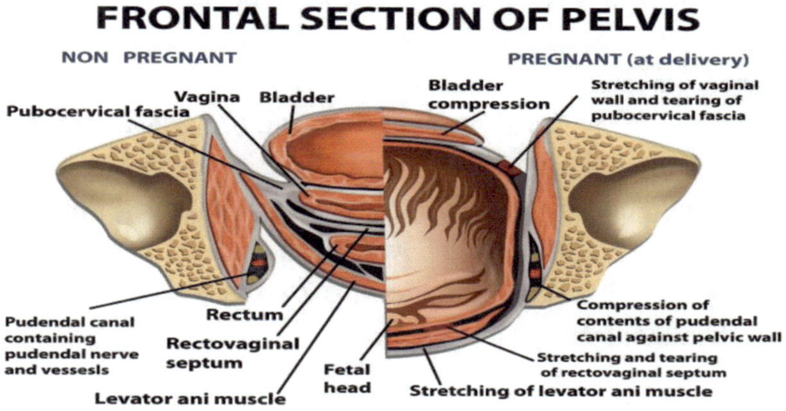

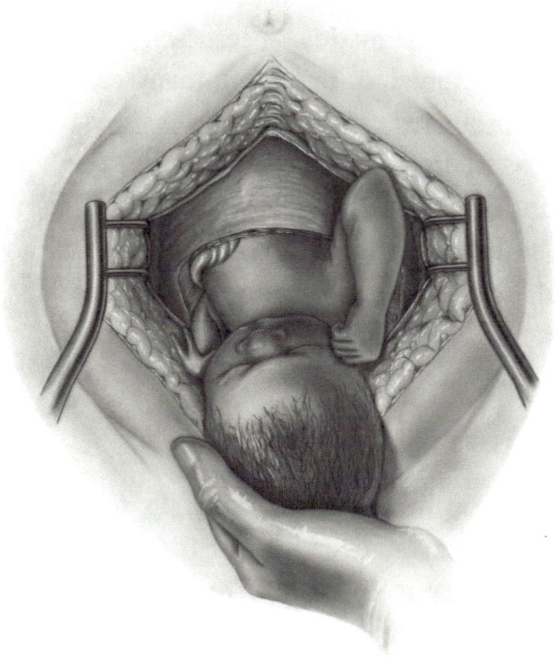

Childbirth, whether vaginal or surgical, can greatly impact the core. Vaginal birth causes extensive strain on the pelvic floor muscles, connective tissue and nerves. Even in the absence of tearing or an episiotomy, dysfunction can occur due to the excessive pressure, stretch and compression that takes place during the 1st and 2nd stages of labor. Many women also face other interventions that increase the potential of tearing and episiotomy, such as forceps, vacuum, and prolonged pushing in the second stage of labor. The act of pushing itself can also stress the abdominal wall, and if diastasis recti has not already occurred, it may occur during the pushing phase of labor. By learning about and connecting with your pelvic floor in pregnancy, you will go into birth knowing how to push and how to optimize your labor so you will be less likely to face a prolonged second stage of labor, a 'stalled' labor or interventions.

A surgical birth involves an incision into the abdominal wall, which affects multiple layers of muscles and connective tissue and therefore leaves behind multiple layers of adhesions that can become the cause of pain and dysfunction. A cesarean birth does not make you immune to core dysfunction. In fact, in many cases, it can leave you even more compromised. You have faced the same hormonal and postural changes in pregnancy along with the weight of the baby on the pelvic floor throughout the pregnancy, and many women who have c-sections have also gone into labor, pushed and then had a surgical birth! Learning proper healing techniques for both vaginal and caesarean births can help prevent or minimize the likelihood of long-term challenges.

Return to exercise postpartum

Many women want nothing more than to get back into their regular clothes and resume or start a fitness program as soon as possible after delivery to lose the baby weight, but the desperately needed core restoration is not even a consideration, and a premature return to impact exercise such as running, high-intensity workouts and the 100's of crunches in the neighborhood mommy boot camp, do far more harm than good.

The first 8 weeks are critical to healing, and knowing what to do and what to avoid during this time will ensure you can get back to the activities you want with a body you are confident in. Doctors and midwives will see you for a 6-week postpartum check-up to ensure the uterus has returned to its non-pregnant state, and this is typically when they give you the green light to get back to your regular activities. In our opinion, this is irresponsible. While the uterus may have shrunk back to its original size, the pelvis and abdomen are nowhere near ready for a return to regular activities. Consider the 6-week check-up as your green light to go see your pelvic floor physiotherapist for a thorough assessment of your core and pelvic floor function, and please refrain from registering for the mom and baby classes. Our slogan is Mommy and Bootcamp do not belong in the same sentence.

Previous injuries

Old injuries, surgeries, strains, and sprains, can all cause compensations and leave your core more vulnerable to new strains, such as those from pregnancy and birth. When you start with non-optimal strategies that have developed from previous injuries and then add the stress and strain from pregnancy and birth, you can end up in an even more disadvantaged position. The preventive exercises in this book and visits to a pelvic floor physiotherapist during your pregnancy are steps you can and should take to help you feel better and stronger before your baby is born.

Fear:

It may seem odd, but fear can affect your core and have a profound effect on your birth. One way it can affect your core is through a muscle called the psoas. The psoas is a muscle that runs from the spine through the pelvis to the upper leg and is the only muscle that joins the top and bottom parts of your body. It is typically tight because of the amount of sitting we do and from the postures we choose. A tight psoas can pull on the spine and thrust the ribs forward. A tight psoas can also pull on the femur head, which causes the pelvis to tuck and tip posteriorly. These both affect alignment in a non-optimal way. One more thing - because the psoas runs through the pelvis, when it is tight, it can limit the amount of space in the pelvis for the baby to move into. This can lead to carrying the baby further out front, which can cause more strain on the abdominal wall. Fear can cause this muscle to be tense, and during labor when you are trying to create the easiest transition into the world for your baby, you need this muscle to be free of fear and tension so your pelvis can allow your baby to navigate into it and out of it.

The second way fear can impact your core is through your pelvic floor. Fear can cause you to hold onto tension in your pelvic floor which can result in chronically contracted muscles, a tucked-under tailbone and pelvic pain. Just as you need the psoas to relax, you also need your pelvic floor to be able to relax and yield and provide space for your baby to move into the pelvis and then into the world. Holding tension in the muscles of the pelvic floor can reduce the space for the baby, meaning a more difficult time during labor.

This may all seem like a lot of doom and gloom, but it is meant to move you to action – actions you will take to prepare and prevent! Going through pregnancy and birth armed with this knowledge puts you in a position of power. You can make informed decisions during your pregnancy, your birth AND the postpartum recovery that put you in the driver's seat rather than just 'hoping for the best'.

Now that we have looked at how pregnancy, birth and life can affect your core, let's delve deeper into the 2 main aspects of the core that are left out of many prenatal education classes – the abdomen and the pelvic floor.

Pelvic floor challenges can result from overuse or underuse of the muscles. Your muscles have been working hard through your pregnancy to try to maintain stability in your pelvis, maintain stability in your spine, keep your organs in place and manage the ever-increasing load of the growing baby. All this while trying to maintain your continence and your sex life too!

When muscles overwork, they can become weak because they never get a break. The reason they start to become overused is that they are trying to pick up the slack from the muscles that are not able to do their job because of posture or alignment changes.

Here are some of the more common types of pelvic floor dysfunction and tips on how to prevent or treat them.

Pelvic Organ Prolapse:

Pelvic Organ Prolapse is another challenge that is even less known and talked about than incontinence. 50% of women who have had children will have some degree of prolapse, and most are unaware due to the few symptoms of this condition in the early stages. Also, 50% of women who have diastasis recti will have some element of pelvic floor dysfunction (mainly incontinence and prolapse). Of note here is that prolapse does not only occur in women who have had children. Pregnancy and birth increase the risk, but it can happen in women who have never been pregnant or had children pointing to other influences such as posture, lifestyle, age, hormones etc.

As noted earlier, one of the functions of the pelvic floor is to help keep the pelvic organs in place. The position of the bladder, the uterus and the rectum is partially dependent on the strength and position of the pelvis and pelvic floor muscles. A weakened pelvic floor loses its ability to provide support which can interfere with the ability to hold the organs in their anatomical position. Unsupported organs will therefore start to descend into and, in severe cases, out of the vagina, which is obviously something you want to avoid.

There are four stages of prolapse: early-stage prolapse, stage 1 and 2, is often asymptomatic, which is why preventive pelvic floor physiotherapy is such a key part of your health care team. When caught at stage 1 or 2, prolapse can be well managed and may even be reversed. Stage 3 is once the organ is at the introitus (the entrance to the vagina), and stage 4 is when the organ is bulging out of the vagina.

Once the organ(s) (you can have more than one organ prolapsing) get down close to the opening of the vagina or out of the vagina, there is no reversing that. Once it's out, it typically becomes a surgical need. This is life-altering. Not life-threatening but very life-altering. Many young women living with prolapse will say, "My body is broken." With the right information and preparation, prolapse does not have to be part of your postpartum body.

Cystocele Prolapse

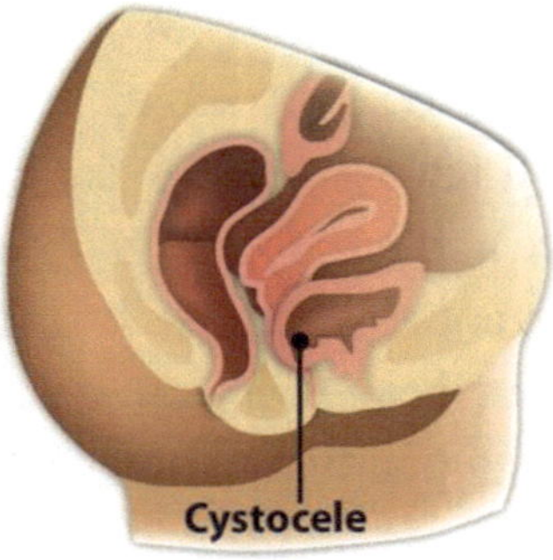

Normal
Female Pelvic Anatomy

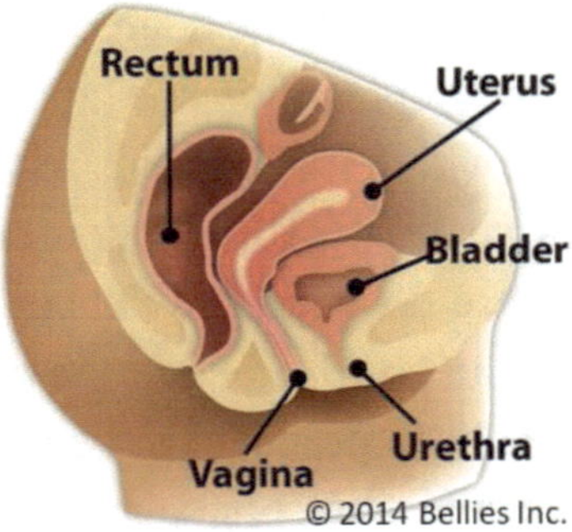

Rectal Prolapse

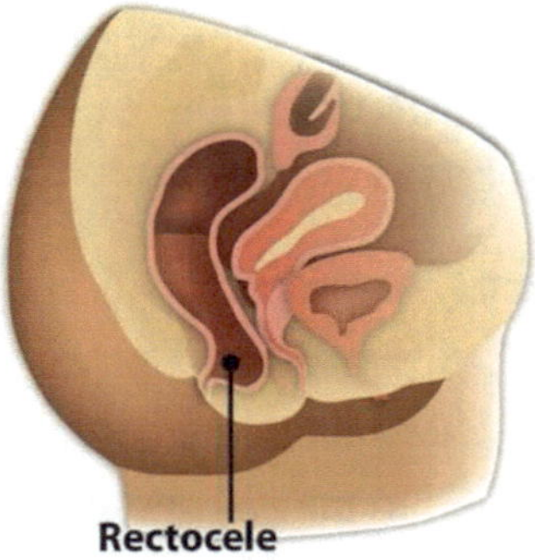

Normal
Female Pelvic Anatomy

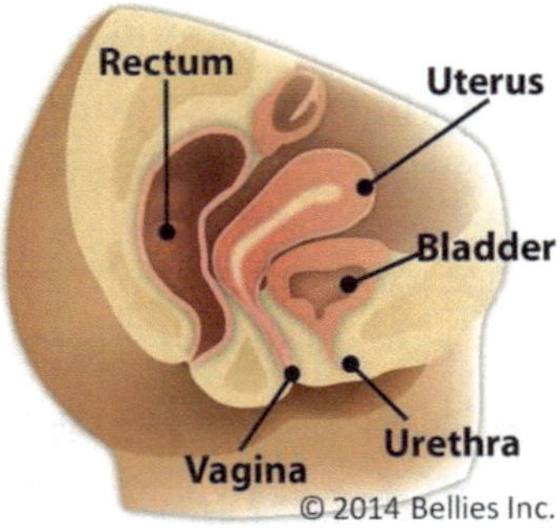

Uterine Prolapse

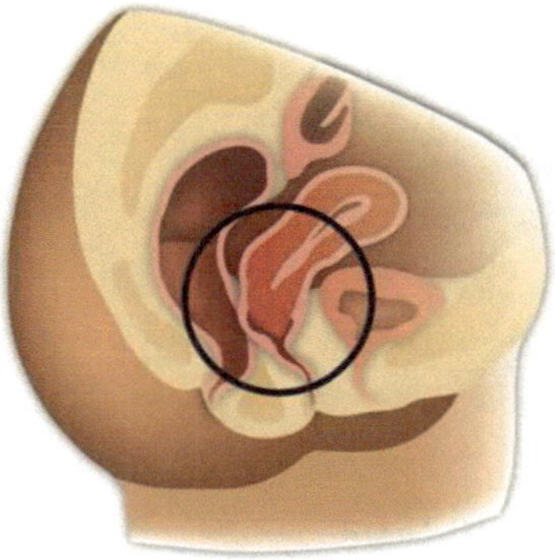

Normal Female Pelvic Anatomy

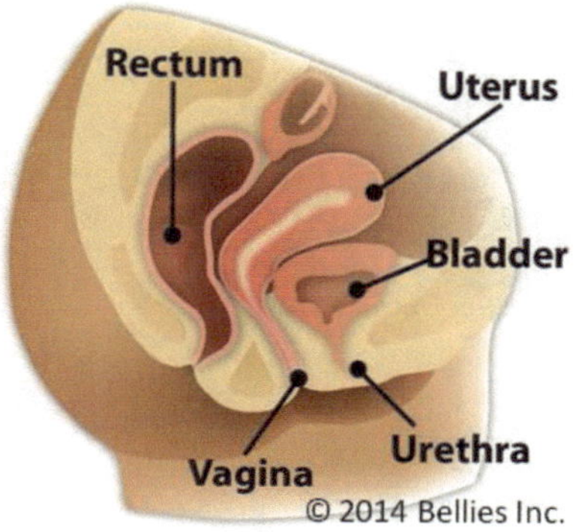

Vaginal Vault Prolapse

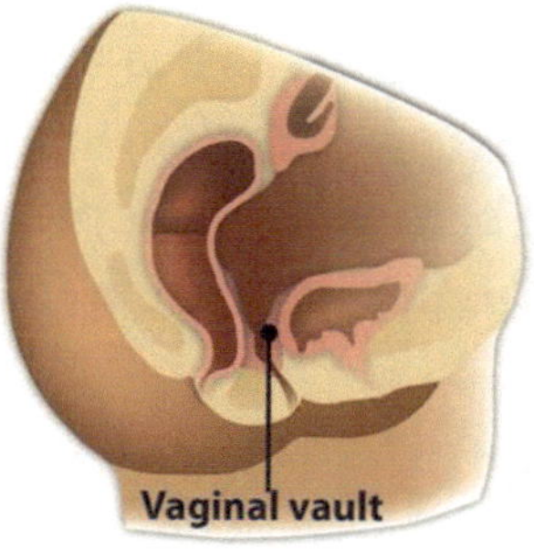

Normal Female Pelvic Anatomy
(post-hysterectomy)

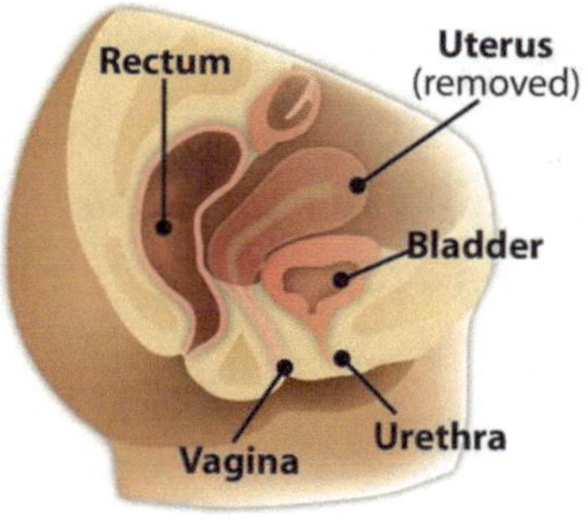

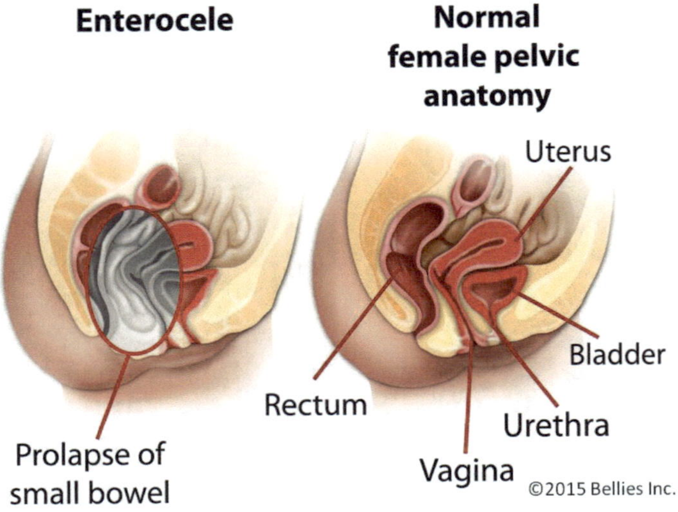

Pelvic Girdle Pain

Symphysis Pubis Dysfunction

One common challenge that can present in pregnancy is pain in the pubic joint. A lot of women report feeling as though they have been '*kicked in the crotch*'. They might find it hard to stand on one leg to put pants on, it may be challenging to roll over in bed or to get in and out of the car. This is called symphysis pubis dysfunction. The pubic joint starts to widen and loosen and become laxer in preparation for the baby. As a result, the pelvis can become less stable and can cause pain at that joint.

Sacro-illiac Joint (SI Joint) Pain

A very common location of pain in pregnancy is the SI Joint - where the sacrum meets the iliac bones. The postural changes in pregnancy can affect this joint, the hormones making the pelvis more 'open' can affect this joint, the added weight on the pelvis can affect this joint and weak or compromised pelvic floor muscles can affect this joint. Note, there are 2 joints - one on either side and the pain can be in one or both sides and can be very debilitating.

During pregnancy, as many as 42% of women will have some form of pelvic pain, with sacroiliac (SI Joint) and symphysis pubis pain being the most common. Wearing a support belt like the BabyBellyBand or the Baby Belly Belt during and after pregnancy can provide relief and help stabilize the pelvis while the function is restored through alignment and exercise. Pelvic floor exercise is critical as it will help strengthen the muscles that support the pelvis and release the muscles that may be overworking or compensating for a weakness elsewhere.

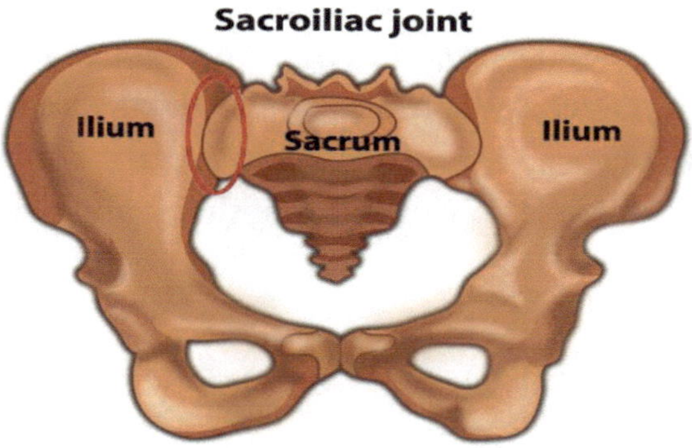

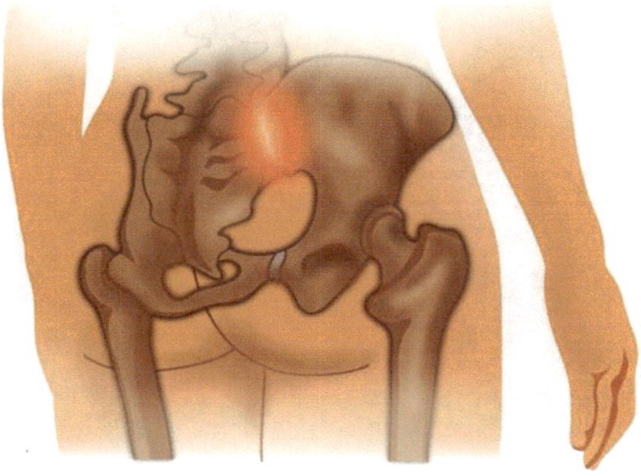

Incontinence

Another challenge and often a common side effect of pregnancy and delivery (notice again that we said common and not normal) is incontinence – the involuntary loss of urine.

There are a few different types of incontinence. Stress incontinence occurs if you are exerting a force like running, laughing, coughing, sneezing, or jumping, and urine leaks out a little bit at a time. Urge incontinence is when you feel like you have to go all the time or feel like you can't hold it and you can't make it to the bathroom in time. Mixed incontinence is a combination of stress and urges incontinence. Incontinence can occur as a result of nerve damage or scar tissue, from overused muscles and from underused muscles, but the good news is it can be prevented and treated with pelvic muscle exercise ideally with a pelvic floor physiotherapist before and after birth.

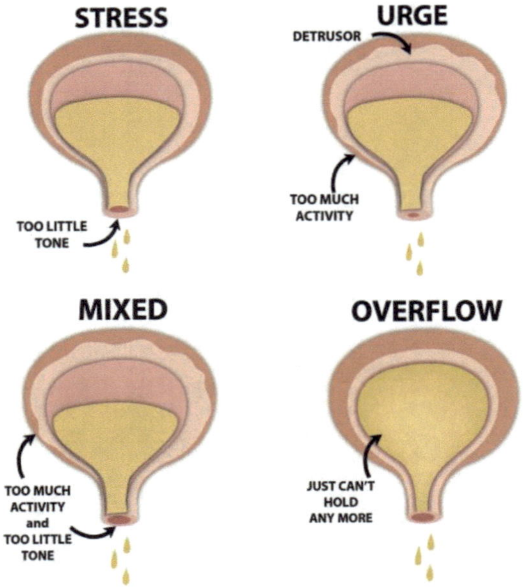

Scar Tissue

Another pelvic floor challenge that can occur as a result of labor and delivery results from scar tissue. There can be scar tissue on the labia and perineum from tearing or if you have an episiotomy. There can also be abdominal scar tissue from a cesarean birth. Scar tissue creates adhesions as the tissue heals, which is natural and needed, but you want to keep the adhesions as mobile as possible, so that doesn't adhere to places you don't want it to and start to cause movement restrictions.

Fascia is the thin white connective tissue that we all have in our bodies. It is a system that envelops muscles but is also interconnected between the muscles. When you have an incision or injury, the connective tissue starts to create adhesions as it heals. A restriction (from adhesions) in the connective tissue can actually create pain in another part of the body as it pulls muscles or organs out of their optimal position. Avoiding perineal tearing or episiotomy is obviously ideal, but working with a pelvic floor physiotherapist postpartum who can mobilize the scar tissue once it has occurred is a must!

Chapter 22: Feeding Baby by Dr Jack Newman FRCPC

Why should pregnant women prepare for breastfeeding?

Most pregnant women focus almost entirely on the birth of their baby, almost to the exclusion of thinking about what happens after birth. They imagine that deciding to breastfeed is all that is necessary and that they will breastfeed. On the one hand, they are right, breastfeeding *should be* simple, not complicated, and it should happen automatically and effortlessly. It should be as easy as just putting the baby on the breast and letting the baby drink breast milk. What more is there to it?

In today's world, however, there are many reasons why a disproportionately large number of women find breastfeeding not as easy as they had imagined; and frequently, there are so many obstacles thrown in their way that they need expert help to overcome them. Why should this be the case?

> *Breastfeeding* ***should be*** *simple.*
>
> *But we have made it so difficult for women to start breastfeeding that up to* ***92%*** *of women experience problems with breastfeeding in the first few days after birth.*

The new generation of mothers is trying to overcome an unprecedented change over two or three generations when babies were *not* breastfed and were routinely bottle-fed formula. Many of today's mothers were not breastfed themselves, and they do not have women in their family or friends to turn to for encouragement or solid advice.

In our society, though most mothers initiate breastfeeding, breastfeeding *knowledge* is not a norm. Bottle feeding formula is common, and it is not impossible for a mother to give birth to a baby without ever having seen babies being breastfed.

These days, there is a tremendous amount of misinformation about breastfeeding, not infrequently coming from health professionals, as well as frightening breastfeeding stories and unethical marketing of formula. So, it is not surprising that pregnant women and new mothers are in a quandary about what to believe.

Formula advertising is so common and so clever that it has become commonplace and an accepted and unchallenged part of our culture. The fact that the formula company advertising is often provided by the mother's obstetrician or family doctor lends it an air of truth.

Births no longer happen normally in an undisturbed way for the vast majority of mothers. Caesarean section rates have skyrocketed in many countries, and birth interventions have become routine. If birth is not natural, how can we imagine breastfeeding would just happen?

It is for these reasons that it is worth reading about breastfeeding before birth and re-reading about breastfeeding once your baby is born.

Resources: Breastfeeding – Starting Out Right (http://ibconline.ca/breastfeeding-starting-out-right/)

Book: Dr. Jack Newman's Guide to Breastfeeding (available on amazon.com and amazon.ca)

What can you do to increase your chances of breastfeeding?

You can plan on as long a maternity leave as possible. Maternity leave in the United States is one of the worst in the world. Many countries offer reasonable maternity leave for new mothers. In

Sweden, Norway and Canada, maternity leave is now 18 months. In some eastern European countries, it is 3 years and sometimes longer.

It has been conclusively shown that the duration of breastfeeding largely depends on the duration of the maternity leave.

Resources: www.thelancet.com/series/breastfeeding

What to Feed the Baby when the Mother is Working Outside the Home (http://ibconline.ca/what-to-feed-the-baby-when-the-mother-is-working-outside-the-home/)

How can you tell whether a hospital or birthing center supports breastfeeding?

There are 10 basic points that the WHO/UNICEF included in the *minimal* standard of care which hospitals should automatically provide to mothers and babies in order to create supportive conditions for breastfeeding. Based on these 10 points, when choosing a hospital, you can ask the following questions:

1) Does the hospital provide information – oral and written – about breastfeeding during prenatal visits, and does this information come from an independent source (not formula company materials)?
2) Does the hospital routinely keep babies in uninterrupted skin-to-skin contact with their mothers for an hour or more after birth?
3) Does the hospital make sure that mothers routinely get skilled help with breastfeeding within 6 hours of giving birth?
4) Is the hospital staff willing and able to provide help with breastfeeding?
5) What is the percentage of babies which are supplemented with formula in this hospital?

6) What are the reasons due to which babies are supplemented with formula?

7) Is formula supplementation routine in this hospital? (It should not be.)

8) What methods other than using bottles or syringes can the hospital staff recommend and show in case a baby needs to be supplemented for medical reasons?

9) Are mothers and babies kept in the same room day and night, and is help available to them whenever they need it?

1) Are mothers and babies encouraged to stay in skin-to-skin contact in bed together during the hospital stay?

2) Is the use of swaddling or wrapping the baby in cloth routine in the hospital? (It should not be.)

3) Does the hospital staff recommend the use of pacifiers or nipple shields? (They should not.)

4) Does the hospital have a breastfeeding support group?

5) Does the hospital not give out free formula samples or formula company literature?

Resources: WHO website:
http://www.who.int/nutrition/topics/bfhi/en/

How are birth and breastfeeding connected?

The events surrounding birth and the birth experience profoundly affect the ease with which breastfeeding begins. Furthermore, hospital postpartum routines following the birth can often greatly complicate breastfeeding. When choosing a place where to give birth, inquire about breastfeeding support and help as well. Many mothers assume that "once you have survived birth, everything else will be a piece of cake". After birth, breastfeeding is just beginning, and with your baby in your arms, you will not have time to study breastfeeding literature.

Resources: Finding a Breastfeeding Support Person (http://ibconline.ca/finding-a-breastfeeding-support-person/)

When do babies breastfeed for the first time?

As soon as you are pregnant, your body invests in your future breastfeeding – growing your breasts before much else visibly grows in your body. Indeed, sensitive breasts and nipples may be among the first signs of pregnancy. Your body then begins to produce breastmilk early in the pregnancy – when you are about 16 weeks pregnant.

When your baby is born, his every movement, his every reflex, guides him towards the breast. Breastfeeding takes care of the baby's needs in a similar way that the uterus, placenta and umbilical cord do during pregnancy: breastfeeding provides nutrition, the warmth of the mother's body, comfort, protection, and regulation of sleep-wake pattern. Thus, the best time for babies to breastfeed for the first time is shortly after birth. And it is not just pretending to breastfeed, in spite of what many seem to believe – they actually drink breastmilk from the breast, and it is important that they do so.

Breastfeeding within the first hour or so after birth influences the amount of breastmilk that will be produced in the upcoming weeks and months.

Resources: BreastCrawl (http://www.breastcrawl.org/)

What should happen when the baby is born?

Babies should be placed in skin-to-skin contact with their mothers immediately after birth, and they should stay there for at least the first two hours postpartum. Skin-to-skin contact has been shown to stabilize the baby's temperature, blood pressure, blood sugar, respiration and heart rate after birth and skin-to-skin with the mother is the best place for the baby to adapt to life outside of the uterus. Babies that are born via Caesarean section, premature babies or sick babies need skin-to-skin contact with their mothers *more, not less* than healthy full-term babies. And healthy full-term babies need skin-to-skin contact too.

Skin-to-skin contact between the mother and baby should be uninterrupted and undisturbed. Hospital routines, such as weighing or measuring the baby, can wait and be done later.

Whether uninterrupted skin-to-skin contact is encouraged, is considered normal and routine during the first two hours after birth should be one of the criteria for choosing a place of birth.

Resources: The Importance of Skin-to-Skin Contact (http://ibconline.ca/the-importance-of-skin-to-skin-contact/)

Is breastfeeding after a Caesarean section more difficult?

Breastfeeding after a Caesarean section is not different from breastfeeding a baby born vaginally. Your body starts to make milk during pregnancy, and your baby is ready to breastfeed as soon as he is born.

What complicates breastfeeding after a Caesarean section are the same things that complicate breastfeeding after a vaginal birth: that is, separation of the mother and baby (mother and baby should be together skin to skin after a Caesarean section too, and the baby should be allowed to crawl to the breast in the operating room), medications are given the mother during birth, difficulty sitting up and walking, the baby being given bottles or supplements instead of the mother having the baby at the breast.

Resources: Book: Dr. Jack Newman's Guide to Breastfeeding (available on amazon.com and amazon.ca)

What are the three things to know about breastfeeding during the early days after birth?

Breastfeeding largely depends on three things:

Continuous skin-to-skin contact between the mother and baby in the first few days and even longer.

A good latch.

Learning how to tell whether the baby is drinking milk from the breast.

Resources: Latching and Feeding Management (http://ibconline.ca/latching-and-feeding/)

What is a good latch?

A good latch is what is called an asymmetric latch. The baby's chin is in the breast, but not the nose, and the baby covers more of the areola with his lower lip than his upper lip.

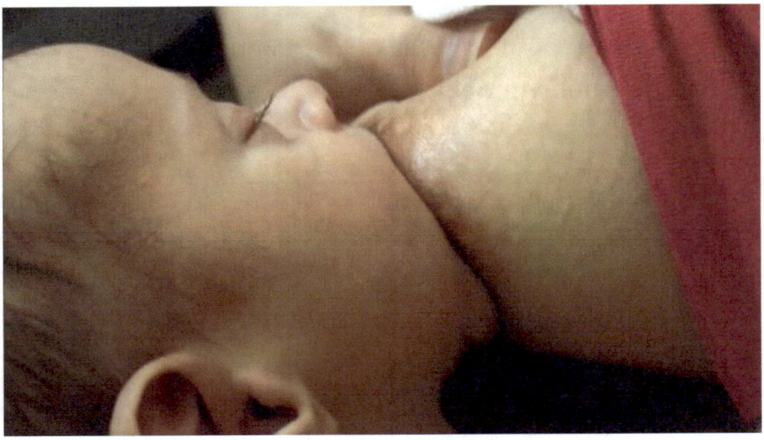

Resources: Can you tell whether a latch is good? (http://ibconline.ca/latch-quiz/)

How do you know your baby is getting milk from the breast?

Many mothers worry their baby is not getting anything from the breast; they worry their baby would starve, and not knowing how to tell whether the baby is drinking from the breast or not often leads to insecurity and unnecessary interventions such as supplementing with formula.

It is possible to know whether the baby is drinking from the breast – the way to tell is to watch the baby when breastfeeding. When he opens his mouth to the maximum, the pause in his chin tells you the baby just got a mouthful of milk.

Resources: Videos: http://ibconline.ca/breastfeeding-videos-english/

Really good drinking: https://goo.gl/56Qrv5

Nibbling: https://goo.gl/z2F7bt

Twelve-day-old nibbling: https://goo.gl/fyocJ2

"Borderline" drinking: https://goo.gl/nd6CHa

How can you help your baby get more milk from the breast?

Breast compressions can be very helpful. When your baby only sucks but doesn't drink, use compressions to keep the baby drinking more milk. Put your hand around your breast and firmly squeeze. It should not hurt. Compressions are like pumping more milk directly into your baby.

Resources: A Method to Increase Breastmilk Intake by the Baby (http://ibconline.ca/breastcompression/)

Why is breastfeeding important?

For centuries, breastfeeding was the common, unrivaled way to take care of babies. This has dramatically changed only in the 20th century, although the wealthy in much of Europe hired wet nurses to feed their babies from much earlier on. Too often, the wet nurse's own baby was fed artificially and not infrequently died of malnutrition and infection.

Since the 1960s, more and more scientific data has emerged, providing stronger and stronger evidence as to why breastfeeding is so important and why there are so many elements of breastfeeding that cannot be provided by artificial feeding. Most recently, The Lancet, the top science journal, published a series of studies documenting the implications of breastfeeding for the present and future health of mothers and babies.

Breastfeeding is the normal, physiological way for babies to feed. Breastmilk is tailor-made for every baby and has a composition that is specific to the needs of the human baby. And each mammal's milk is specific to the needs of its offspring. The primary function of breastfeeding (breastfeeding is much more than the milk, being a close physical and emotional relationship between the mother and baby) is to help the baby's brain to develop and achieve its full potential and for the baby's gut to develop the right kind of microbiome (bacterial flora in the digestive tract) and, essentially to lay the cornerstone of the baby's health. While providing the nutrition the baby needs, it also plays an important role in the development of the baby's immune system. Nearly half of all diarrhea episodes and one-third of all respiratory infections would be prevented with increased breastfeeding rates. There is growing evidence that breastfeeding provides protection against obesity and diabetes later in life.

Breastfeeding contributes to the development of the baby's brain and his intelligence. The baby's being breastfed significantly contributes not only to the baby's current health but also his future health and his academic performance, long-term earnings and productivity.

In all countries of the world, rich and poor alike, breastfeeding plays a significant role in providing nutrition and maternal and child health and survival. High-income countries lose more than $230 billion annually (0.53% of GNI) due to low rates of breastfeeding.

Breastfeeding is important for the mother's health too. For each year a mother breastfeeds, her risk of developing invasive breast cancer decreases by 6%. Breastfeeding also reduces the risk of ovarian cancer. Current rates of breastfeeding prevent almost 20,000 deaths from breast cancer each year.

Resources: www.thelancet.com/series/breastfeeding

> *Nipple shields do not offer the real solution for any of the problems they are sometimes recommended for:*
>
> *Not for sore nipples*
>
> *Not for non-latching babies*
>
> *Not for premature babies*

How do babies learn to breastfeed?

Babies learn to breastfeed by breastfeeding.

Mothers learn to breastfeed by breastfeeding.

Consequently, mothers and babies do not learn to breastfeed by bottle feeding. Nor by syringe feeding. Nor by sucking a pacifier. And the same applies to using nipple shields. Do not take any of these for an answer to your breastfeeding problems. If you are having breastfeeding issues, do not accept any of these "solutions" as the way to go.

Resources: http://ibconline.ca/

When should you worry?

In the first few days, your baby needs attention and help with breastfeeding if,

- the baby is crying much of the time
- the baby is sleeping more and more. Babies may be sleepy from medication used during labor and birth, even if given by epidural, but should become less sleepy as the time after the birth goes on, not sleepier
- the baby is not drinking breastmilk from the breast
- the baby is not latching on to the breast
- the baby is constantly on the breast but does not drink
- the baby still has only black stools – meconium – by the 3rd day after birth, certainly by the 4th day
- you have sore nipples or breasts

Resources: Book: Dr. Jack Newman's Guide to Breastfeeding (available on amazon.com and amazon.ca)

What are NOT the reasons for supplementation?

Supplementing does not make sense if you are told you must supplement for the following reasons:

- "because there is no milk in the first few days after birth" (there is)
- "because your baby was born by Caesarean section" (your baby can breastfeed immediately after being born)
- "because your baby is born heavy". (That babies over 4 kg (8lb 12oz) or more need to be supplemented is a myth. Furthermore, the notion that a baby born "heavy" is at risk for low blood sugar is also a myth if the mother is not diabetic.)
- "because your baby does not settle" (it is possible to help a baby breastfeed well and to show a mother how to put her baby to sleep)

- "because your baby slept longer than 3 hours" (this baby needs to breastfeed well or get help to breastfeed well, but if the baby has been consistently drinking well at the breast, he does not need to feed at least every three hours)

Resources: Book: Dr. Jack Newman's Guide to Breastfeeding (available on amazon.com and amazon.ca)

> When supplementing is mentioned, people tend to automatically interpret that as "formula". If supplementation is truly medically necessary, there are other options:
>
> 1) Mother's own expressed breastmilk
> 2) Donated breastmilk
> 3) Glucose water (ideally mixed with the mother's own breastmilk) in the first 2 to 3 days

How can you tell what good breastfeeding help and advice is?

Good breastfeeding help means you get the help that leads to making breastfeeding work long-term. So, you can ask questions such as: "How does this advice help my baby drink breast milk from the breast?" "How does this help my baby learn to breastfeed better?" "Does this teach me and my baby skills necessary for breastfeeding?"

> *Breastfeeding is a relationship, breastfeeding is more than getting breast milk from the breast.*

And one more thing, breastfeeding and rules do not go well together. If you find you are being told rules and numbers (such as the number of minutes your baby should spend on the breast or the number of millilitres your baby is supposed to drink), find someone else to ask.

Here are examples of bad breastfeeding advice:

- Offer one breast only at each feeding. (This can lead to a decrease in milk supply. The mother should "finish" one side and then offer the other. If the baby is full, the baby will not take the second side.)
- Breastfeed for 15 or 20, or any number of minutes, only. (Limiting the time the baby spends on the breast can lead to the baby not getting enough milk from the breast.)
- Your baby is lazy. (Babies are not lazy, they simply respond to the flow of milk from the breast; if the flow of milk is slow, a baby may fall asleep.)
- You can tell whether your baby is getting milk if his ears wiggle. (You can't, the real answer to whether your baby is getting milk from the breast is the pause in the chin.)
- Weighing your baby before breastfeeding and after tells you how much breastmilk your baby got. (Wrong. This tells you nothing and can falsely reassure you or bring about panic for no good reason. Why? Because too many mothers are so worried that they will fail the test, that the letdown reflex is inhibited, and they do fail the test.)
- You should wake your baby up to breastfeed. (This does not help. Instead, you should put your baby skin to skin with you and wait for him to wake up on his own and then use the opportunity to breastfeed him.)
- Breastfeed 8 or 10, or any number of times per day. (There is no number set on how much or how often your baby can breastfeed.)

Resources: Finding a Breastfeeding Support Person (http://ibconline.ca/finding-a-breastfeeding-support-person/)

You should continue breastfeeding if:

- Your baby has jaundice.
- Your baby has hypoglycemia.
- Your baby lost more than 10% of his birthweight or any other arbitrary number (7% is also popular, also based on no science).
- Your baby is sick (there are very few conditions when babies cannot be breastfed, and a sick baby needs breastfeeding more, not less).
- You are sick (there are very few conditions when the mother cannot breastfeed). Take the baby to bed with you and keep nursing.
- You need to take medications. If you need medications and you are told you cannot breastfeed, look further. Medications are almost never a reason to stop breastfeeding.

These situations are also not reasons to supplement your baby with formula. You should make sure your baby is drinking well at the breast.

Resources: Jaundice (http://ibconline.ca/information-sheets/breastfeeding-and-jaundice/)

Hypoglycemia (http://ibconline.ca/hypoglycaemia-of-the-newborn-low-blood-sugar/)

Maternal Illness (http://ibconline.ca/breastfeeding-and-illness/)

Medications and Breastfeeding (http://ibconline.ca/breastfeeding-and-medications/)

What should breastfeeding mothers eat?

There are no special dietary requirements for breastfeeding mothers. There are no foods to avoid, as a rule. Just like all other people, breastfeeding mothers need normal, healthy and nutritious food. There is no need for any special diet.

Exercise – Breastfeeding does not mean you cannot stay active or keep fit. You can exercise. Worries about decreased milk supply or babies refusing to breastfeed because of different milk taste are a myth.

Weight loss – Breastfeeding usually helps mothers lose weight over time. This is normal and expected. There is no reason why you could not lose weight during breastfeeding.

Resources: Book: Dr. Jack Newman's Guide to Breastfeeding (available on amazon.com and amazon.ca)

WHO postpartum materials, section on Nutrition: https://www.ncbi.nlm.nih.gov/books/NBK304191/

Do you need to buy something special to be able to breastfeed?

Under normal circumstances, you do not need anything to be able to breastfeed. You only need your baby and you. If breastfeeding gets off to the best start and is going well, you do not need anything else.

Mothers are often told to buy all sorts of unnecessary equipment in order to breastfeed. There are countries in which breastfeeding has become a synonym for pumping, and every woman is expected to buy a pump. This is not only not necessary, but it is also a waste of money. Pumping takes the joy out of breastfeeding, and a pump is not something you should buy just because you will be breastfeeding. You also do not need to buy formula or bottles "just in case".

Resources: Read the chapter on "Breastfeeding Devices" in: Dr. Jack Newman's Guide to Breastfeeding (available on amazon.com and amazon.ca)

How often should a baby breastfeed?

Babies should be breastfed whenever they show signs of readiness to breastfeed. There is no limit to how often or how much a baby can or should breastfeed. You can go back and forth from one breast to another several times to keep the baby drinking milk. Breastfeeding is a relationship, and it provides much more than just breastmilk – it provides closeness, intimate contact, a sense of security and well-being. It is also for these reasons that babies want to breastfeed at night even when people say they "do not need food" at night. Breastfeeding is not just "food".

Resources: Book: Dr. Jack Newman's Guide to Breastfeeding (available on amazon.com and amazon.ca)

What can you do so you do not spoil your baby?

There are a number of things that do not spoil your baby: breastfeeding your baby as often as the baby wishes, holding your baby in your arms, carrying your baby, co-sleeping with your baby, spending time with your baby, putting your baby to sleep by breastfeeding the baby, offering the breast when the baby is upset or crying, calming your baby down when crying and responding your baby's crying.

When should you wean your baby?

The baby's brain, the baby's gut, the baby's immune system, all of the baby's body and the baby's relationship with his mother develop for a long time – not just the first weeks or months of life. The WHO has shown how significant the 1,000 days of the baby's life are as a window of opportunity for laying the foundations of the baby's health and well-being.

The WHO recommends that breastfeeding should be part of the baby's life for a long time. There are three distinct phases in breastfeeding:

The first 6 months – during this time, the baby should be breastfed exclusively, without being given water or any other food.

From 6 months to 2 years – during this time, breastfeeding should continue as usual, and solids should be introduced and added to breastfeeding so that both breastfeeding and eating normal food become established during this time.

From 2 years on – during this time, both breastfeeding and eating food are established. Toddlers stop breastfeeding when they are ready, usually around the ages of 3 – 5 years.

Resources: WHO website: https://thousanddays.org/

Breastfeed a Toddler – Why on Earth? (http://ibconline.ca/breastfeed-a-toddler-why-on-earth/)

When should my baby start eating solids?

There are signs of readiness that can be seen in babies that indicate that a baby is prepared to eat food. Most babies are ready to start eating food at around 6 months of age. Babies at this age have the ability to begin trying out food – the same normal, healthy food that their parents eat.

Babies starting to eat around 6 months do not need “special baby food”. They do not need commercially produced baby food. They do not need baby cereals or “follow-on formula” as part of introducing food. Babies should be learning to eat family food. Commercial baby foods are a waste of money and not always safe.

The time when the baby starts to eat food is a time of introducing water from an *open cup*. Babies do not need to “transition” from breastfeeding to bottles or sippy cups, or any other special cups designed for babies. The purpose of introducing the baby to eating and drinking is to show the baby how to eat normal food and how to drink normally, the way adults do.

Resources: Breastfeeding and Other Foods: http://ibconline.ca/breastfeeding-and-other-foods/

How can you tell a health provider is supportive of breastfeeding?

Support for breastfeeding means looking for ways breastfeeding – meaning feeding your baby at your breast – can be made to work. The approach of health providers who are supportive of breastfeeding is one where they see breastfeeding as a priority and can include breastfeeding in everything that is done with the mother and baby. They know the mother and baby to be one inseparable unit that needs to be considered together, treated together and kept together.

Such health providers not only verbally say that breastfeeding is important, but they are also able to take practical steps to ensure that breastfeeding continues even in difficult situations.

They are able to help with breastfeeding or recommend someone who can help. They do not keep any formula company materials displayed or hidden in their waiting rooms or offices. And do not offer you samples of formula or infant feeding information pamphlets that come from formula companies.

They believe that breastfeeding problems can be overcome, and if the mother or baby is sick, breastfeeding is essential to their treatment plan and to make them feel better.

Resources: How to Know a Healthcare Practitioner is not Supportive of Breastfeeding (http://ibconline.ca/how-to-know-a-healthcare-practitioner-is-not-supportive-of-breastfeeding/)

What are the challenges women sometimes encounter?

Breastfeeding problems are frequently the result of birth interventions, separating mothers and babies after birth, unnecessary supplementation of babies and bad breastfeeding advice. *Most problems are preventable by getting off to the best start possible,* carefully choosing the place of birth, carefully selecting the people to ask for help and knowing where to turn for breastfeeding information.

If you are experiencing breastfeeding difficulties, do not wait for things to get better; seek good breastfeeding help as soon as possible. Breastfeeding problems are much easier to solve at 8 days than at 8 weeks.

Here is a list of the most common problems that some women may be faced with:

1) *Breast engorgement on the 3 – 5 day postpartum.*
2) *Sore nipples and sore breasts.*
3) *A baby who does not yet latch.*
4) *A baby who does not get enough milk from the breast.*
5) *A baby who does not gain weight.*
6) *A baby who cries for prolonged periods of time or is fussy.*
7) *A baby with "reflux".*
8) *A baby who has a tongue tie or a lip tie.*
9) *A baby who is fussy, pulls away from the breast, and breastfeeds for a very short period of time.*

Breast engorgement 3 to 5 days after birth:

Painful engorgement 3 – 5 days postpartum is not normal. When the mother's milk "comes in", the mother normally may feel some fullness, but she should not have painful swelling of the breast. (I use the term "comes in" because it is commonly used and understood, but in fact, there is milk from about 16 weeks into the pregnancy. The milk production *increases* about 3 or 4 days after birth.) The only reason that such painful swelling of the breasts would be considered normal is the history of postpartum policies over the last 150 years which resulted in limited breastfeeding (2 minutes/side the first day, 5 minutes/side the second and so on) and frequent separation of the mother and baby. In this day and age, engorgement has become worse because of the intravenous fluids most mothers receive during labor and birth and frequently afterward the birth of the baby.

Painful engorgement 3 to 5 days after birth is due, basically, to the baby not breastfeeding well during the first 3 days after birth. A baby is not getting milk simply because he has the breast in his mouth and making sucking motions. One can tell if the baby is actually drinking by watching for the pause in the baby's chin as he opens his mouth to the maximum opening. A really good drinking video, https://goo.gl/VSxqjE, shows a month-old baby drinking very well at the breast and is here so that the very obvious pause is easy to see. Ten-hour-old baby https://goo.gl/IFi4Ml shows a baby just born 10 hours before who is also showing those pauses, but as there is normally much less milk in the first few days than at 1 month, say, the pauses are shorter.

There is enough milk in the first few days, but the baby has to get that milk. If the baby does not seem to be getting much milk, then improving the baby's latch http://ibconline.ca/the-asymmetric-latch/ and using breast compression http://ibconline.ca/breastcompression/ will almost always increase the baby's intake of breastmilk and prevent painful engorgement.

But what if the baby doesn't latch on and drink? This frequently occurs because the mother's nipples and areolas are swollen with fluid, much of which comes from the intravenous fluids given during labor and birth as well as after the birth. Prevention would be useful, and the amounts of fluids given routinely given to mothers during labor, birth and after could be considerably reduced.

Reverse pressure softening can reduce the swelling of the nipples and areolas and makes it easier for the baby to latch on. See the video Reverse pressure softening: https://goo.gl/NfWMyF.

Sore Nipples:

Pain during breastfeeding is not normal and should not be considered normal. If the mother's nipples hurt, then something is wrong, and that is most often when the baby's latch is not as good as it could be. True, some skin diseases affecting the nipples can also cause painful nipples. These include eczema and psoriasis, but these are unusual situations and should have been treated before the baby was born.

So, why would the baby's latch not be as good as it could be?

The latch: How a baby takes the breast, the way of putting the baby to the breast matters. If the baby takes the breast and, the mother has no pain and as well, the baby drinks from the breast, the latch is good. If the baby takes the breast and the mother has no pain, but the baby is not drinking well, the latch is probably not good. This is what a good latch looks like, at least from the outside: http://ibconline.ca/the-asymmetric-latch/

The use of bottles and pacifiers can affect the baby's latch. A nipple shield definitely interferes with a baby's latch because, in fact, a baby on a nipple shield is not latched on at all. http://ibconline.ca/nipple-shields/ The use of artificial nipples in the immediate postpartum period may be especially disruptive of the baby learning to latch on well and may be a factor in the baby refusing the breast and causing the mother sore nipples.

A tongue tie is a frequent cause of sore nipples. A baby with a tongue tie cannot latch on well.

A decreasing milk supply, http://ibconline.ca/decreased/, can also result in nipple pain. When the flow of milk from the breast decreases, the baby tends to slip down on the nipple and/or the baby will pull at the breast.

So how to treat sore nipples? The best treatment is always prevention. Prevention gets short shrift in our society because one does not always appreciate sore nipples that didn't happen. But it's still the best treatment. And what is that treatment if sore nipples occur? The understanding that breastfeeding should not hurt and good help as soon as possible to make sure the baby has a good latch as soon as possible after the birth http://ibconline.ca/the-asymmetric-latch/and making sure the baby gets milk well http://ibconline.ca/breastcompression/.

Our All Purpose Nipple Ointment could help considerably with sore nipples. Any physician/nurse practitioner/midwife (midwives in some jurisdictions) can prescribe our **ointment** (All Purpose Nipple Ointment (APNO)). **However, the ointment is a stopgap measure only.**

And if the mother does have sore nipples? Fix the latch, and make sure the baby is milk well from the breast. Avoid artificial nipples.

Sore breasts:

To repeat: If breastfeeding hurts, something is wrong. And that goes for sore breasts as well. Pain may also radiate from the nipple to the breast and thus give the impression that something is wrong with the breast.

The vessels of the nipple may go into spasm, likely because of trauma to the nipple, and this, too, may cause pain that radiates into the breast. The absence of blood flow to the nipple will cause the nipple to turn white, and then the blood flows back, and the nipple turns back to pink, and the mother will experience the pain of a throbbing nature.

But the breast itself may develop a blocked duct, mastitis or, on occasion, an abscess. And both a blocked duct and mastitis are usually quite painful. If there is no painful lump in the breast, there is no blocked duct or mastitis. Another reason needs to explain pain in the breast without a lump in the breast. An abscess is not necessarily painful, but it may be. It is often quite tender if the area is squeezed.

A blocked duct and mastitis are both due to a milk duct being obstructed and the milk collecting into what feels like a lump in the breast. Both conditions are, essentially, the same thing, and the treatment is the same.

However, when milk supply decreases, this too can result in the baby pulling away from the breast before the breast is well drained (babies will often pull away from the breast when the flow is slow). Not draining the breast because the baby pulls away early may result in blocked ducts, mastitis and even, under certain circumstances, a breast abscess.

A blocked duct and mastitis often will go away without any treatment except continuing breastfeeding on the painful breast, ideally in combination with adjusting the latch. Continued feeding will almost always result in a more rapid resolution of the blocked duct and mastitis.

Are antibiotics always necessary in case of mastitis? Not always, probably not even most of the time. Most of the time, both a blocked duct and mastitis will resolve on its own and do not need antibiotics. I will usually recommend that the mother hold off on taking antibiotics for 12 to 24 hours. If the blocked duct/mastitis starts to improve in that time, chances are it will continue to improve only with continued breastfeeding. If the blocked duct/mastitis is worsening over the next 8 to 12 hours or is not improving in 24 hours or so, antibiotics to which the usual organism, *Staphylococcus aureus,* is sensitive should be used. This means that amoxicillin or erythromycin, which many physicians prescribe, are *not* appropriate.

An abscess is treated with needle aspiration to make the diagnosis and then a technique described in this article Radiology 2004 abscess https://goo.gl/PtLbMQ. This procedure is done by an interventional radiologist who maps out the abscess with ultrasound and then places a catheter to drain the abscess. The mother continues breastfeeding on the affected side without interruption, so it is important that the catheter is not placed so close to the areola that the baby cannot latch on. Our experience with this procedure is described in this chapter Sore breasts https://goo.gl/reRyIX from my book Dr. Jack Newman's Guide to Breastfeeding.

When the baby does not latch on:

There are several reasons why a baby might not latch on after birth, the most common being that the baby is not given the opportunity to latch on. It has been known for decades that if a baby is put on the mother's chest, skin to skin, immediately after birth, babies who are not affected by medication given to the mother during labor and birth will crawl to the breast and latch on all by themselves.

However, there are many ways this normal behaviour is interfered with. As mentioned, some babies will be disoriented or too sleepy to crawl to the breast due to medication, even in an epidural, that the mother will have received during the labor and birth. In addition, the large amounts of intravenous fluids so many mothers receive during labor and birth may result in the mother's nipples and areolas being swollen and making it difficult for the baby to latch on to the breast.

Commonly, with most hospital births, babies are suctioned at birth with a catheter that reaches deep into their trachea, the idea being to clear the baby's airway. Not only is this completely unnecessary in the vast majority of newborn babies, even when the baby has passed meconium in the uterus, but it actually causes disruption of the normal reflexes that facilitate the latch.

Separation of the mother and baby and giving artificial nipples to the baby also may result in a baby not latching on.

True, some babies are born with abnormalities of the mouth and lips. Babies with a **cleft palate** may find it difficult to latch on, but many who have cleft palates can and do latch on. In fact, experience suggests that the reason many babies don't latch on is that they are not given the opportunity to latch on. Mothers are often told that they might as well not even try to breastfeed a baby with a cleft palate. Of course, if there is not even an attempt to latch the baby on, then one thing is sure: the baby won't latch on (though sometimes babies fool us – they start searching for the breast, find the breast and do latch on). An isolated **cleft lip** should not be a reason for the baby not latching on.

Tongue ties alone should not cause the baby difficulty with latching on unless the tongue tie is very tight. But combine a sleepy baby with the mother's swollen nipples and areolas, and other factors mentioned above and a tongue tie may become a factor in the baby not latching on to the breast.

What should be done to get the baby to latch on? First of all, do not panic. Neither should the hospital staff panic. What a baby cannot do immediately after birth, a baby can do a day or two later. But it is best to avoid feeding the baby with a bottle during this time. The mother should express her milk by hand (much more effective than a pump which may, in fact, increase the swelling of the nipples and the areolas), and this milk be fed to the baby by spoon or cup. Bottles should be avoided. A tongue tie should be looked for and released as soon as possible, as soon as it is diagnosed.

Increasing the mother's milk supply helps. Various herbal remedies, such as fenugreek, blessed thistle and moringa, seem to work. More milk means faster flow, and babies like faster flow.

Once the milk increases significantly after 3 or 4 days, many babies will latch on without any difficulty at all. It's important to take advantage of this moment by not waiting too long to get good help. Too often, the mother believes her troubles are over with a nipple shield and will not seek help early. A nipple shield is not a good idea. For an expose on nipple shields http://ibconline.ca/nipple-shields/

The baby is not getting enough from the breast

There is the occasional woman who is unable to produce all the milk the baby needs. And most women who have had breast surgery with the incision around the areola or breast reduction surgery also may have decreased milk supply on that side. But in most cases, mothers whose baby is not getting enough from the breast have followed advice about breastfeeding that makes no sense. For example: feed the baby on just one side at each feeding, so the baby gets the high-fat milk, feed the baby 15 minutes on each breast and all such rules. Rules and breastfeeding do not go together. Knowing how to know a baby is getting milk from the breast and when a baby is not getting milk at the breast is the first step in understanding why rules don't work.

Domperidone can help increase milk supply and milk flow. We start with 30 mg (3 tablets) 3 times a day and sometimes go up from there in two steps, first to 40 mg (4 tablets) 3 times a day and then 40 mg (4 tablets) 4 times a day, or 50 mg (5 tablets) 3 times a day (for convenience).

And if the baby is truly not getting enough from the breast?

Supplementation with **a lactation aid at the breast** will allow the baby to continue getting milk at the breast, even formula, if it is given as a supplement. I strongly believe that breastfeeding is much more than milk. It is a relationship, not just milk.

Here is a video showing a baby being supplemented with a lactation aid at the breast Inserting lactation aid, English text: https://goo.gl/PL8HKH Notice that babies respond to the flow of milk.

What about Reflux?

I believe strongly that reflux, or more accurately "gastroesophageal reflux disease or GERD," does not occur in healthy, exclusively breastfeeding babies. This diagnosis is made principally because physicians are marketed by pharmaceutical representatives who offer just what the doctor ordered for all the breastfeeding problems that the physician does not understand. So medications for "reflux" are selling like hotcakes. The fact that they rarely do any good is beside the point, the baby will eventually get better once they start food.

Incidentally spitting up is not necessarily bad. For more information https://goo.gl/ApYPib

And for a full discussion of "reflux," http://ibconline.ca/reflux/

Why do babies cry?

The most common "false cause" of crying is an ear infection. This is a very convenient diagnosis for the doctors as it gets them off the hook for figuring out what the real problem is. "Ah, a red eardrum; the baby has an ear infection." Except that a baby who cries may have a red eardrum from crying. This is not to say that ear infections do not happen. Of course, they do. But to make such a diagnosis, the eardrum must be seen to be bulging outwards, not just red.

In the vast majority of cases, however, babies cry because they want more milk. And they may want more milk even if they are gaining weight very well. The growth charts, even the World Health Organization growth charts, are relatively rough indicators of how the baby's weight is over a period of time, not some measure of how much milk the baby is getting. If the baby is crying, the baby should be fed.

If the baby is crying for a long time because the parents can't believe he still wants to breastfeed, he may be so upset as to refuse the breast even if he does want more milk.

Tongue and lip ties:

Often, the first question that comes up when I am speaking on tongue ties at conferences is, "Are there more tongue ties now than there were 50 or 100 years ago?" I doubt there has been a true increase. What might explain why more tongue ties are being diagnosed is:

More mothers are breastfeeding, so the issue comes up more frequently, particularly when mothers have difficulties with breastfeeding. 2. More physicians, nurses in postpartum, midwives and lactation consultants are aware that tongue ties may interfere with breastfeeding. 3. Mothers used to be wrongly told, "It's normal for nipples to hurt for the first few weeks, but then the pain goes away." Well, the pain going away after a few weeks was true for a few mothers, maybe many, but certainly not all. Quite rightly, more and more mothers are not accepting that "it's normal for breastfeeding to hurt" myth. If breastfeeding hurts, the baby's latch is not what it should be.

It is important that every newborn baby should be checked for a tongue tie as part of the routine physical examination soon after birth. It's not diagnosed just by looking at the baby's tongue because many tongue ties will be missed. The fact that the baby can stick his tongue out over the gums does not rule out a tongue tie. What really helps diagnose a tongue tie is checking for upward mobility of the tongue by having an index finger on each side of the frenulum and lifting. What exactly is enough or not enough mobility is a real diagnostic problem.

As far as **lip ties** are concerned, they do seem to cause difficulties in some mothers, in particular, causing sore nipples. If the breast moves back and forth under the baby's upper lip, if the baby's upper lip blanches or creases, and if the mother has soreness under the baby's upper lip, these are taken as indicators of a significant upper lip tie.

Resources: A book dedicated to explaining solutions to breastfeeding problems: Dr. Jack Newman's Guide to Breastfeeding (available on amazon.com and amazon.ca)

What about premature babies?

Premature babies need breastfeeding and skin-to-skin contact more, not less than full-term babies. For premature babies, being breastfed or not, being skin to skin with their mother or not, can truly be a question of life and death and profoundly influences their health, present and future and their prognosis. Yet, it is a paradox that it is these babies who are most often presented as babies who have to "wait" before being given a chance to be breastfed. Or their mother is told these babies need to first learn to bottle feed before they can breastfeed. Breastfeeding premature babies is often reduced to asking the mother to pump breastmilk but feeding the baby at the breast is not only neglected but often seen as dangerous and unreliable. If your baby is premature, you are likely to need expert help and support so that you can breastfeed.

Can premature babies actually breastfeed? Yes, they can, but in most neonatal intensive care units, they are not given a chance. From very early after birth, most premature babies are subjected to anti-breastfeeding protocols and procedures. What are these?

1. Supplementing breastmilk with so-called fortifiers. Fortifiers are made with cow's milk and are given this name, so parents (and the neonatologists) think that the baby is not getting formula. Some very small babies may need fortifiers, but fortifiers can be made with human milk. Once the baby is no longer fed by a nasogastric tube, the baby can breastfeed exclusively, and it is likely no fortifier will be necessary.

2. In much of the world, it is thought that a baby cannot go to the breast until the baby is 34 weeks gestation (still 6 weeks premature). It is thought the baby will get tired at the breast, and breastfeeding is more tiring than bottle feeding, so the mother is told the baby must learn to feed from a bottle first. This notion is false and based on the notion that babies transfer milk from the breast, essentially that they pull milk out of the breast. But this is incorrect. Babies do not transfer

milk from the breast; mothers transfer milk to the baby. For more about how "who transfers milk" misleads us into wrong notions of how breastfeeding works, http://ibconline.ca/who-transfers/

In fact, from work in Scandinavia, we know that many babies start going to the breast and latching on by 27 to 28 weeks gestation, and many are actually breastfeeding by 30 weeks gestation.

3. Although most neonatal intensive care staff believe that skin-to-skin contact and Kangaroo mother care are important for premature babies, often skin-to-skin contact is very limited, often no more than an hour or two a day in total. And then back into the incubator. However, we have very good evidence that a baby is much more stable in skin-to-skin care than in an incubator. His body temperature is more stable, and his blood sugar is less likely to fall; his heart rate, breathing and blood pressure are more normal and more stable. Kangaroo mother care also increases the chances of the baby being breastfed significantly.

Resources: Breastfeeding the Premature Baby (http://ibconline.ca/breastfeeding-the-premature-baby/)

Kangaroo Mother Care for premature babies (http://www.kangaroomothercare.com/about.aspx)

Can adoptive mothers breastfeed?

Throughout centuries women have breastfed babies other than their own. Therefore it is not surprising that adoptive mothers can breastfeed. We have had considerable success in helping mothers who were not pregnant to produce milk and breastfeed their adopted baby. It is not only newborns they can start breastfeeding; it is possible to start breastfeeding toddlers. Mothers can also re-start breastfeeding babies or toddlers who were once breastfed and then weaned. Adoptive mothers can breastfeed even if they cannot themselves have children and have never breastfed before.

Resources: Breastfeeding your Adopted or Surrogate Baby (http://ibconline.ca/breastfeeding-your-adopted-or-surrogate-born-baby/)

Can mothers of twins or multiples breastfeed?

Twins and multiples can be breastfed, and while there may be useful "logistical" tips, there are no special requirements or methods needed to breastfeed twins or multiples.

Is it possible to breastfeed during pregnancy?

It is common for mothers to breastfeed during pregnancy, and there is enough scientific data to show that this does not increase the risk of miscarriage or cause problems for the pregnancy. Many women continue breastfeeding both their older child and their newborn after birth.

Are breastmilk and formula the same?

Formula companies' advertising leads people to believe that formula is similar to breastmilk, using in their marketing campaigns words such as "inspired by breastmilk" or "closer than ever to breastmilk". Their marketing is well-thought-out and plays on people's deepest wish and vain hope – that something other than breastmilk could magically turn into … well… breastmilk. It doesn't.

It is because of formula companies' marketing practices that formula is not used the way it was intended – as emergency nutrition to save lives in situations when all possibilities of breastfeeding have been exhausted. Inappropriate marketing practices have caused formula to be overused and to be used unnecessarily by convincing people that using formula is just like breastfeeding. Additionally, due to formula marketing, donated breastmilk is being marginalized and used far less often than formula when supplementation is medically indicated.

However, breastmilk is only produced in the breast of humans, and other mammals produce milk designed to support the growth and the needs of their own young, which may need to grow at a different rate, whose brains develop differently and who use different methods of taking care of their young, such as leaving them alone sitting in the grass or in a warren for long periods of time.

Thus, formula and breastmilk are biochemically entirely different. Moreover, while formula is typically dried powder to be reconstituted with hot water, breastmilk is full of living cells, white blood cells, stem cells, immune factors and antibodies, macrophages, vitamins, minerals as well factors entirely specific to breastmilk only, which cannot be found anywhere else. The protein composition of breastmilk is not comparable to cow milk, the former being composed mostly of whey, the latter of casein.

The formula is made from cow milk (or sometimes soybeans). The reason for that is not that cow milk would in any way resemble breastmilk, simply because cow milk is widely available in the Western world and is available in large quantities, thus suitable for mass production. In fact, cow milk and breastmilk couldn't be more different. Cow milk, intended for a calf with four stomachs and a large body to grow quickly while being left to sit in grass or hay, cached, is nothing like breastmilk meant for a human baby with a fast-growing brain who is in need of constant physical contact with the mother and needs frequent breastfeeding and lots of interaction and attention to develop its full potential.

Resources: Read a detailed analysis of the topic in Dr. Jack Newman's Guide to Breastfeeding (available on amazon.com and amazon.ca)

Is breastfeeding the same as bottle feeding?

Breastfeeding – feeding the baby at the breast – is a different method of feeding babies from using a bottle. First of all, breastfeeding is a relationship between the mother and the baby, and there are different mechanisms that contribute to the baby's brain development as a result of not just drinking breast milk but sucking at the breast. Breastfeeding regulates and normalizes the baby's body: it helps increase or decrease the baby's body temperature, regulates the heart rate and breathing, reassures the baby of the mother's presence, calms down a crying baby and helps put the baby to sleep.

The facial muscles involved in breastfeeding are different from those involved in bottle feeding. The movement of the tongue is different in both. The shape and texture of the breast and nipple are different in breastfeeding and bottle feeding. No bottle looks like the breast nor functions like the breast. No bottle imitates the way the baby breastfeeds. Despite marketing claims, there is not and never will be any bottle that makes switching between breast and bottle easy.

There are other methods of supplementing a baby who, for medical reasons, needs to be supplemented – the superior one being the use of lactation aid. If the baby truly has to be fed off the breast, cup-feeding is a better approach than using bottles.

The use of bottles is so firmly ingrained in many people's minds that they imagine that babies who are weaned need to use bottles. Instead, they can use an open cup and eat solids normally without ever using bottles.

Resources: Cup feeding (http://ibconline.ca/finger-and-cup-feeding/)

Lactation aid (http://ibconline.ca/lactation-aid/)

Chapter 23: Early Labor and Tips

Most people go into labor on their own.

Labor does not often start on its due date.

I believe the baby has their own birth journey set.

Labor can start at any time of the day or night.

Many times people or babies need *help* to deliver.

There is no way of knowing how long early labor will last.

Babies often get themselves stuck on their journey down.

Labor can start in the middle of pregnancy or after your due date.

We expect that the first labor will take a much longer time than a second.

Author's Note ~ For the Labor Partner: Thank you! You may be a partner, a friend or a family member. Your biggest tasks are to be gentle and attentive, do not leave the birthing person alone if possible. Give comfort when it looks like they need a hug or encouraging words. It may be hard for you to know what they need because, most often, the birthing person will not know what they want. Keep the birthing person hydrated and make sure they take bathroom and rest breaks. Encourage them to keep up with labor tricks (to their comfort level) and get active with them by dancing around the living room or in the delivery suite, stomping down some stairs or going for a long walk, doing all acupressure points and often. Your journey may be long, but they will be so grateful they had you to help them through this time.

Author's Note: This book talks mainly about hospital births. Please note that all of the birth tricks and everything you will experience will be the same, no matter *where* you deliver.

What if your baby wants to come earlier than their due date? Labor can start any time, any day, most often between 37 to 42 weeks. Many people are caught off guard when their baby decides to come early, they go to the hospital because they seem to be having early contractions, to find out they are in active labor. Surprised and with no preparations the partner might scramble home to put together a hospital bag, some try to find and buy a car seat and many have no idea about their birth wishes, they have not thought about that 'yet'. To alleviate some of the chaos, you should have had some conversation and thoughts for your Birth plans, what you want to take in a hospital bag and have items ready to pack, and diapers already purchased at home all by week 36. There is peace of mind by being prepared early, but either way be assured, you will be well taken care of at the hospital.

The Cervix seems to be very complex. I have been with and watched many clients in labor go through a lot of discomfort when the cervix is thinning (called effacement). On the other hand, people seem to have already had *some* thinning of their cervix without even knowing or feeling any contractions, but this is not as often. If your cervix does not dilate fully after many long hours of labor, it might indicate you will need some help getting the baby out. However, after hours in labor and finally at 10 cm, you should naturally have the urge to push the baby out. A vaginal exam should only be done by your primary care provider, the person looking after your delivery, i.e., a doctor, midwife or nurse at the hospital. Before but especially in labor, when a cervical exam is done, it gives the care providers important information on your progress. It does not tell us if or when you will dilate to 10 cm and/or how you will deliver, for example, vaginally or with a little bit of help, in the operating room.

Note: Near the end of pregnancy, possibly week 38 or 39, your care provider may have asked if they can do a vaginal exam. This information gives them a starting point for 'where' your cervix is. You may be told your cervix is closed, posterior, long and firm. Then as you start to have some contractions, it begins to change, and then it will be confirmed whether you are in early labor or having Braxton Hicks, which does not necessarily change the cervix. This is useful for when labor starts and then changes with the progress of your labor. They may, at this time, ask you if they can do a stretch and sweep. This would be when they examine the cervix, they take their finger and, in a circular 'sweep' of the inside of the cervix, essentially 'strip the membranes', which can often bring on contractions.

The Uterus houses the placenta, where the fetus/baby develops and grows in the birth sac, which is filled with amniotic fluid that helps keep the baby safe and protected as they float about and grow. The umbilical cord inside has two arteries and one vein; one end is attached to the placenta, and the other end is attached to the baby on their tummy. It provides oxygen, glucose and nourishment to the baby, then removes waste and carbon dioxide from the baby.

When labor starts, the uterus will contract at the top and in a downward motion to push around the baby's body towards the birth canal and vagina. Then after delivery, the uterus will expel the placenta and birth sac. It may take a few weeks for the uterus to get back to its pre-pregnancy size.

What Does Early Labor look like? For many people, early labor is a gentle process and not particularly uncomfortable, and you can expect to go through many different sensations. If this is your first baby, it *may take several days or longer*. If you suspect that labor is starting, but you are unsure, a great way to confirm this is to go for a long walk for at least an hour or more or find some stairs, do 10 to 20 sets of stairs, lunge at the bottom and walk up and when you come down **drop** each foot or separately bounce vigorously on an exercise ball or dance in your living room, *or* a combination of all. Then take a rest break from all exercise, have a shower or bathtub, and possibly lay on the couch or sit on the deck of your home enjoying nature. If contractions slow down or stop, it is most likely you are having Braxton Hicks contractions or possibly very early labor. Typical of early labor:

- Irregular contractions.
- Intensity will stay the same; that does not get too much stronger.
- Contractions do not change even after being very active for several hours.
- Contractions tend to stop when you take a relaxation break.
- Having a tub or shower can make the contractions slow down or stop.
- There are no signs of mucus or bloody show.

Reasons for a slow start of labor:

- The baby's head is not in the pelvis.
- The baby's head is not in an ideal position.
- The baby has a large head and can not descend into the pelvis.
- Sometimes, we never know what the hesitation is with someone's body, even after you deliver.

Your labor is as unique as you and your baby, you may have some similarities to other birthing people, but the path to your baby's birth will be individually yours. There are many tricks to help encourage a stronger contraction pattern. The 'marathon' starts slow and easy. You will have discussed, ahead of time with your family members, doula and care providers, techniques on how you wish to stay calm and allow the birthing process to play itself out. Some coping skills you want to use, for instance could include, massage, tub or shower, music, visualization, and the use of your TENS machine; all of these should be in your birth plan.

You should not be thinking of going to the hospital until you know you are in very active labor. Ask your helpers to be with you when needed and ask for tips from Care Providers. Stay at home where you are comfortable and try to get yourself into a really good pattern of active labor! Double up your time doing all of the Birth Tricks!

Braxton Hicks, commonly known as false or practice contractions, can start in the third trimester. These 'contractions' confuse many people into believing labor has started. The only thing that this gives you, is an idea of what early labor and real contractions are going to feel like. It can be very frustrating because you are so excited for your labor to start. Typical of Braxton Hicks;

- Contractions that never become regular and are easy to manage.
- You may be feeling random or sporadic tightenings that stop and start.
- The feelings last from 30 seconds to 2 minutes but never get strong.
- They can last for days or weeks before labor actually starts.
- The feeling is mild enough that you do not have to go to the hospital, *but* you can not sleep.
- They seem strong enough, you are breathing and working hard, but then, they stop.
- They usually make little or no change to the cervix.
- You believe you are in early labor and get excited to meet the baby.

If you are told that your contractions are Braxton Hicks, try to stay positive, your labor will start soon enough.

Natural Ways to Induce Labor: (The first point 'Having sex' should not be done if you are having an induction of labor by Cervidil)

- Having sex can help to ripen or soften and prepare the cervix for dilation, as semen contains prostaglandins. It may cause the uterus to contract.

- Nipple Stimulation can help to start or increase stronger contractions. This can be done by rubbing the nipples for 10-minute intervals at a time, with breaks, stimulating the nipples releases the hormone Oxytocin in our body. Add kissing, cuddles and caressing, or anything similar to what got you pregnant; this will help get all your birthing hormones working for you.

- Acupressure points should be done by constantly repeating them until you deliver and should be carried into postpartum. If you are having trouble doing these by yourself, ask for help or delegate someone that can first practice and become efficient at them. During early labor and onwards, you will be surprised with the results.

Induction of Labor is when the body has not spontaneously or naturally started labor. The reasons are many and unknown, but your care provider will suggest that you need some help. Possibly you are over your due dates, or you are in your late 30s or older, or you have high blood pressure or gestational diabetes, the baby's head is not in the most ideal position, the baby is OP; there can be many different reasons. Induction is very specific for each and every person and different in subtle ways because there are two people involved, the birthing person and the baby! Care providers may come up with unnatural ways for this for a medical induction.

Prodromal labor can be frustrating and tiresome! Very similar to Braxton Hicks, it tricks you by thinking you are working hard and getting closer to having a baby. If the pattern of contractions is random or does not progress into a regular pattern where they get stronger and longer, they are not making the needed change to your cervix. Prodromal labor can happen to anyone, and it does not matter that you have had a baby. I have seen clients have prodromal labor that can last for a couple of weeks, which can and will exhaust you, mainly because you are excited, but the false contractions do not allow for a good night's rest.

Consult with your care provider when you are confused or unsure about what is happening to you, or you believe labor is getting more intense, or if you are having doubts or concerns of any kind. Going in for a vaginal exam will tell you if the cervix has started to change or not. Now more than ever, you need to be doing all the labor tricks vigorously, but as long as you are comfortable doing them. Stay hydrated, eat smaller meals with some hot spice and then take some 'time out' to have a bathtub or shower and try to rest. Sleeping may be difficult, but it is essential! If this goes on for some time, it exhausts you, and then it can compromise how you will cope during labor and especially when you are pushing your baby.

(First Stage) Early Labor:

Up to 20 hours, approximately

Contractions will last 30 - 50 seconds

When they start, they can be 5 to 20 minutes apart.

Contractions are often random, with dilation of 0 - 3 cm.

Author's Note: How dilated the cervix is will define the different stages of labor. These are very subjective, and there are subtle differences in print and with different practitioners. For instance, you may be told you are 3 to 4 cm; this is because each practitioner 'feels' with their fingers, and it can be very subjective. Know this, you start with no dilation (your cervix is closed), and you can start to push at 10 cm, the magic number that brings you your baby. Try not to get too wrapped up in the number of your dilation. Your body will work in its own time frame, and your body will most definitely tell you when you need to start pushing.

Early Labor: The beginning of the birthing process is when the uterus starts to contract; this is when you will experience mild contractions that should start spontaneously, and they will be irregular, lasting 30 - 45 seconds in duration, anywhere from 5 to 25 minutes apart and are easy to breathe through. Your cervix may have a slight dilation, or most often, it is closed - no dilation, but it will gradually start to soften, thinning out to nothing (paper thin) and open to 10 cm. (Note that the cervix will continue to open to pass the baby through).

Contractions help your baby to position themselves and put pressure onto your cervix. This phase can last for 8 -12 hours, but for a first pregnancy, it can be longer. These contractions are easily managed at home, and it is better to stay in the comfort of your home, where you have access to a shower or tub, food, and music. There is no rush to get to the hospital until you are well established in a regular pattern of contractions that have been lasting many hours. During the day, you should get very active with all the birth tricks, then follow all suggestions for ways to relax and take some rest in the evenings. Over many hours, the uncomfortable contractions gradually become regular and increase in intensity; they will not stop when you rest or sleep. This is a really good time for the birth partner to practice all pressure points and massage techniques, be very encouraging and tell the birthing person how well they are doing.

Most often, people's labor starts at 40 weeks pregnant; it is usually spontaneous and ends with a vaginal delivery. Your body and your baby are in full command, so try being proactive and get labor started a week or two before your due date. You can achieve this by doing the labor tricks and using acupressure points, and see an acupuncturist a few times.

If you are having an uncomplicated pregnancy, you should spend most of your early labor at home until your contractions start to increase in frequency and intensity and you are no longer coping. *Stay at home as long as possible, laboring in your own environment, where you can eat food and beverages, listen to music or tv, bounce on a ball, and find a quiet place to meditate with as many helpers as you need or want.*

Early contractions may feel like cramping or tightness or possibly some pelvic pressure. There may be some blood or mucus discharge, called a bloody show; this is normal *if there is not too much blood.* This happens when your cervix starts to thin out and soften. You may have feelings of lower backache, cramping and pelvic pressure or tightening. Any lower back ache will indicate that the baby is not in an ideal position. It is very important to get on hands and knees and do all of the tricks to move a posterior baby before they get stuck in the pelvis. It is very common to have random and mild contractions at this time in labor.

The uterus is above the vagina and between the bladder and rectum, which is why you feel 'bum' pressure when your baby gets very low and closer to delivery (their head comes down and over the rectum). If the bladder is full (like an inflated balloon), it can *hold up* the baby from descending farther down, it is often difficult to relax on the toilet and void, but you should be reminded to try often.

When taking a break, you will need to have some distractions, for instance, going for dinner or to a movie, enjoying with family and friends, and trying to forget that you are in labor. All the people that want to help you should be advised to come by and help to keep you comfortable with acupressure or massage, feeding you well (with spicy food) and laughing and enjoying the company. This will help to distract you for a while from the early 'nigglings' of early labor.

Author's Tip: People talk about the 'pain' of labor, and many people fear pain. I can feel the pain from a broken bone, but I am not sure it equates with labor. There is no break, only a baby wriggling their way into the world. That wriggling can be very distracting. Labor is a mind game, but there are many coping skills to help you progress and meet your baby. A reminder to review techniques in the Vision, Birth and Affirmation section.

It is really fascinating that the perceived pain vanishes with the contractions at delivery (the pain from your contraction stops after the baby delivers). Then, shortly after you meet your baby, the memories start to slowly melt away after a few months, and before you know it, you start thing about how wonderful another sweet baby would be. Your birth team should be using all of the affirmation, massage and acupressure techniques and helping you to relax into the experience of meeting your baby. I hope these coping skills will resonate with you.

Breathing techniques for Labor: I hope you have mastered the 'big breathe', if not start now. Practice by sitting down in a comfortable space, be still and try to relax. It may be easier to focus if you close your eyes and think of something very special to you, *a new baby, perhaps*? Then take a very deep breath in, hold for a couple of seconds, then release and blow the full breath to the floor. You need to have three long breaths for each and every contraction, it brings much-needed oxygen into your body, but most importantly, it helps you focus on something other than contractions. Make it your mission to focus totally on each breath, in and out, repeating the breath over and over. It is easy to become overwhelmed in labor, so when you notice that you are tense and holding your breath, stop, focus on your breathing, and bring yourself back to calm and normal breathing. Having a good rhythm of breathing is very beneficial for your entire labor. Then when it is time to start to push, you will change your breathing. You can ask your birth partner to gently remind you when they see you tense up.

Ramp it UP: You need that active, strong and continuous contraction to make a change to your cervix. To distract people from their contractions, some of my favorites would be strolling in a park. There are so many pretty things to see, plants, flowers, other people, and breathing fresh air. If you live in a warmer climate, walk on a beach or find a place that has gentle hills to walk up and down. A favorite fun place while being with clients is walking around the mall. First and foremost, you can do this on any old rainy day. This place has perks, and there are benches to sit on when needed, a lot of fun things to look at and window shopping. You can buy beverages and food, and there are toilets. Be creative and think of other similar activities that can take your mind off of your contractions. Anything that keeps you walking as long as possible is a great distraction in early labor. Every time you need to stop and breathe through the next contraction, I will do acupressure points on the client's back, bottom or shoulders. It is important to keep your birthing person hydrated and voiding in all activities.

At any time and only if you are up to it, to increase contractions while resting, you can have sex IF your water has NOT ruptured, and/or nipple stimulation to help stimulate contractions. During the day, get up and move around, become and stay really active. Do the more aggressive tricks in early labor, as much as you can possibly manage, just need to MOVE!

- Long walks
- Squats
- Tahitian hip shake
- Visualize
- Affirmation

- Nipple stimulation
- Stomp around
- Lunge
- Wiggle hips
- Lean against the counter
- Listen to and dance to your favorite music
- Change birth tricks positions often
- *Many* sets of stairs
- Acupressure points - especially Spleen 6
- Exercise Ball and bounce vigorously and figure 8 motions

Continue for as long as you are still comfortable doing all tricks and hopefully until you deliver! These movements will put more pressure from the weight of the baby onto the bag of waters, and hopefully, they will break, but if nothing else, it will help the baby's head to put pressure onto the cervix to dilate, making contractions stronger, leading you towards a shorter delivery. All of these activities should put you into a nice pattern of active labor.

**If something does not feel right or hurts, please stop doing that particular trick or exercise and contact your care provider to advise them you have some pain (other than contractions).

For a Break: When you are laboring at home, keep lights low or use candles in the bathroom and/or all throughout your home, or have the sun and a nice comfortable fresh air breeze coming in through the windows. Play your favorite music throughout your home and dance your way from room to room by swinging your hips, both vigorously or gently. Watch tv or a favorite funny movie while sitting on a ball or in other laboring positions; this helps to distract you. Short breaks of rest are very effective, and when you wake up or get up, it can give you more energy. Start gently and continue all birth tricks. Repeat this every day *until* you are in good active labor.

Use water standing or sitting in a shower and let the water rain all over you, or spend time in the tub, to help you relax. You may have a birthing tub in your home, or you have access to a pool in your yard or a beach (ocean water and the salt content helps you float). Have your birth partner sit beside the tub and pour cups of warm bath water on your tummy with every contraction. When your body is enveloped in warm water with low lighting, listing to meditations or favorite music will give you time to have a much-needed rest between your contractions. Make sure that in a tub or shower, the temperature is not too warm; very warm will cause you to overheat, but more importantly, the amniotic fluid will become overly warm, and babies do not like being hot.

When the evening is approaching, and you have been gently laboring all day, and now you are getting tired, and contractions are random and very manageable, and you can still smile and carry on having an easy conversation. You may feel that you want to settle into your bed to get some rest because your labor is not very active yet. Have a spicy meal to aggravate your gut, which will hopefully give a stronger contraction. Try all meditation and/or relaxation techniques, have your partner give you a massage and settle in for a nice rest or nap; it is better than staying up all night. Lack of sleep is going to be the biggest factor in how you can cope during active labor. If you are still having irregular contractions, I highly suggest you take the night off!

Or if there is no indication of slowing down labor and contractions are getting stronger, you will most likely be laboring all night, and your body may take on a worrier stance. Try to be mindful of taking rest breaks if you can. You do not need to stick to all of the aggressive birth tricks, you just need to sustain yourself until you become more active and want to go to the hospital. Your focus should be more of a ‘how can I continue coping at home’ using all comfort measures, tub or shower. Sleep is your biggest barrier to the longevity of labor, but you will find the energy and focus on pushing on through. You can do this!

Whether you want to try to rest or you are going to be up for the night, and you need help to sleep or alleviate some pain, it is suggested by many care providers to take Tylenol and Gravol (ask them for the correct dosage). This can help reduce some of the pain and for you to relax and help to become drowsy. You can watch a movie or just go to bed early and try to rest between labor pains.

Author's Note: Many times, a client tries to be more active by staying up all night and doing birth tricks with little rest. They go into active labor the next morning, and because they missed a full night of rest, they are exhausted. It makes for a very long day, and into the next night, when they end up delivering, a day later, *you* are bound to be totally exhausted. You can miss some of the fun of meeting your baby because you can barely hold your baby or stay awake. Labor is a mind and body game, and it is important to take breaks or some sort of relaxation to give your body a chance to rest; many people are in shock when they are finally IN active labor.

Comfort Measurements for the birthing person;

- Do not stimulate the senses as the evening gets closer.
- T E N S machine (take it to bed with you).
- Keep lighting low.
- Use a warm blanket (to wrap around their shoulders).
- Warm rice packs.
- Listen to your favorite gentle music.
- Big gentle long breaths.
- Enjoy a cup of camomile tea or similar.
- Massage tips from Paula Jaspar.
- All acupressure points.
- Positive encouragement.

- Touch, a hug or caress, hold hands, be near to your partner
- It is very important to get *some* rest rather than trying to continue into the night and use all your energy. Exhaustion sets in fast after one night of no sleep.

People can be…

- very sensitive and will decline any touch.
- at times, they prefer a certain area of the body massaged.
- prefer a particular position.
- become frustrated with slow progress.
- become very focused on their labor.
- do not want any stimulation; they prefer quiet.

Contractions will increase their intensity. Try to change positions often and find your new favorite place when the baby moves and you get closer to delivery. No matter what happens, keep trying everything.

TENS: If you haven't already, you can try your TENS machine. Have your birthing partner put the pads on your back. It is very effective in early labor, especially when you are trying to have rest breaks, or this is effective as a general pain reliever and for distraction. Wear it when you go on any walks or are doing stairs. Take it to the hospital with you; many people use it until they are getting close to delivery. When you want a break or want to go into the water, have someone peel the pads from your back and attach them back onto the same plastic card that they came on; you can re-use them as often during labor as you want. Have extra batteries; you may expect to use the machine for a long period of time or several times during labor.

*Do not use it in a shower or tub.

Visualization is easy for you to carry all the way through until you deliver. Visualize your perfect and peaceful birthplace. Envision a favorite spot or place on this earth; a hot crackling fire, wrapped up in your favorite comfy blanket; the scent of fresh baking; watching the snow gently caressing the tops of the trees outside; family get-togethers. Have your favorite pictures in front of you or on a cell phone or a tablet/ipad to look at. In early labor, your birthing helpers can remind you of your favorite place to visit or vacation. I suggest that they tell you a story. You can focus on your partner's face!

Author's story: At one of the births, a partner started talking to the birthing person about how they loved to be on a row boat, on a beautiful sunny calm day, and rowing across a lake. The partner talked about this for hours, and it put the birthing person into their own special space every time they had a contraction. So talk about what your aspirations are for your baby; talk about a hike or walk in your favorite park or favorite place to vacation because these are your personal thoughts, places, and ideas that can help you to daydream during your contractions.

Music can soothe and put us into our favorite place and take us back in time. No matter what you are doing in labor, it is easy to listen to music anywhere. It can be fun music that makes you get up and dance or can be gentle and relaxing while you rest time with an epidural. Have a few different music playlists, one for the calm of early labor, then more upbeat and exciting for the pushing stage. Your favorites that are easily accessible for any stage of labor. I suggest clients to bring a portable Bluetooth speaker and play music where ever they are laboring, walking in a park or dancing in your delivery suite.

Meditation: You can use a script that is downloaded to your cell phone or tablet. HypnoBirthing is a favorite that comes to mind or Buddhist chanting. Anything that can clear your mind and allow you to relax.

Water is very relaxing; a tub or shower can relieve stress and pain from your body. I know this from being in a tub with one of my own births. The nurse told me it was time to get out, which I said I didn't want to, but they told me I was going to be delivering my baby if I didn't get out (except that they were not doing water births back then). So, for my clients, I will always ask the nurse that is going to assign us a delivery suite if we can have a room with a tub if possible, knowing many of my clients want to labor in water and if they are trying to have a water birth.

Comforting positions for early labor and active labor: When your baby is well positioned, your contractions will increasingly become more intense and become closer together. This progression causes the cervix to open and does not stop until the baby is born. When your cervix is 10 cm dilated, you will be able to start pushing and birth your baby. Getting into all positions for the entirety of your labor and rotating positions often is really helpful when your helpers remind you to change up often. Then you can add to the mix acupressure points and all massage techniques.

Some positions that are helpful and you will find some relief from are:

- Side-lying with pillows between your legs, from the knee to the ankle.
- A small hand towel under the ankle of the leg that is lying on the bed helps relieve hip pain.
- Hands & knees.
- Sitting on a birthing ball.
- Lunging.
- Slow Dancing with your partner.
- Water.

Birth Tip: When labor starts, you will be distracted and focusing on your labor and working very hard. It will be difficult for you to make decisions or tell anyone your wishes. Allow your birthing partner to advocate for you as needed, so you can totally let go of everything.

What does an OP (posterior) baby mean for labor? Many people complain about how intense and more painful 'back' labor is; the pain is down in their lower back, with the baby's head and back resting on your spine. Regular contractions in the belly are difficult to manage with this extra discomfort and inability to manage your labor. It is essential to help the baby move out of the OP position as soon as you feel any back pain before or during contractions.

A posterior baby WILL make your labor longer and more painful. You will be able to feel their movement from their hands and knees in the front of your belly button. Most importantly, if the baby gets stuck while they get lower into the pelvis, you may not be able to deliver vaginally. You will need some kind of an assisted delivery, and often that will be forceps or by cesarean section. Prevent this in early labor by moving your baby!

Once in labor, the combination of labor pain and back pain can be debilitating, and it may lead you to want some help by having an epidural.

If you are curious to see what your belly looks like, stand sideways and look at your belly in a mirror. An OA baby will give your belly a nice round appearance from top to bottom (because you are seeing the long back, head to rump). With an OP baby, you will see that the top of your tummy has a bulge and a bit lower, the tummy has a visible indent, then lower where your baby's head is, will have a bulge. The side view of your belly will look like a peanut that is still in the shell.

You should not be feeling the movements of the baby's legs and arms out front. They should be on one side or the other of your tummy. As a reminder of this position, look at the image of a posterior baby, OP, in the Cervix & Vaginal exams document. You need to move your baby!

Author's Tip: *I do not recommend starting any birth tricks if you suspect your baby is in a posterior position. You run the risk of getting the baby stuck in the wrong position, which will lead to interventions.*

Do you know if the baby is more left-side lying or right-side lying? If you believe the baby is LOP left occiput posterior, your baby is lying off to your left side and looking at your belly button. You want them to rotate from the left side to the center of your tummy so they are looking at your spine.

While getting into any of the positions below, you can either place the palm of your hand at the side they are lying, and gently put a small amount of pressure and massage the baby's bottom toward the front and center of your belly. Or put a bag of ice on the side where your baby's body and bottom are, and leave it for a few minutes. You can usually feel the baby move because they do not like the cold. If the baby does not want to move, do not keep trying, the baby may move during labor, or you will have a chance later on as you get closer to delivery. Find pictures of the acupressure points that work best to help relieve back pain. BL60, SP6, BL67.

Similar to being on hands and knees on the floor and doing the 'wash the floor'.

You can go into your bathtub or a shower and get down on your hands and knees (with towels to support your knees) using a warm shower, raining down over your back, and then start to wiggle your bottom randomly, gently and vigorously.

Sitting on a ball or chair, legs wide apart, lean with your tummy forward and hanging over. Sit as long as you are comfortable.

While standing, lean over a kitchen counter and brace your folded arms on the countertop. This will help to relieve some of the discomforts of a posterior baby. In this position, the only place for them to move, because of the weight of their body, would be sliding forward toward the front middle of your tummy.

Do the 'Shake the Tree' from Birth Tricks until the baby moves off your spine. Once moved, the back pain will also go away. When your baby is in a more ideal position, your labor should become more active fairly soon. Use a rebozo or do the double hip squeeze (chapter from Paula Jaspar). This should relieve some or all back pain by helping them to get off your spine.

Pelvic tilt is done by doing the Cat/Cow Yoga position. Start by kneeling on the floor, hands on the floor and shoulder-width apart, your knees directly below your hips. Breathe in deeply and curve your lower back, then bring your head up, tilting your pelvis up like a 'cow'. Exhale deeply and bring your abdomen in, arch your spine and bring your head and pelvis down like a 'cat'. This can be repeated several times and often or until the baby moves.

After moving their baby, many clients can go about their labor, feeling that they can cope much better with 'just' labor contractions.

When the baby moves, I highly suggest you get onto your exercise ball and bounce your baby deep into the pelvis.

Author's Note: *If the baby is stuck, and it is too difficult or impossible to move a posterior baby, and after you have tried your best, then you will have to wait until you are fully dilated. The care provider may be able to move them manually. (This procedure will require an epidural)*

Author's Story: *My client asked me to meet them at the hospital. They were trying to have a VBAC, and they were having their second baby. At 2:00 p.m., the client's cervix was 2 cm, and the head was still high -1/-2 meaning the head was not yet engaged into the pelvis. For several hours, it was hard to know exactly where the baby was lying,* *the baby was moving around quite a bit in their tummy. We actively did acupressure points all afternoon. In the early evening, the client had a shower for 20 mins. At 8:00 p.m., we walked the halls for a 1/2 hour. Then when we came back to the room, they were so tired they laid in bed. At this point, I could tell where the baby was so we used a peanut ball, and I gave them a 45-minute foot and lower leg massage.*

10:00 p.m., another vaginal exam because their labor started to get very active. The cervix was 4 - 5 cm, -1 and LOT (left occiput transverse). They got up to pee and they thought they needed to poo but did not, then they got back to the hospital bed. 10:27 p.m. The client had an epic contraction that was really intense which prompted them to ask for an epidural but they were sounding pushy, (my thought was they where most likely fully dilated and would want to start pushing soon). The nurse and I had been thinking the same thing, that the client needed another vaginal exam, before they give the order for an epidural. The Nurse did another vaginal exam at 10:50 pm. The client was fully and the baby was very low in the pelvis. 11:03 pm baby was born!

After delivery, this Client said in a quiet voice

and a big smile on their face ~~ No Pain, No Gain!

Author's Tip: *Use a peanut ball (it looks like a peanut) or improvise. Lay on one side. The ball is between the legs, the hip (of top leg) should be moved slightly forward and upper leg dangling over the top of the ball. The lower leg at the knee, slightly bent toward the buttocks. Stay in that position for fifteen minutes, then turn to the other side for 15 minutes. If there is no change, try doing both sides again. The peanut ball works very well to move the baby. Add to the mix, acupressure points.*

If the baby is transverse lie: This means the baby is lying sideways in your tummy. Top of their head on left side and their bottom on the right side of your tummy, (or visa versa). They can be lying with their face looking up to the ceiling, or the opposite lying with head facing down towards the floor. Usually an ultra sound will show that baby is in this position, many times it is not found out until you are in labor. If your baby's head is not near or in the pelvis, might be cause to ask your care provider, to feel for baby's position to confirm where they are. When baby is in the position you will go to the operating room for caesarean section.

SROM Spontaneous Rupture of Membranes. There is no predicting when your waters will break, it can happen at any given time, often before labor or during labor with your contractions or at the end when you are pushing baby out. When your amniotic fluid releases during labor and you are having contractions, your baby's head will move down a bit, closer to the cervix and that helps bring on stronger contractions and helps the dilation of the cervix. There will be a sudden increase in contractions which often challenges people, it can be over whelming at times. It is important to have your birthing helpers remind you to breathe, deep and long, and blow to the ground and then verbal reminders that 'you can do this' or 'this will bring baby to you sooner' lots of encouragement. When the waters break, it feels like you pee'd your pants.

If you are at home you should call your care provider, to inform them that your water has broken. If you are at the hospital and the nurse is not in the room when this happens, tell them as soon as they are back. The care provider will want to confirm if it is indeed a rupture of waters and if not, is it possibly be a Hind Leak, which is a bit different and not your waters breaking. This may be a tiny amount of fluid and care providers treat this differently, they are not as concerned that contractions have not started, yet.

The birth sac, where the amniotic fluid cushions baby starts to get old, (in your 40th week) and a small break higher up inside your body, has a small tear. This usually happens with some pressure from the baby inside, that stops leaking altogether and is not the same as your water breaking.

When waters have broken, you should need to wear a panty liner or sanitary pad, depending on how much fluid there is. Your baby's head should come down a bit further into the pelvis and may block some or most of the leaking, from the amniotic water but you can expect to continue leaking until you deliver. Many people are concerned that their baby will not have enough water in the birth sac by delivery, amniotic water is made by baby swallowing and then peeing this same water, and they will continue this process until delivery.

Call care providers when your water breaks.

Bleeding of any kind, you should call your care provider ASAP.

If water breaks and labor contractions do not start? When you have a leak or gush of water, you will advise your care providers about the amount of water (half a cup or perhaps a tablespoon) and the color of the waters. You may be asked to come into the hospital or their clinic, so they can confirm that your waters have broken with a litmus paper test. They usually will want to check for any dilation of the cervix.

There may be some obstacles or concerns that arise when your contractions do not start after your water has ruptured, the risk of infection in the womb, that can increase significantly after 24 hours of rupture. When contractions do not start in the first 18 - 24 hours, your care providers will advise you to come to the hospital for an induction. Then once you are at the hospital, they will start protocols for an induction; this would be specific to each individual and your medical history.

Lightening is a term for when your baby 'drops' deeper into the pelvis. Some people feel this, most do not, your family and friends may comment that your baby looks 'lower' and/or you may have been wondering why all of a sudden, you can eat a bit more food, and you can breathe easier. This may happen, but not always when you have a SROM. This scenario should help the baby to naturally drop a bit lower into the pelvis.

Birth Hormones are produced in our body and help our body to get ready for labor and birth. They help start our contractions and when we have to face stress or pain, but especially when we are in labor, then the delivery and pushing the placenta out. They are important to prepare the baby for labor and being outside of our body, to tell our body that when the baby suckles at the nipple, to make milk. Most importantly, it signals to our brain that when we see and hold our baby that we "fall in love" with them so easily.

Low levels of these hormones can slow or stop labor or can make for a longer labor, or it may be that we have difficulty bonding with our baby, which will lead to postpartum depression issues. It can lessen the chance of excessive bleeding after the placenta has delivered, thus the shot of oxytocin at delivery and possibly other interventions.

We tend to have higher levels of all of these hormones as we get closer to the end of pregnancy, then it may take up to twelve months after delivery for them to stop or be clear from our body. The body will slowly start to get back to a normal, or its pre-pregnancy state. This time is challenging with a new baby and recovering from labor and into your post partum months.

Endorphins increase as we get to the end of our pregnancy and the delivery. They are produced for us to better response to the pain and stress in labor, the hormone help us to stay calm and helps in relieving some pain. High levels can make you feel alert and happy after birth, and is believed to strengthen the parent/infant bonding. If you have low levels of endorphins it may cause your labor to feel more painful and more difficult to tolerate labor. This can lead to more interventions. After delivery it can contribute to the feeling of depression that many people have called post partum.

Adrenaline known as the *fight or flight* hormone, it helps 'to ensure our survival'. When we feel threatened or stress or have fear and extreme pain, it is produced to help ensure our survival. Levels are increased during labor but if too much is produced it can slow or stop contractions and our labor. It may cause distress too baby, and can create a sense of panic and increasing pain to the birthing person. All of which can result in you having interventions.

Prostaglandins help promotes cervical ripening and encourages the cervix to soften and stretch in preparation for childbirth.

Oxytocin is known as the 'love' hormone, it also has a lot to do with getting pregnant and fertility. It is secreted during sex, after ovulation and during labor, birth and chest feeding baby. It creates nurturing and loving feelings. It stimulates contractions during labor and birth, and it causes the uterus to contract and leads to the separation of the placenta from the uterus (which reduces interventions).

During pregnancy we can enhance the body's natural production of hormones by staying calm and putting yourself in a comfortable and safe environment. Do all of the things that help make you relax and release stress and stay confident in your environment by taking very good care of yourself, as your body progresses further into labor, your delivery and the first year post partum or frequently called the Fourth Trimester.

When trying to start labor or increase contractions, nipple stimulation is a great way to release Oxytocin into your body and create contractions. Sex might be the last thing you would think of at this stage of pregnancy; however, when you have an orgasm and/or when sperm (which has a high amount of prostaglandins) is released, it should help 'ripen' the cervix and help start labor. Being proactive in helping your body to start labor by Week 40 reduces the need for induction because after this time, your care provider may be asking you to consult with an obstetrician to help start labor with drugs or, if you are in labor, give your labor a boost.

Author's Tip: Boundaries and Privacy regarding your body and personal space. Some clients in labor that have had some unpleasant past experiences can be triggered in labor and that can result in stalling or stopping your labor. If this is you, please have a conversation with your primary care providers for ideas that will help you to achieve a more effective and shorter labor. It will also be beneficial for your birth helpers to be aware (of some) so they can be prepared to help you to their fullest.

- When triggered, what do you do?
- What are you not comfortable with?
- Are you uncomfortable walking *into* a hospital?
- What fears do you have surrounding pain and medications?
- Maybe you would prefer only female providers?
- What will you be comfortable wearing during labor if you go into the tub or shower?
- Do you *not* want your birthing companion to 'see' some part of you during labor or when pushing?
- Will you have any triggers or flashbacks of trauma that might stall your labor?
- There may be a time you would like to be in a tub or the shower, or you will be asked to void in the bathroom, or during labor when you are pushing, and you pass gas.
- Does your partner have a problem seeing blood or gooey things or procedures like needles and having blood drawn because they could faint or pass out?

- Talk to your care providers before labor starts about how they can keep you 'feeling safe' and with certain procedures to be done respectfully, for instance, vaginal exams.

I have seen people walk into the hospital, and something triggers a past issue or trauma, which slows down their labor. If you know that you have triggers, convey them to care providers and birth helpers, so they can be extra sensitive, give you extra calming care and help you to cope.

A Primip is a person having their first baby. Your body will work at its own pace, and it usually takes longer to get through the first stage of labor which can take several days. Your uterus starts by having contractions, and your cervix is usually closed and tight or has a slight amount of dilation. It can take many hours of labor for your cervix to dilate to 10 cm. Then you will start with a very slow and long push time that hopefully will move the baby down farther into the birth, which can last several hours. A normal labor for a first baby can often take several days.

A Multip means you are having another baby, and even if you had a cesarean section or forceps or vacuum delivery, *you labored,* and your body remembers the birthing process. Your labor may have had a slow start, but once you get to 4 - 5 cm, your cervix can dilate *much* faster (like turning on a light switch) to fully dilated; this can also make for a faster descent for baby. It is usually easier to cope with stronger contractions that are clumped in that shorter time frame. You will remember parts of your previous labor and that you got through it! You should be ready to go to the hospital sooner in your labor. I have had many clients wanting to push as they come in, breathing heavily through the hospital doors. Often pushing can be as quick as 4 or 5 pushes but not always. I equate a multip's labor as a roller coaster ride, it goes fast and is over quickly, and this is most often the case. You may be able to push less and breathe the baby out. Things to have your partner remind you of:

- "This will be over soon."

- "You are almost there."

- "You are dilating faster this time."

- "You are so strong."

- "You are doing this."

- "Our baby is almost here."

Author's tip: It is much healthier for you and your baby to labor even if you are having a scheduled cesarean section.

Author's birth story: When I was pregnant with my fourth baby, I was at my regular doctor's appointment. I was told I was already 5 cm, with no indication of labor. I went to lunch with my Mum and delivered five hours later, I had approximately 3 hours of labor.

Author's story: My sister-in-law telephoned me in the middle of the night, sitting on the toilet, asking me about the sensations they were feeling. I was at their first delivery, which was fast, and by listening to the sounds they were making, I gently told her to wake up my brother, get their toddler and go straight to the hospital asap! My brother drove up to the Emergency entrance, where she was whisked up to the delivery suite in a wheel chair. My brother waiting for our mum and sister to get to the hospital to take the toddler back home. I raced into the delivery suite **just** as my sister-in-law had delivered. Both my brother and I missed the birth. But there was no toilet birth!

Author's story: A multip client texted to say they were in labor and were going to the hospital. I got a call half an hour later, on my way to the hospital and was told the baby was delivered while she had been sitting on the toilet. The ambulance had not yet arrived to take them to the hospital. I was not needed, so I turned my car around and went home.

Author's note: I have had so many clients that I meet at the hospital, and after the vaginal exam, are 4 - 5 cm, then 40-ish minutes later, they want to push. They are re-examined and are fully dilated. Some times we do not have time to go anywhere, the baby is born in a small assessment room (set up for deliveries) and sometimes, we rush to the delivery suite and deliver there, just in time!

Author's note: Not all Multip births are fast. In fact, they can be fairly slow (but not the norm to be slow). There are many reasons regarding the length of labor and pushing and why they are different each time; having a different baby; a bigger baby; a different partner, the baby may not have a similar head size or shoulders as other babies. I have had many clients that have had a long prodromal labor, and it can be frustrating - just like the first time!

Surprise your Baby is coming fast! I have had many client's that go into labor, then their dilation progressed so fast, they had to call an ambulance to come and take them to the hospital. Some did not make it and were delivered at home. Most times, the paramedics whisked them off to the hospital just in time. If the baby decides they are coming early, call your care provider, or if birth seems imminent, call the operator '0' or emergency line '911'. They will stay on the telephone with you and give instructions until help comes to you. Place the birthing person onto a clean and flat space, either bed or couch or a blanket under them on the floor. Have your door unlocked, so the emergency personnel can come into your home, you will not want to leave your partner. If help is on the way, try to ask the birthing person not to push, but to breathe. They should pant or blow lightly for as long as possible. It may be intense, but hopefully, someone should be there soon.

If you believe you can get to the hospital in time, have a couple of towels under the birthing person, make the automobile warm as you drive, and be on speaker phone with your care provider or the 911 emergency person. They may ask you to pull over at any time if they (the emergency person) feel the baby is coming, and then they will give the driver direction for what you should do to catch your baby.

While **laboring at home with children or pets,** consider having someone come now to your home to look after them, or have a trusted person, take them to their home. I have seen both children cry and animals whine, they 'hang around' wanting your attention and comfort, because they sense you are in distress but do not understand what is happening to you. Your labor can slow down or stall if you are worried about family and pets. The sooner you can relax, without distraction, the sooner you can focus on your contractions and breathing. Your family can come back to your home, after you have left for the hospital, or when you have delivered or when you come home from hospital.

Get last minute preparations done, for instance calling your support people to tell them labor has started, or maybe you need them now, or tell then *when* you might want them to arrive. Pack any last minute items for the hospital, for instance; the Labor Aid, the popsicles in the freezer, and snacks and drinks for the birthing helpers.

Birthing Partners and Helpers: You are going to see a different person than you are used to while this person labors and delivers this baby. All of the following are common and normal for a birthing person to experience during labor.

- Doubt that they will get through labor.
- They want to give up.
- They are sad or feel like crying for no apparent reason.
- They can not let go and allow the birthing process.
- They are very tense.

- They are afraid of the 'unknown' of labor and pushing.
- They are in a lot more pain than they ever thought.
- They feel out of control or out of their element.
- They feel very overwhelmed.

You know them so well. Here are some suggestions that should make your participation easier for you to help them cope during their labor. Try doing all or as many of the following as possible;

- You stay relaxed and calm. You can always ask for guidance from the care providers.
- Be gentle and give effective touch by acupressure and massage.
- Stay close to them, be at their side or near their face, as often as possible.
- Give a gentle hug that helps them feel well-supported.
- Hold their hand or arms gently and caress.
- Talk to them with stories about the dreams and wishes for the new baby.
- Give them positive encouragement.
- Ask them often to have a drink or popsicle (stay hydrated).
- Remind them every hour to void.
- Try different positions and places to lay or stand.
- Show them you are interested in what they are doing or feeling.
- Distract them in any way you think is best.

Conversation: The birthing person will be able to focus on your words by listening to your voice during every contraction. Start by having a continuous one-sided dialogue going on. Talk about future plans with your new baby or the birthing person's favorite vacation, anything to distract them. When the contraction stops, remind them to take sips of fluid or help them change position, then with the start of the next contraction, start the same conversation again. As labor progresses, in addition to the conversation should be closeness, touch, acupressure and massage.

My client's partner went back to the same story, with subtle changes. It revolved around being in a canoe, on a lake and on a sunny summer day. It was interesting how they embellished the story to keep it fresh. It happened that this was the birthing person's favorite place.

Hydrate! It is one of the most important and challenging tasks for the partner, because the birthing person thinks they do not need to or forgets to drink fluids. Both in early and active labor, they need to drink plenty of fluids, a full glass of water per hour. Use a travel mug or exercise container, anything that is easy for them to hold and has a straw. This makes it easier while laboring at home or in the hospital, when they are in a shower or tub, walking, and laying in a bed. I would suggest for every contraction or second contraction to, give them a sip of fluid or ice chips.

Being de-hydrated as you get farther into labor can bring on complications and can compromise your endurance while affecting how the baby reacts to the labor. Suggestions for hydration are Labor Aid drink recipe or coconut water, water with emergen-c, frozen fruit or popsicles. It is also very important to remind them to take a bathroom break at least once every hour.

Author's Note: *Labor is a team event. Help the birthing person through labor by respecting the time it takes and that they need to be totally focused on themselves.*

Food in early labor, eat spicy food to aggravate the gut and irritate the intestines, which will cause your uterus to contract. Nibble on small amounts of food and easily digestible foods until you no longer want to eat.

NOTE: Your stomach takes a break in *active labor*, it does not digest most food or smoothy-type drinks. It is common for people to feel nauseous and many will vomit anything that they put in their tummy. It is typical that most people in active labor do not want to eat anything, until the baby delivers and then they get their sensation of hunger back.

Author's Story: A client called me, they were a bit before their due date but in early labor, wanting to know if they could go outside for a drive, I said yes of course! They wanted to make sure their baby's car seat was installed properly, and our fire department will check baby car seats for people. They happened to meet another couple from their prenatal class at the Fire Hall and talked for awhile. My client was having contractions, they told me that the distraction was very good at keeping their mind off of their contractions, so you should try to find some fun distractions in early labor.

Timing contractions: It is not necessary to time contractions that are irregular and random, it means you still need more time to labor at home. When contractions start to become regular, or the pain has ramped up substantially, you can start to use your contractions app, (or download one now). Contractions should become '511' meaning 5 minutes apart, lasting one full minute, and this pattern has been at least one hour or more, and you are no longer smiling or talking through any contractions, because they are very uncomfortable and much stronger. You should only be focusing on your contractions, similar to being tunnel vision, or all encompassing.

Labor at home as long as possible, stay in the comfort of your own environment and move around at your leisure, this can help you dilate faster. You may want to go to the hospital at this stage, but with the help from your labor support people you should be able to stay home longer. When I am at a client's home, I usually wait for them to tell me they want 'something' else, which may be the nitrous oxide or an epidural because they are no longer coping with contractions. They may be feeling the sensation they want to poo which means they may want to start pushing out baby soon, so we call the care provider to tell them how labor is progressing, and advise them that the client wants to come to the hospital. For a primp we would wait for the sensation of wanting to poo, that will mean your baby is getting very low, and that labor is progressing, and you should call the care providers to give them the heads up, with this and anything you feel is important. If you are a multip and you are starting to feel the poo sensation, phone the care provider *as you are getting ready* to go to hospital. It can be tricky but most often it is recommended to go to hospital right away.

Calling your Care Provider If you want to confirm that you are in early labor or tell them you are becoming more active or to ask for suggestions, or if you think you want to go into the hospital. You should start by tracking your contractions for at least an hour or more (the 511 timing). By listening to your voice over the phone, care providers can usually tell how you are coping and whether it is time to come to in, or not. They will ask you, how *often* contractions are; how *long* the contraction last; and how *strong* they are; so have that information handy, in addition 'when' contractions started, and another possible question, 'out of '10' how strong you consider your contractions are feeling?'. They will also want to know if there has been any discharge of waters from your vagina. If they suggest you stay home a bit longer, ask them for help and suggestions, to better cope at home.

People that are in early labor should not go to the hospital, unless something significant has happened, like bleeding or extreme pain, not if you have light and irregular contractions. You should be calling your care provider anytime with questions. Here are some reasons you should call straight away:

- If your waters break and you are *not 37 weeks yet.*

- If you are feeling warm, your temperature is over 38 degrees or higher.
- Your amniotic water breaks, or you are leaking water (you will need to wear a pad in your panties). They will ask 'how much' water leaked. They will want to know if the fluid is clear. *If not*, they will ask what color the fluid is. Light or dark of either green, brown or yellow (the color indicates that your baby has had a bowel movement inside, and it is called meconium). You should expect contractions to start or pick up substantially because of the break.
- Your water breaks, *and* you are in active labor
- If water breaks, but contractions have not started yet. Then if no contractions start over the next few hours, your care provider may want you into the hospital for a vaginal exam and may suggest helping to start your labor.
- If you are GBS+ and your amniotic water breaks, and if you are not in labor, they may give your body 24 hours to start contractions. If they do not start spontaneously, you will be asked to come to the hospital for an induction of labor.
- If you are GBS+ and amniotic water breaks and you are in labor, the care provider may ask you to come into the hospital for a dose of antibiotics and a vaginal check.
- If you are not feeling your baby move for a period of time. The baby should move at least 3 times in an hour.
- If you are exhausted and not coping very well with contractions.
- If you see blood clots in the toilet (bloody show), take a picture if you can, and send it to the provider OR be able to tell them how big the blood clot was 'the size of a coin or plum' OR if you are **bleeding** of any kind call them straight away!

You may be sent home if your contraction pattern is irregular or not strong enough to make significant changes to the cervix, even though for you, they feel strong. Because you will be spending enough time at the hospital once you are in an active pattern of labor and then the time after, when you are delivered, you should be staying at home as long as possible, in the comfortable in your own environment being relaxed, this will defiantly help to dilate you faster. You are clearly working hard, it can and will exhaust your energy, keeping you up most of the night and day, and you will find it difficult to rest or nap. It can be frustrating and disappointing waiting for labor to pick up and as you wait for your cervix to start too dilate.

After arriving at the hospital, the care provider or the nurse will put you in an assessment room, put monitors around your tummy to listen to baby. After a vaginal exam and if you are less than 4 cm you will be asked to go home and labor there. It can be very deflating that you have been working so hard for so long and your cervix is not ready for admission to the hospital.

They may offer to give you a needle in your bottom with morphine and gravol, and then send you home to rest. This medication should give you a four to six-hour window of some or total pain relief. It should start to work within 20 minutes, so go straight home. It will make the person feel very drowsy, and they may need help going upstairs. They should be put into bed or on a couch upon getting home to rest. When the medication wears off, they are most often (but not always) in a very active labor. Expect them to be in much more discomfort, and you will be coming back to the hospital quickly.

- You should not be doing any birth tricks at this time.
- You may be feeling the excitement of meeting your baby disappear.
- Being sent home can confuse you and brings the though and fear of your body not being able to do what is needed to go into active labor that progresses to delivery.
- It is imperative to hold on to the positive, and there can be other ways to start labor and deliver if needed.

If you do not want or decline the morphine and gravol, before you leave the hospital, find out exactly where your baby is and how to move them if moving the baby is needed. This should be your new starting point for when you get home. Do all the birth tricks to move the baby and then bounce them down deeper!

More importantly, every person is different, and it may take a few more days before active labor starts. Be gentle on yourself and try not to stress. What might help you better is to do the opposite and relax. Often, patience is our best friend. Take the night off, go out to dinner or have a romantic, spicy dinner at home. Take gravol, a relaxing tub, a gentle massage, have some fun in bed, and rest!

If you are in active labor and are more than 4 cm, you will stay and progress to delivery.

Breathe! Big & Deep Rhythmic breaths IN, then Blow to the Floor. Do this breathing technique UNTIL you are pushing!

Author's Fun Fact: Some of my clients are professional athletes and extreme workout enthusiasts; they have a dedicated workout routine that allows them to take their philosophy into their labor, where they can endure that 'Marathon Attitude.'

Simplistically put: run fast like a bear is chancing on you, have a team that can *cheer you on* with each lap, especially when you get close to the finish line, and remind and encourage the person by saying, "You can do this!" as often as it takes

~

My Moto in life and especially in Labor - ***Breathe and Believe***

I believe in you. Stay focused while Breathing

This is all about meeting your baby!

Chapter 24: Labor

Labor is a Labyrinth

There are many ways to *start* labor, then many ways *to* labor

There are many twists and turns along the birthing path

Expect surprises during labor, it is not an easy journey

There is no simple one easy way to have a baby

Labor is one of the *hardest* things you will go through

Thankfully there are many ways to deliver your baby

There are many reasons why your labor might change

Labor and delivery have no rules and do not know time

Your labor will be different each time with each new human being born

Labor is a force of its Own!

How will I know this is Real Labor? Labor is a progression of contractions. Once started, they do not stop, they move on to the next one, and they are regular until the baby is born. The Uterus starts contracting, and the early sensations are usually mild, irregular and short in duration. For a primip (first baby), it can take many hours to dilate the cervix and then a slow push to move the baby down farther into the birth canal, and those can last several hours. Many hours of contractions that build and gain intensity grow stronger and come closer together, which ends with delivery. Most often, they are strong enough to help push your baby down into the birth canal; combined with your strong pushing, you will birth your baby into the world, and the Care providers will put the baby into your arms.

What I wish I was told about Labor and Delivery:

- That labor hurts! Labor can be long! Labor is exhausting!
- Sometimes, there is grief, anxiety and fear.
- Sleep is your biggest barrier to the longevity of a slow-progressing labor.
- Laboring with your first baby can take several days; a second baby is usually faster.
- There is no time frame for an induction, it is usually long, but it can be fast.
- The length of labor is totally up to your body and the baby.
- Labor and the process can be a bit of a mystery and very surreal.
- The hardest workout of your life.
- It is life-changing.
- It is the most enriching, happiest and most fulfilling memorable day OF YOUR LIFE.
- Uncontrollable sensations of miraculous love and joy.

Breathe! Big & Deep Rhythmic breaths, then Blow to the Floor,

Do this type of breathing UNTIL you Deliver.

Fight or Flight Is a natural response for many people when they have moments of anticipated danger that they can feel and they need to either protect themselves or turn and get away as fast as possible. They can become fearful and stop, become frozen in the moment, or just run away. Our body 'does' what it believes is best, depending on how it perceives the situation. This is common with many people as they go through labor; it can literally stall labor because you are so uncomfortable about your well-being that labor becomes scary, and you want OUT of labor. I have seen people that do not want any kind of touch, or they become distant and want total quiet to focus and concentrate on their next contraction. All of this and more is normal and necessary, the birthing person's needs come first, they will be back and will be present - after the delivery when the baby is in their arms.

Try to help the birthing person stay open and present and in the moment, and the birthing partner should be available to offer encouragement with soft words, gentle touch and reassurance; you know them best. It is important for the birthing person to know that they can rely on their birth team and partner to recognize and then do something to help them at the moment so they can respond accordingly. Often, labor triggers past experiences that have been very traumatic and in addition, people can have feelings of exposure, being in labor by having their naked bodies exposed to others. When there are experiences from your past, it is essential to have tools for the partner to use to bring you back to 'birthing'. If you can mention to your team that there was something in your past (without divulging too deeply), it helps them to take better care of you during your labor.

How long is labor? Labor is different for every person, and there is no set time frame for labor. There are many factors that can come into play and influence your labor. For instance, the size and shape of your pelvis; the position and size of baby's head; is the baby's body in a favorable position; how you and baby tolerate the labor; is baby's head down far enough and applied to the cervix for it to dilate. Once a good pattern of labor starts, then dilation of the cervix should also occur. These following times and dilation estimates are not an exact measurement, just a guideline.

If this is your first labor and birth, 'you are a Primip' labor can be slow and take several days for your body to start a regular pattern of contractions; you are getting very excited or possibly anxious because things have not started. Now until you deliver, during the day, be diligent and do all birth tricks as often as you can. Birth tricks are your go-to until the baby delivers!

You may not be getting any sleep or rest, or relief from contractions. Evenings should be about taking a break and resting in any way that works best for you. Sleep is your biggest barrier to the longevity of slow-progressing labor and how you cope. It is essential to find rest in the form of napping and relaxing. Have someone give massages as needed and try all relaxing techniques. Most importantly, DO NOT worry about time.

For a multip, it means you are having a second or more babies; expect the active stage to be much faster. I explain to clients that they may go from 4 cm to fully, just like turning on a light switch; once turned on - the light is bright, well 'baby is going to be delivered very soon'. Our anxiety level is less, and we remember what we did as we go through the labor again, and how well it worked the first time.

(First Stage) Active Labor:

More intense contractions and are frequent & longer

Frequency 45 - 60 seconds

2 - 4 minutes 5-1-1

Dilation 4 - 8 cm

Labor is:

- Contractions do not stop until the baby delivers.
- Contractions, when they start, become more regular as your labor progresses.
- Contractions get stronger, longer and closer together.
- Contractions do not stop when you take a relaxation break.
- Showering and especially a warm tub should encourage more contractions.
- You may see mucus, a bloody show, and your waters may leak or break; this is normal.
- Start to keep track of contractions once there is a rhythm to them.

Active labor and your contractions are coming at regular intervals, lasting approximately one minute long. During active labor, your cervix will dilate to fully (10 centimeters). On average, the cervix is expected to dilate 1 cm every 1.5 hours of labor. Active labor can last from 4 to 8 hours or more. Your contractions will become stronger and closer together and regular, either 411 or 511, meaning your contractions are four to five minutes apart, lasting a full 1 minute long, for at least 1 hour, and your cervix will start dilating to 10 cm. It is difficult for anyone to predict exactly when you will become fully dilated to 10 cm, but that will be when you can start the push. Pushing can take several hours.

Contractions usually start easy and manageable for many hours, and possibly for a day or two. The contractions will gently ramp up, you will get used to the easier ones and then, they gain intensity and become very strong, and come closer together. Once your body establishes a regular pattern of contractions, this will continue to increase and get stronger. They do not stop when you rest or try to sleep. They end when your baby is delivered.

Call your support team if you have not already. You should have your team of birth helpers: partner, family member, friends and doula should be arriving for support and encouragement. Set up a time for your other children or animals to be picked up from school or activities and stay at your home with a designated caregiver or go for fun time elsewhere.

Active labor is a natural transition from early labor, which started mild and is now stronger and more intense, making it difficult to breathe and at times, you might start to involuntarily fight the laboring process. Pain from labor can be intuitive. It gives us important information when we feel pain and how we should respond. It can tell us to move and find a more favorable position to relieve pressure from a heavy baby that is moving inside. You may want to go to your Birthing place. It can be a difficult time until you get into this new rhythm and/or learn how to manage your stronger contractions. Some relief measurements might include times to relax with massage and acupressure points, and they can be used randomly and/or continuously to your comfort. Breathing techniques are essential, use the big inhale and big exhale. Some may be thinking it is time to consider help with pain management, ask your birth helpers to advocate for you, and ask about options for pain relief.

If you have decided to have a natural birth with no drugs, know that, it is absolutely okay to change your mind in labor, to try the nitrous oxide (gas) or have an epidural

Hydration and Food It can be common to have an upset stomach. You should stick to foods that are easy to digest, and small amounts, soda crackers or a piece of bread, to calm the tummy are best because the stomach in active labor may not digest food (you will bring it back up). Getting closer to Transition frozen fruit, possibly grapes or fruit that is squeezed and frozen into popsicles, is a good way to have some natural sugar for energy (this is not recommended for anyone that has Gestational Diabetes). Otherwise, stick to clear juices and lots of water; it is very important to keep hydrated and for you to keep your energy up. When you 'forget about food,' it tells us that you are in a more active labor pattern.

Author's Tips: A special mention, because recently it has happened a few times with clients. If there is a chance during labor you might have a C-Section, possibly you are trying a VBAC or other reasons that you may end up in the operating room. You will be asked if you have eaten anything in the last 6 hours. When you say yes, you had a cracker or a few nuts or whatever, you will not be allowed in the operating room until it has been a full 6 hours afterward the last time you have eaten (time to fully digest). It might be best practice to go on a clear diet during your Active labor stage (and honestly, most people do not want to eat anyway).

Many people try to have a bowel movement with no success because, it is your baby's head is getting lower into your pelvis and giving you this full feeling in your bowels.

Embrace all of these sensations; they are normal and safe, and soon, when you are fully dilated, you will change your breath and actively push the baby out. But until that time, it is essential to breathe through every contraction, big breaths in and long breaths out, repeat and repeat. If this is hard to do, your helpers will be there to keep you on track.

With more pressure coming from the uterus and the baby's head putting pressure onto the cervix, you may have a SROM, spontaneous rupture of membranes, or possibly a leak of fluids, and if this happens, you may feel the baby 'drop' further into your pelvis and you may have a feeling that baby is lower and experience more intense contractions or intense pressure in your bum. But you should be able to breathe a little easier.

You will work hard and long using the birth tricks, but you must take time to have some rest when you can. The partner can distract the birthing person by starting a one-sided verbal conversation, as they will be listening to you while working hard with each contraction. Encourage the person to visualize, by talking about their favorite place and or vacation, or what the future with this new baby might look like. Being prepared with pictures for them to look on a tablet or phone for a visual effect. Encourage deep breathing and relaxation techniques especially give a massage and acupressure points, while the person listens to you.

At home, it is good to stay in touch with your care provider and check in when something happens that you are unsure about and if you need to ask for advice regarding how to take some rest or cope when labor becomes too overwhelming.

Birth partners should endeavor to be attentive to all of the birthing persons' needs and try to give what is requested, or more importantly, to come up with what they feel the laboring person might prefer, i.e., for snacks or hydration or comfort. Try all different ways to distract and reduce pain by using position changes and acupressure or encouragement. This should be done at any and all times in labor as needed.

- Keep the person hydrated and then bathroom breaks
- Know where the puck bucket is
- Acupressure for hours
- TENS, as long as you want
- Massage for hours
- Change positions
- Touch should always be gentle and caring
- Hugs, kisses holding hands are encouraged
- Remind them to breathe big and let it go!
- Sway or dance to music
- Visualization techniques
- Storytelling
- Hold a leg when pushing
- Stay up all night with you (unless there is an epidural, then everyone sleeps)

Birth partners should show respect, be kind, and stay calm with the birthing person by:

- Encouraging words and reassurance that 'you *are* doing this!'
- Asking how they can help you.
- Asking if you need something.
- Remind you not to worry or not to be afraid.
- Telling you a guided story.
- Asking how they can change things for you to feel better.

- Preventing you from getting out of control; it can be hard to bring you back to calm.
- Do they understand procedures? Then find a nurse or doctor for clarification.
- How do they feel about being offered a procedure? Epidural or C-Section etc., ask the care providers to step out of the room so you can discuss between the two of you.

It is very important to check in; every person feels and perceives things like anxiety very differently. When people are in the constraints of a hospital room, they can feel they do not have the space to breathe, and then anxiety seeps in. If this happens, ask yourself:

- What is my body or inner system trying to tell me?
- What is upsetting me at this moment?
- Is it loss of control, feelings of fear, pain, or vulnerability?

The partner should be watching for changes in the birthing person. What does their face and eyes look like? People can hold IN their baby; they literally hold in by pulling up their shoulders or squeezing their butt cheeks. While standing, I giggle their hips or their bottom with every contraction; it is similar to the 'shake the apple tree'. Furrowed brow, tightly closed eyes, a frown, quick or shallow breathing, clenched jaw? We want the opposite, so do some of these simple and easy things that will help to release oxytocin;

- pressure points to release stress
- warm blanket
- sips of water
- eye-to-eye contact
- smile
- tender touch

A grounding exercise might be to: stop, sit and close your eyes; Breathe, long inhale and a long release. Be aware of yourself, and with each breath, start to hum or make a quiet sound. Explain to someone and ask for help to make *you* feel better.

It is difficult to address how you or the partner will be in labor, was there fear as you walked into the delivery suite, or are you concerned about how or when baby will deliver or a big question Can You Do This? Best practice if either of you is overwhelmed, talk to the care providers; they may be able to come up with a solution or a way for you to make a decision. They are always there to help you. There might be times that the partner needs to get food or beverages (the birthing person will NOT like *you* partaking in the same room); their senses are very sensitive. Or if you are exhausted and need some rest, care providers can bring blankets for you to rest.

Bring some Tylenol for the birth partner in case they get a headache. The hospital does not give medications to anyone else but the birthing person. I have had so many partners that have had a headache in the hospital.

Labor Positions: All movement helps your baby move lower, which shortens your labor. Try all these positions. You may be surprised they feel good, and you will find your favorites; there is no right or wrong. Try not to stay in one position for too long. Changing frequently is very good for helping the baby to move. With almost any position, try to sway or wiggle your hips. Note ** two stars means this is also very good for when you are pushing.

- **Acupressure or Massage: If you enjoyed this in early labor, you will love it now and all throughout labor, as it is very effective, especially during the pushing stage. All throughout labor, this is very effective, especially pushing. This should be done with gentle hands, as the birthing person's body and skin are very sensitive; it is on high alert to touch and massage.
- *Walking, squatting, and sitting on a ball will not feel so good when the baby is low in the pelvis.

- **Lean over the countertop or table, and do all pressure points on your back and your bottom.
- **Partner standing or sitting in front of you, lean forward and rest your arms on their shoulders or waist - sway your hips.
- **Being on hands and knees on the hospital bed and raising the head of the hospital bed so you can kneel against the back of the bed OR standing beside the bed leaning forward against the bed with a pillow under your head.
- **Kneel on the bed for cat/cow position (on a floor is too sore, or use blankets under knees).
- **Semi-reclined to your comfort, resting in this position on a bed or couch, open your legs wide, bend your knees, then legs resting on bed or couch (with a towel for support under each knee), heels together and vacillate wiggling your bottom then stop and relax.
- **Lunge (clients love this) is often done in the delivery suite by putting your foot on a chair (that is secured against the wall), then holding on to the chair arms and lunging deeply, do both legs and for as long as it feels good.
- **Side lying with a blanket between the legs and a small hand towel under the bottom ankle that is resting on the bed (to take the pressure off the hip). This helps if the baby is coming fast and takes the pressure off the sacrum and coccyx or hemorrhoids.
- **Counter pressure on the back is when you put the heel of your hand or a tennis ball (or similar) against the lower back during a contraction. You may be asked to press harder (but mind not to be too aggressive). You also may have to do this in any position they are in - when they complain about pain.
- *Squat on the floor, on the bed or with a squatting bar that attaches to the hospital bed. Your legs should be apart but still be able to support you, lean against a squatting bar or your partner or sit on a Birthing chair (if available).

- **Sit on a toilet with your legs wide apart. This is similar to squatting, and for as long as you are comfortable! This is the best place to be, you do not overwork your legs or arms, and you can take sips of water and pee all at the same time. This gives the baby a wider pelvis to come through. Stay in this position as long as you can and go back to the toilet often to labor.

Relaxing in labor: By getting comfortable and reclining on the couch or bed, add the use of an electric heating pad or warm up a hand towel in the dryer, pour warm water from the kettle or tap onto a hand towel, wring out excess water, and wrap it up in a puppy pad (the ones you train a puppy to pee on) then wrap the tape around the package to hold it together. Put a warmed pad on your sore back in conjunction with the use of your TENS machine (if you have one). Placement suggestions are given on the instruction pamphlet. Note that you should be using the same spots you use for Acupressure points.

Author's note: I have seen some clients that do not want ANY touch at all during labor, so you must respect that. Just be present and stay close to them.

Cold: When the birthing person is working very hard and getting through each contraction, believe it or not, a very cold wet face cloth on the back of and/or front of their neck, upper chest, forehead, and under the chin is very beneficial, in bringing down the heat their body is generating. People are working very hard during their contractions and can overheat, and I find all my clients love a cool cloth. It can be used in Active labor and especially during the Pushing stage.

I take a cloth, put cold water on it and wring it out. When it gets warm (from the birthing person's warm body), I swing it around in the air above my head with my hand. This helps it to cool down. In the past, I would use a container of ice and cold water. However, there is usually nowhere to place the container down in the delivery suite. And it can be uncomfortable to place your hand in the ice water, and it makes a mess. More importantly, the laboring person may not want you to leave their side to tend to cool down the cloth. Ice chips in a cup with a spoon or ice water is very effective. Often they do not want any sheets or blankets over themselves, they throw it to the floor, and some even prefer to take off the hospital gown and walk around naked because their body is warm from working so hard.

When calling the hospital to advise the care providers you want to come in, they will ask a few important questions:

- Starting with your name, if you are a primip or multip, how many weeks are you?
- Has your water broken? If so, what color was the fluid and how much?
- How long and often are your contractions (you will have been tracking them for at least one or more hours).
- How are you coping, or are you coping?
- Why do you want to come to the hospital?
- Do you want advice (over the phone) on how to cope better at home, or are you struggling?

It may be that you want reassurance or to have drugs (morphine and Gravol) and be sent home, or if you are dilated enough that you can stay and have an epidural.

The hospital staff will be listening to *the way you sound* while talking and if there is a change during a contraction. Both your voice and your breathing will have changed, and the Care Provider can hear if you are struggling or whether you can continue to *talk during a contraction***.** They will be trying to assess how you are coping, and you should stay at home longer or come into the hospital for an assessment.

At the hospital, they will:

- Assess the cervix by doing a vaginal exam.

- Monitor your tummy and listen to the baby's heart rate, this tells them whether the baby is coping with the contractions (by the dips or accelerations in their heart rate).
- Take your blood pressure.
- Find out how long the contractions actually are and how often they are coming.
- Do your contractions feel like they are stronger than before?
- Specifically ask how you are feeling and what you need.
- Do you want help from morphine and Gravol and be sent home?
- Are you looking for reassurance that you are "*doing well in this moment*"?
- You may want to go to the hospital in the hopes of staying for pain management, such as an epidural.

For a **Primip,** it might be reassuring when you talk to the Care Provider on the phone, and they can answer all or some of your questions. They are good at advising if it is too early for you to come to the hospital and giving suggestions for coping. It is always better to stay at home in the comfort of your own environment for as long as possible an hour or a few more hours can make the difference in dilation. It can be tough coming to the hospital and then being told you are 2 cm and not in active labor yet. The drive home is deflating, and you feel disappointed and wonder how much longer can this all be. Many people feel a sense of security and comfort from *being* at the place where they are going to deliver.

The time and length of contractions will vary with each individual. As a primip, you will go by the '411' formula. Contractions are regularly every 4 minutes apart, lasting *at least* 1 minute long or longer, for over 1 full hour or more.

For a **Multip,** it can still be confusing, but most often, you remember from your previous labor how you coped and that knowledge on how you dilated slowly or quickly. You may be admitted if you appear to be in very active labor. With a vaginal exam, your cervix may be 3 cm or more. Your cervix can dilate very quickly, and then your pushing and delivery are expected to be faster than the first. It would be unsafe for you to be sent home, especially if your first birth was fast. Your care providers will expect you to dilate faster and then deliver quickly.

The time and length of contractions are regular at '511'. You should contact your Care Provider. Contractions that are regular and every 5 minutes apart, lasting *at least* 1 minute or longer, for over 1 full hour or more. If any of the following happens, you need to call the care provider straight away:

- IF you feel any 'bum' pressure or you have a sensation of pooing, call and advise the hospital. They will most likely ask you to come straight to the hospital!
- By calling the hospital, they can be ready for you when you come in and are trying to push.
- You should always call the ambulance if the Baby is *coming!*

What to expect when you are admitted to the Hospital: Everything at this time is going to seem overwhelming and give you the feeling of being out of your element. The contractions are so strong and coming so close together. These are very normal sensations, and the care providers understand you are having many conflicting emotions and working very hard. They are very dedicated people that are trying to take care of your well-being and will help you with suggestions for an easier time during this stage of labor.

You are probably huffing and puffing through your contractions and not paying attention to anything else. A clerk at the hospital will ask your partner for your personal information and will go through the process to admit you, and they will need to confirm that your telephone number and address are all correct. If in active labor, the questions are usually too much for you, so let your partner answer questions and give labor timelines. You may be asked the following;

- Need your Medical card and your ID.
- Any surgeries, what was the procedure, when and where.
- Have you been out of the country in the last year?
- Any allergies or medications that you are taking?
- Asked about contractions, how often are you contracting - when did labor start?
- If your waters ruptured, when was that, and what color was the fluid?
- Has there been any bleeding or blood show, if so how much

You will be taken to an assessment room unless you are having signs of an imminent delivery. If that is the case, you will be put in a wheelchair and taken straight to the delivery suite. I have seen people coming through the hospital doors and trying to push. They go into one of the assessment rooms that are ready and set up for impending deliveries.

In the assessment room with a nurse, you will be hooked up to the monitors to start tracing your contractions and to determine how often and how long they are. They will listen to the baby's heart rate while being hooked up to the monitors for approximately half an hour. The nurse will watch for *how* your baby is coping with contractions and determine how active you are in labor. You will have your blood pressure monitored and temperature taken and the staff are watching to see how you are managing through each contraction.

The care provider or nurse will give you a vaginal exam to determine how dilated your cervix is. To be admitted, your cervix should be 4 - 5 cm, and you should be clearly in active labor; otherwise, you will set home. You should be feeling;

- Contractions are regular, strong and very intense.
- Contractions can make you feel out of control and difficult to cope with.
- You are focused and breathing heavily through contractions.

- If your water has broken, contractions can be very intense.
- You may feel a lot of pressure in your bottom.
- You may be asking for help with pain management for the contractions.

Some things that are not done in the hospitals where I work:

- They do not give people Enemas.
- You will *only ever* be given a shave, down where an incision will be made if needed because you are going in for a cesarean section.
- They would make you lay on your back (only as needed with an epidural or on monitors).
- They would assume you want an Epidural or Drugs; you may want to labor without them.
- They will not randomly Break your Waters.
- They will never automatically give you an Episiotomy.

After being admitted, your delivery nurse will come and get you. They will ask if you can walk to the delivery suite, most people in very active labor will prefer going there in a wheelchair, but there are many that would like to walk. Your nurse, who will be staying with you in the delivery suite, will be asking you some questions about your wishes for delivery, whether you want to be in a tub or shower or neither. They will ask about the medication you take and about your labor so far. This is a good time for the birthing partner to ask questions like, where is the water or ice machine, or where is the bathroom? Or where you might be able to take some rest or sleep during the night? They are very accommodating and happy to answer questions and can give you a quick tour of the ward, but they are there to look after the birthing person.

*Note ~ Please advise your nurse if you are modest, it is important for you to be comfortable and that your wishes are respected. You will be wearing a flimsy hospital gown and, for a vaginal exam, will have a sheet over you from the waist down, which is lifted upwards from your feet. It can distract the birthing person, and it is essential that you feel relaxed and that you are in a safe and supportive environment as you go further into your labor. People need to let go and allow their body and baby to labor and deliver.

*Note ~ at the hospital and using a tub or shower for pain relief, I would suggest you use the hospital gown or bring a big shirt or sundress. Do not bring a bathing suit; they are too difficult to get off when you get out of the tub to push.

On the other side of the coin, people often do not want the feel of clothes on their bodies, and walk around naked, which is also totally fine.

Control: There is no room for control in labor! Just let it go, and your body will know what it has to do, it may have had a tough time getting started, but once it gets active, it is best to allow all sensations and give yourself into the process. I see many and most people go into a 'birth trance', and they thrive! When you feel you are in a safe place, with knowledgeable people to guide you, the birthing space is quiet or you are playing your favorite music, and you are given suggestions to move in specific positions. Let go of the process, go within yourself and find a place where you can let your body navigate through the labor stage on its own. Try not to 'think' about having control; there is no such thing. Your body and baby are working well together already.

Who is allowed to be at the Birth: You are in charge. If this birth is private and only you, your partner and Care Providers, then don't be afraid of tell others that. If you believe family or friends will just show up at the hospital, and do not want anyone in the birthing suite, tell the staff that they are not wanted. Most often, they will not allow people to come into the delivery suite.

If you have changed your mind about giving permission OR you haven't told the persistent person yet, that they can not come to your birthing place. I tell my clients, "Don't tell them you are in labor'. Avoid answering most texts and some calls a few weeks before the day of labor. This way, those persistent family and friends will not suspect when you do go into labor. Sound sneaky? Good it is, but this can be a very private time for most people. The time in the first few hours after delivery is extremely important for new parents to *bond* with your baby. Not having to talk to others or have them holding your new baby may sound selfish, but once you meet your baby, you will appreciate that you had *the most precious time meeting your baby for the first few hours.*

I have taken pictures of my client's birth for years with permission. Clients love their birth pictures, it truly is a once-in-a-lifetime moment, unless you have another baby, BUT then it will be a different baby and different delivery. My question to clients is ~ do you want pictures that are above or below the waist? Above the waist means just that, baby on the chest, and I will try to make sure that the nipple is not in the shot! Below means the birth and everything, even *the* delivery!

If you want to take your own pictures, that is great but very difficult, especially at delivery. You should not ask anyone to use a camera; it can be difficult to learn how to use it properly in the moment, just the cell phone's camera. Ask your Doula; they might be the best for taking pictures. Nurses and care providers have so many things to attend to and are simply not available. Getting a few pictures at delivery with both parents in the pictures and then pretty much the first hour is awesome. Or you may have hired a professional photographer to be at your delivery.

Use your phone or let someone else use your phone or camera (if I use my phone, I transfer pictures before I leave the delivery suite, then delete them). I love that with a phone camera, you get a time stamp for each picture. It can be hard for someone else to use your camera because they are busy with your own tasks during delivery. There are many precious moments in labor, during delivery or after birth. It shows us how strong you were and gives you a glimpse of what you really did during labor because we will forget most of the moments during your labor.

I take many random pictures throughout labor, and I love to catch the emotion in the face of the birthing person. Some perfect pictures might be:

- During early labor - active labor - delivery - the first hour.
- Walking down the hall to the delivery suite.
- Stop for a contraction, leaning against the wall.
- In the wheelchair to the delivery suite.
- When the pair embraces or has a kiss or holds hands.
- The partner is doing pressure points.
- The person is having a very strong contraction - the grimace.
- Expression to most anything in labor.
- Laboring in the tub.
- The person is pushing and in different pushing positions.
- The face as they deliver.
- The partner 'helping' catch the baby.
- Partner cutting the cord.
- Baby's head as they are delivering.
- Picture of the clock on the wall at delivery.
- The first reaction from parents 'seeing' the baby for the 1st time.
- Baby's reaction when they hear you talk.
- Baby is placed near the nipple, and watch what they do.

Many more pictures at the first 1-hour baby check-up:

- Head-to-toe health check by the Doctor (excluding the Dr).
- Measuring baby.

- Weighing baby.
- Partner putting a diaper on baby.
- All pictures of you, your partner and the star of the show, the baby.
- Sometimes, after delivery, the Doctor or Midwife will give their permission for a group picture with the baby.
- In the hospitals that I attend, pictures of the birth team or other staff, especially for procedures, for instance, cesarean section or forceps, are not allowed.

Staying at the Hospital: Carry on with all techniques that worked best for you in early labor at home, unless you need to have an IV placed or need to be on the monitors. You will be able to walk the halls at the hospital, and use a birthing ball, (if you know your hospital does not have balls, ask if you can bring yours from home (ask your care provider ahead of time). The birthing person may be feeling a sense of relief because they are at the place their baby will be born, this usually helps them to relax, and this can help their labor to progress. They may find that they have different sensations and more intense contractions. As you settle into the hospital, try everything that you did from home and if there are some specific positions that might help.

If a specific position or massage does not seem to be working at home, you may be surprised that when you try it later on in labor, it is beneficial. If you have not already, start to use any Meditation script, a popular one is 'HypnoBirthing'. You will have practiced this in the third trimester. Music, Relaxation techniques, and position changes are both relaxing and active.

Warm water: If you have access to a shower or a tub in your birthing suite, this is a great place to labor for a long time, especially in *active labor and transition*. It allows you to float or have the shower head raining on your back and/or tummy. It reduces the pain from contractions, the release of an overworked body, and legs from standing, walking or climbing stairs. Your back from the pressure from a posterior baby or the weight of the baby, shoulders, relax and ease sore muscles just by getting off your feet and the gentle warm water.

If you can have a shower, you can sit on a ball or stand or if in a warm tub, you can lay and float on your back. If on your hands and knees, put towels under the knees to soften where you are kneeling. Have your birth partner or someone else pour warm bath water onto your back, stomach or shoulders; they can use a large cup or small bowl or shower head. The water should be warm and comforting, but not so warm that it overheats you or the baby. Also, have your partner do some acupressure points that are easy to access. With lights down and staying hydrated, you can visualize while listening to a story from your partner or just by listening to favorite music. You can also use nitrous oxide, the gas, if needed. I also encourage people, just before they get out of the tub or shower, to void their bladder (if they can). It seems to be easier while in water.

Note: the partner would benefit by bringing a bathing suit or similar so they can stand beside you in a shower.

Author's tips: *If your waters have broken, consult with your care provider. They may not want you in the tub. Try to stay in as long as you can, maybe until you are fully ready to start pushing. If allowed, it is nice to start pushing in the water, then get out and deliver on the bed.*

Be Active in Labor: Without an epidural, you should be able to try all or most of the regular birth tricks. Your focus should be on being upright or sitting on a birth ball; gravity will definitely help the baby to move lower. In all upright positions, vigorously and over-exaggerate all of the birth tricks, any position that you can move into, and keep changing positions to give baby help for them to move.

Epidurals take away the PAIN during labor: Many people say they want a natural birth, which means they are trying for no interventions, no epidural and no drugs! After many many long hours, if you want an epidural or need one, *you will get one!* You will have decided you want relief from the constant and strong contractions, or you are exhausted and not coping well. I have explained the procedure for epidurals in the Procedures chapter.

Something to keep in mind, my experience with clients at other General hospitals that do deliveries, is they share the anesthetist with all other departments that go to the operating room, and the wait can be much longer for the doctor to come in to see you. This can make for a long, frustrating and painful time waiting for relief.

I explain to clients, IF you know you will want an epidural, ask for it when you start to think about having one, do not wait until you are struggling. At the birthing hospital where I work, we have access to an Anesthetist fairly quickly, if, for some reason, there are a couple of people that have asked for an epidural before us, it can take some time for the doctor to come to our room. Fortunately, that is not often. The procedure, from deciding you want an epidural to total relief can take up to 45 - 60 minutes. (Ask your care provider to advise protocols for your hospital and average expected wait times.)

Talk to your nurse or care provider when you are getting more uncomfortable that you would like an epidural, the nurse will site the IV in your hand or lower arm (if not already in place) then the nurse will request the epidural from the Anesthesia department. The nurse will get you up to the bathroom and have you prepared and sitting on the bed for the Anesthetist when they walk in the room.

The epidural has a few really amazing perks, it helps you cope more efficiently through contractions. It helps you release and relax all of your muscles, which helps the baby to come further down the birth canal. I see people 'hold' their baby in because of old trauma, fear or anxiety and from the pain of contractions, all of which have stalled labor. It is helpful for releasing stress and anxiety from the discomfort and pain of contractions, it helps you get closer to pushing and birth. It is helpful to reduce pain during the repair of the perineum. It is essential if you are going into the OR, for a procedure to help the baby out. You might wonder if there is a cut-off, are you too far along in labor? I have seen people, for a variety of reasons, have an epidural at 9 cm.

Every person metabolizes the drug used in the epidural differently; some can have freedom from pain and/or the ability to move around to stand, walk, bounce on a ball and position themselves to push. With an epidural, your mobility may be challenged, you may have the feeling of *heavy legs*, and your body does not support you, and it makes it hard for you to stand and walk to the bathroom to void. You may have difficulty or limitations with laboring tricks and position changes and positions for pushing and squatting. The upside, you will be comfortable and have a change to rest or sleep until you are fully dilated.

If you know you will have an epidural for a planned Cesarean section, it is important to understand the procedure, so you will be given a consult with a doctor for the anesthesia. They explain the procedure and check your spine for any natural spinal curvatures or discuss whether you have had a back injury.

If a person has settled in and are now relaxing with their working epidural because you are most likely very tired from being in labor for so long. You should get them tucked into the bed with a warm blanket (from the hospital warmers). By doing this, they can fully relax and nap or just rest and let the contractions work their magic so you get fully dilated. If you have forgotten to bring an eye cover, I suggest a small folded hand towel to place over their eyes and, in addition, turn the lights down in the room. Then music with ear buds to bring extra calm. To soothe the tired and sore muscles while resting, have someone give a massage or the feet and legs and/or do acupressure points.

You will need an epidural if you are having a procedure, such as a rotation of the baby in the delivery suite, forceps, vacuum or Cesarean section, in the operating room.

The basics of how an epidural is placed is explained in the 'Procedures' chapter.

Difficult Voiding: The hardest thing to do in labor is to void, it is not easy in labor, especially as labor progresses it can be hard to know whether your bladder if full but it is essential for you to have hourly trips to the bathroom or more often as needed. It is also difficult to void because of the baby's head in close proximity, and there are a couple of tricks that might help to relieve yourself; try them all, whatever works best for you;

- Leave the bathroom light off or turned down. Take a moment to breathe and relax before trying to void.
- Turn on a facet so you can listen to running water.
- Blow bubbles through a straw into a glass of water.
- Rinse the perineum with a squirt bottle filled with warm water.
- In a shallow bowl of warm or cold water and on the toilet, place your hand in the water.
- Have some essential oil, peppermint and breathe it in a few times, or I will put a few drops into the toilet as the person sits.
- When you are in the bathtub or a shower, try to void just before you get out.

When you have an epidural and are resting, the nurse will ask you to void, and they will do a step test to make sure your legs will support you when you stand up and try to walk. Epidurals are notorious for giving you a heavy feeling in your legs, and it can be difficult to lift your leg while lying on the bed. If you pass the step test, you will get up, and as you walk to the toilet, you will have someone support you on either side to ensure you do not fall on the way there and back and to help you sit and get back up from the toilet.

If you do not pass this step test, you will be confined to the bed because it is not safe to get up. If you still have hours before you are expected to start pushing, they will not want to do an In and Out catheter several times. To prevent infection, they will suggest a catheter that will stay in until the baby's head is low enough. They will take it out for you to start to push. The care team will advise having a catheter placed that stays in and continually drains the bladder until your cervix is fully dilated, and then take it out before you start to push. The bladder can slow down a baby's descent when it is full; it is like having a balloon in front of the baby's head. This will make it harder for the baby to wiggle their head past the bladder and descend.

You may be offered a bedpan, and I think I have seen it work a handful of times; it seems that sitting on a bedpan in the delivery suite feels really awkward; a tip, you can ask your team to leave the room while you try.

If pushing is imminent, the bladder needs to be drained, but you can not support yourself to get to the bathroom, the care providers will ask if it is okay to drain the bladder by using an IN and OUT catheter it is just as it sounds, clean the area, place the catheter in, drain the bladder, catheter out, and you can start to push.

When you know you are going to have a Cesarean section or other procedures in the operating room, and it is not an emergency, you will have a catheter placed in the delivery suite before you go to the operating room.

(First Stage) **Transition**

Duration 60- 90 seconds

Frequency 2 - 3 minutes apart

Much more intensity

Dilation 8 - 10 cm

Transition is when the cervix dilates from 8 cm to 10 cm. Very intense contractions are approximately every 1.5 - 2 minutes apart and last 60 - 90 seconds in duration, and the intensity of contractions is much stronger. Coping can be totally different than what you have experienced yet. This is when many people have nausea and/or vomit, have chills or become overheated and shaking because of how hard the body is working.

Baby's head is lower: If it is coming down over the rectum, there is a mounting pressure in your bum, which gives you the feeling of wanting to have a bowel movement. You will have an overwhelming feeling and strong urges to push, or you may be involuntarily pushing. It can be a frightful time that you have to push, but exciting knowing you will soon meet your baby!

Author's Note: This baby has a short distance, in terms of centimeters, to come through the pelvis, then down the birth canal. The time for a first-person pushing can be from 1 hour to 4 hours, and that is with very strong pushes from you. The body's tissues have to stretch, and at the same time, your body has to release and allow the baby out; this is a lot of long and hard work pushing.

A multip should have an easier and shorter time during transition for their push. Your body will 'remember', and the uterus and the birth canal will open more efficiently, making it a shorter push.

Think like an athlete, you are at the end of a marathon, and the finish line is just in front of you. With an amazing cheering team in your birthing suite, it can be a huge game changer. It is time for you to hunker down and PUSH! for however long it takes. For a Multip, it may take 20 minutes (but not always). For a Primip, it may take 2 - 5 hours.

Author's note: I am amazed by the transition and pushing. I have seen many people birthing strong, where no drugs or interventions were needed. These people get to 10 cm and believe in their support team and allow the team to guide them with strong and long pushes. Then their inner spirit roars up and takes over, or they could be excited to finally meet their baby. Where ever the burst of energy comes from; it is truly needed for the last and most important part of your labor.

(Second Stage) **Pushing**

Duration 60 - 90 seconds long

Frequency 2 - 4 minutes apart

Intensity at its highest

Dilation 10 cm (fully dilated)

Pushing can be long, from 3 to 5 hours for a primip

Pushing can be short and fast, from 5 minutes to 1- 3 hours for a multip

Contractions will end with the birth of your baby

The care provider will do a vaginal exam to ensure your cervix is fully dilated, 10 cm and 100% effaced, which is your green light to start pushing. They also feel for the baby's position and how far down the baby's head is in the pelvis. When they tell you there is still a rim of the cervix, they call it a 'lip'; this means there is a small part of the cervix that needs to thin out before you can start to push. The care provider may try to slide the cervix over the baby's head during a contraction, but if it slides back, you will be asked to wait. It is not safe to start pushing, as you risk damaging the cervix when you push too early, not even a wee bit.

You must wait for the baby to naturally come a bit lower, and this can be a huge challenge to relax through the strong contractions. You can try to change your breath by panting or blowing away the contractions. When the lip is in the front, you need to go onto your hands and knees for approximately fifteen to twenty minutes; this puts the weight of the baby's head onto the section that needs to be reduced. If uncomfortable, take a few minutes break, in another position and then back onto hands and knees.

If you can not tolerate being on your hands and knees, try a more comfortable position, side-lying, with the help of a peanut ball, depending on where the baby is (left or right). Also, do the appropriate acupressure points on the buttock, specifically BL32, on the dimples of the back or Spleen 6. Put the person on the same side as the cervical lip; you want some pressure to help it to melt away. This helps the baby move down through the birth canal and then deliver.

If you are feeling that something is different or have increased sensations in your bottom, your baby has possibly moved, and care providers will check again. It has often been encouraged to have an epidural to help the birthing person relax so the sensation of pushing is quenched, and it helps you to breathe through the contractions again.

When you are near the end of labor, and your body is tiring, and contractions have spaced out or are not as strong, Spleen 6 pressure point and nipple stimulation are my two favorite tricks for increasing contractions. Spleen 6 may have helped to start your contractions for labor, and now, this pressure point will help increase the number of contractions at this last stage. I will sit at the end of the bed because it is easy to access the person's toes. If I do not have access to both feet, I will ask the partner to help by them doing one side, and I have the other (I feel it works best with both sides receiving pressure at the same time. I do Spleen 6 for approximately one minute, then break for approximately 20 seconds and redo the pressure point for as long as it takes for the contractions to pick up on their own. I can sit at the feet for a good half hour if needed, and I will also offer to give a massage on the feet and lower legs by vacillating between both pressure points and massage. I will wait until the next contraction should have started, then start the pressure point for a full minute and try to repeat when the next contraction is expected. Another option is nipple stimulation which is only done by the birthing person *or* the partner, and this is done by rolling or rubbing the nipples. I have seen partners that will suck on the nipples, and then there is good old fashion ~ kissing.

Your uterus has created strong contractions and has pushed your baby downwards. That pressure has made a change to your cervix to dilate to 10 cm. The uterus has been doing all the work, but now you will gather all your strength and energy to help push. The cervix will slide over the baby's head as you and your uterus will push the baby lower, and they will be born. When being told you are fully dilated, a huge euphoric feeling takes over that helps to get you to the end of this birthing journey. It can also be overwhelming. It seems that your contractions are more manageable, and you find it invigorating when you are told you can start pushing. For a couple of contractions, before you start to push, there is a lot of adrenaline going through your body that will help you to finish labor and delivery your baby. You will need all of your energy, reserve, and determination to push your baby down and out.

At this time, I encourage clients to take a few minutes to clear their heads, relax and focus before the push, hydrate and then take a bathroom break, to try and relieve themselves.

Sitting on the toilet while having a few contractions and having some practice pushes into the sensation (like having a bowel movement). The pressure in your bottom is the baby moving lower and over your rectum; these are safe feelings. People that practice on the toilet can help the process; the position is perfect, especially because you are very relaxed. You will need all of your energy, reserve, and determination to push your baby down and out. You may be exhausted, but there is an adrenaline rush that people have during this time.

The pressure feels like you have to poo. Think of this sensation as your friend. It tells you the baby is very low, and you need to try and relax your bottom as the sensations grow and your baby gets closer and deeper in the birth canal. I see people hold up a baby, and they physically fight the urge and hold the baby in. You should stay on the toilet to void and practice pushing, and you will not see anything comes out. If in a bed with an epidural, the catheter will be taken. The room will be set up for delivery.

Without an epidural, you will know exactly when your contractions start and end. However, with an epidural, you may feel any tightenings. Most often, with a good working epidural, you have no sensation when contractions start. Your care provider can put their hand on your tummy to feel when the contraction starts and stops. We only want you pushing during a contraction because it is the most powerful time, with both you and your uterus working together. For a first baby, this pushing time can be several hours. For any other babies you push, you should expect the push time to be substantially faster.

This is the last part of your labor, the end of the marathon and you have been laboring for many hours and most often you are exhausted. Baby is being gently pushed by the uterus, slowly down the birth canal, opening and stretching and (hopefully) the baby will fit through the pelvis and then through the perineum. It is essential for you to push hard when you are told to. You will need to dig deep into your energy reserves for the pushing stage.

A first baby will slowly make their way down the birth canal, and with very strong pushes, the head literally rocks back and forth, until baby's head passes under the pubic bone. This time can be lengthy, your body releases and opens, allowing baby to descend. The time can be exhausting, as you push for many hours. When baby is just under the pubic bone, they will stay and birth is usually imminent.

The push for your first baby (primip) can be on average 2 to 4 hours approximately.

There are many factors that can influence the outcome of this stage, the more obvious because of a very long labor are:

- Your uterus may be tired
- Contractions are spaced out
- You are exhausted from a long labor

Breathing changes when you start to push. You will take three breaths during one contraction. Each breath will be a very big breath in. It is very helpful for someone to count as you have each contraction. The count can be from 10 down to 1 **or** from 1 up to 10. It is interesting that people have a preference for counting up or down. When the contraction starts;

I explain that you will change up from breathing and blowing through contractions to a different way and push very strongly.

- 3 breaths and 3 pushes for each contraction.
- Each Breath is BIG, filling your lungs, then HOLD for a count of 10 as you PUSH.
- Designate someone to count for you.
- Quickly release by blowing the breath away.
- Immediately take the next breath.
- The push is exactly like when you feel constipated and pushing hard.
- Curl around your baby - Chin to Chest.
- Focus on pushing into your bum, just like a Poo! Yup.
- Breathe in Big and Deep - Hold the breath.
- Each contraction push is Long and Strong every time.

Pushing is most effective when each and every push is strong and long! You will be encouraged to push more and more. Baby is working hard, and they need all of your strength to help them. This is a team event! The stronger you push, the shorter time until you deliver. For each contraction, you will always curl your head forward and put your chin to your chest. When in a lying position, your partner can help to support you behind your head by putting their hand behind the pillow you are laying on, at your neck but supporting the weight of your head, in a forward position. Supporting your curled head so you do not wear yourself out, from holding your head forward and pushing. Focus on a strong push. You will push in different positions but with the same push strategy for each contraction.

While waiting for your next contraction, approximately 3 minutes, have an ice chip or a sip of water. You can have someone place a cold cloth over your brow, your upper chest area, or behind your neck, you will be working very hard, and it is extremely refreshing. You may consider some energetic music for encouragement.

Big Breath ~ PUSH ~ Blow Breath 3 times for one Contraction

Repeat until your baby is 'Crowning' then you change to a pant

- Wait for the natural urge of the Push sensation.
- Feel your tummy. If firm, start to push.
- Waiting for the next one, totally relax and breathe deep.
- Try to push stronger each time you push.
- With an epidural, your care provider can put a hand on your belly till it gets hard.
- It helps when you can curl around your baby, Chin to Chest.
- When you push ~ go stronger than the last one.
- For encouragement, reach down and feel your baby's head as they are crowning.
- For encouragement, look in a mirror at the foot of the bed to see how much progress you are making as the baby's head starts to show.

Doula Trick: When any of the following happens while pushing, I ask my client to shake and wiggle their hips vigorously, even if they are laying on a bed. This is similar to the 'Tahitian dance' for approximately 20 seconds at a time, this can help baby to move, often we see that the heart rate goes back to normal, the birthing person is encouraged to do this for about 5 minutes, if it does not rectify what ever is going on with baby's heart rate, we change positions. Do this in between contractions. It also helps to loosen muscles in your bottom, (we do not want you to clench or squeeze the bottom). This helps baby move and bring on more and stronger contractions.

- You are laying on the bed for more than an hour.
- You need to increase the number of contractions.
- When pushing, the baby's heart rate drops.
- Helps the baby's head slide through the pelvis.
- They are laying on their cord.
- Tahitian wiggle.

To encourage contractions that are less frequent, you can release your own natural oxytocin, by kissing your partner, rolling your nipples or Spleen 6 pressure point.

When pushing you need support from behind the head: If lying down have your partner support behind your head, by putting their hand gently behind your neck and lower part of the head. You should always endeavor to curl around the baby. You will take your hands and hold the backs of your legs, knees should be very wide apart. You will push in different positions but the same breathing and push strategy with each one.

Carry on with early labor breathing and visualization until delivery.

Different pushing positions - try all positions; you may find some feel better than others. Have someone close to support you as needed. Move and change positions often. With an epidural, you may be restricted to staying in bed because you have heavy legs, and they do not support you. Most positions are flexible, whether you are laying or standing. Labor will change and ramp up as the baby moves and tries to descend.

These positions will help the baby to go through the pelvis and may relieve some back pain.

- The partner can help the birthing person to be held and supported in an upright position (if possible) to sway their hips. If not, then they can sway their hips sideways on the bed.
- Floating in the tub.
- Lunge with one foot up on a chair, footstool or crouch.
- Kneel on hands and knees (cushion under knees for support) or the cat/cow yoga position.
- Lean over a bed (at home or hospital).
- Swing hips (dance slow or fast).
- Rebozo for hanging on to (or a sheet).
- Squat and lean on a birthing bar that attaches to a Hospital bed.

Sitting on a toilet (in hospital) when you are fully dilated this is an advantage and encouraged while you are pushing that can bring good results! Sit with wide legs, there will be pressure in your bottom, but not the pressure that you are sitting on your baby. It makes a lot of room to help baby make their way downwards, and you can usually void your bladder. This is ideal position for you to try to push.

**At HOME Do not push without an exam, if you are on the toilet, and if sensations feel very strong, like you need to have a bowel movement. You may just have to grab your baby as they deliver in the toilet. Have someone call the care provider or possibly the emergency number for an ambulance.

Positions as you get closer to delivery. This is a really good time to find a focal point, someone's face, that you can stare at. At someone reminding you how and when to breathe. You need:

- To be in a comfortable birthing position

- Freedom to move
- To move continuously as needed
- To stand - Hands and Knees - Lay down - Legs wide and supported
- Music to inspire you for the end of your long birthing time

Rebozo, OR if you do not have one, you can use a sheet. This is good when you want to relieve pressure from a sore back or when the baby is not in an ideal position and to open the pelvis.

- The rebozo wrapped around your back, the support person in front of you, holds on to both ends of the wrap, OR you lay down, and the person stands above your hips. Either way, they giggle the rebozo sideways, back and forth across your back
- Wrap the rebozo around your back and around their back while they hold the ends tight and allow the birthing person to rest back or above a chair or on a chair
- Get onto hands and knees OR lean against a birthing ball, with the rebozo around the baby tummy, if two people, one on each side and each holding on each end of the rebozo. Jiggle the tummy back and forth. If one person stands above you, their feet on either side of your hips and behind your bottom
- Wrap a knot with both ends of the rebozo - open a door, put the knotted side over and above the door and close the door, then let the birthing person hold onto the rebozo and lean forward and allow their back to gently swing back and forth or a to give the back a long stretch
- Shake the Apples with your head resting on a pillow, on the floor, in a kneeling position, so your bottom is higher than your head (knees can be elevated on a piece of furniture by using a couch or footrest). It works well in an almost upside-down position (with very solid support on either side of the person). The Rebozo goes around the tummy, and the person standing above and behind you will hold the ends of the

Rebozo, then shake the Rebozo briskly back and forth. Similarly, if you do not have a Rebozo, you can use a sheet folded up OR put your hands on the person's hips and vigorously shake their hips as the person on the floor braces themselves in place.

Squatting: *This position is beneficial for helping the baby descend further into the pelvis before and especially during the pushing stage.* The use of a birthing chair or squat bar or squatting on the floor helps your pelvis to relax and to open and then for you to push the baby downward. The exercise ball may not be comfortable on your bottom but try it, it allows you to bounce your baby lower, and the swaying motion helps them navigate downward. If you are comfortable doing squats and can hold that position on your own, do them often and stay for as long as possible. While squatting and with a wide stance, sway your hips, then add a *full lean forward* in the squat.

The squat bar can be added to the birthing bed in the hospital. You may need help, to move up and onto the bar, especially if you have an epidural. The bar will support you, do not use if your legs become tired or if your legs do not support you with an epidural. If you can change to a birthing chair or lay back down on the bed. Many hospital beds have different positions, for instance you can bring the head of the bed fully upwards, and be in a sitting position, then the bottom of the bed should also have the ability to move down. If both options are used it can become some what of a chair, at the point for pushing you can put your legs up on the birthing bar in a 'sitting' position push.

The birthing chair (does not have legs) and can be used on the hospital bed, or on the floor. This is a similar squat position but very good if you have an epidural and can not support your legs to stand (your team will help you onto the chair), this helps the baby's descent. You have a nice wide open stance, no pressure to your bottom, and if you have an epidural, it will support you, while pushing. The birthing chair is similar to a toilet and squatting which is ideal for a baby that is making their way downwards. Or on the bed and laying sideways and with help to lift and or support your leg onto the squat bar, is another great position for pushing.

I have been with clients that push on a birthing chair. Then they lean over and catch their baby! It is extraordinary to watch.

Care Providers will ask if they can help stretch the tissues while you are pushing? This is done wearing sterile gloves, the care provider will use lubricate gel, they will put the gel onto the area. With both hands they gently stretch the tissues of the bottom part of the perineum. It is effective in helping relax and stretch the area where baby's head will be coming through.

Each time you are asked to let your body do the work, you will be asked to stop pushing and pant (or not push at all). This is the time *not to have an aggressive push,* you should be encouraged to let go and allow *only* your uterus do the work! You will have been pushing strong, now when the head is about to deliver we need a *slow and gentle push through the perineum.* Slowing down your push allows your vaginal tissues time to stretch rather than tear.

For the curious and to stay motivated, you might ask if you could feel the baby's head between your legs or look and see the head in a mirror.

Delivery is Imminent: *Gentle pushing and panting when the baby's head is crowning; you will be asked to pant*!! When the contraction starts, you will be having slow and deep breathing. During the peak of the contraction, you will feel the urge to push strongly. It is important to take shallow breaths in and exhale, using short 'huff' noises. With every push, you will do 3 huffs as you breathe out and then another breath in. Keep your chin up; it makes it easier *not* to push. Often people can be out of control at this time and keep pushing too strongly. If the push is too strong at the end, it gives the effect of the baby bursting out of the perineum, the results in a very bad tear. You will end up having a second or third-degree tear that will need a big repair. To prevent this, list to the person asking you to Pant Pant Pant! The care provider and support people will remind you to pant. Low *humming* as opposed to a scream. Screaming does not work to push your baby; it may feel like it releases pain, but if your birth helpers can help you to focus on the next push by humming and then start to breathe, it helps you control the next push. You do not need to scream and have sore vocal cords for the next few days. Breathe and pant three times, repeat and repeat.

Huff Huff Huff, or silently Blow Blow Blow (just use your breath)

If you do not have an epidural, the Ring of Fire is very real. When your perineum is stretched to the limit, it truly feels like it is burning. This is also when your baby is almost delivered.

Your care provider will put a warm compress on your perineum to relax and protect the tissues from tearing as the head delivers. There will be guidance to stop pushing when the head is crowning, and you will be asked to gently breathe your baby out (to ensure less tearing). Your baby's head needs to gently and slowly stretch the tissues, then deliver.

Fun Fact: When you are in close proximity to a room where a birthing person is without an epidural, you can tell by the sounds they are making, their screams and loud grunting that they are pushing with each contraction. This is when I go and close the door to our room. So my client does not get frightened by the screaming loud noises.

After your baby's head is delivered, the rest of the baby's body will follow shortly. The baby's airway will be cleared if necessary. If you've had an uncomplicated delivery, your health care provider will put baby on your tummy and will wait a few seconds to a few minutes before the umbilical cord is cut. Delaying clamping and cutting the umbilical cord after delivery increases the flow of nutrient-rich blood from the cord, back to the baby. This increases the baby's iron stores and reduces the risk of anemia, promoting healthy development and growth.

LABOR stalls care providers will watch and monitor both of you all through your labor and especially in the later stages of labor. How you and your baby are tolerating the labor. There are many reasons why your cervix does not dilate to 10 cm:

- If your baby or you are not responding in the usual way expected in labor.
- Labor is not progressing, and contractions slow down.
- The cervix does not dilate to 10 cm, and nothing has worked so far to increase the dilation.
- The baby's position, OP (not the most ideal position), and they will not turn.
- The baby's head circumference is too big.
- The baby's head is Asynclitic, which is not an ideal position.
- The baby is tired and not tolerating labor.
- You are tired and not tolerating labor.
- The baby may appear to be in peril.
- Baby is squeezing the cord.
- The cord is around the baby's neck or other parts of their body (more than once).
- The baby has a hand up by their face and is not descending far enough for delivery.
- The head is not applied to the cervix.
- Pelvis is 'Lucy' shaped (looks like a heart) and will not fit the baby through.
- Baby gets tired and shows signs of stress.
- Bags of water are still intact; the care providers will suggest AROM.

You may not deliver your baby vaginally; there are many reasons or complications that are often not known until the baby delivers, usually in the operating room.

Many time there are interventions taken to find out what is happening and to increase contractions or assess your labor. The whole team of care providers, will come into the birthing suite to try to assess and find out why. You and your baby will have been closely watched and monitored all through out your labor. If you or baby are not responding very well or progressing the expected way, that the birthing person does not dilate to 10 cm they can not push out a baby. There is the operating room that your Care Providers will recommend you to have your baby - via forceps, vacuum or a cesarean section.

AROM: Artificial Rupture of Membranes is when the bags of water are still intact and when contractions have slowed down, and care providers want to augment (increase) contractions or expedite delivery. The result is to artificially release and/or break the amniotic fluid from the sac, that is, keeping your baby's head from coming down farther into the pelvis resulting in increasing your contractions and making the needed change to the cervix. The Care Provider first will examine the cervix to see if it is at least 5 cm dilated and then have a good feel of where the baby's head is positioned and if it is well applied to the cervix or not. The conditions should be ideal so the cord can not slide out when the waters are released.

The person will lay on their back, legs bent, heels together, and knees apart, the same position as a vaginal exam. The care provider takes the amniotic hook (it looks like a long plastic knitting needle), puts the hook between their two fingers, and inserts fingers up towards the bag of water. They wait for a contraction or two and then 'hook' the bags of water in the hopes of popping the sack. It may take a couple of times because the bag is strong but not too difficult to pop. There is usually a small amount of fluid, approximately 1/2 cup, and then after the bag of water is released, you should have a smaller amount of fluid discharge with every contraction.

The baby's heart rate is watched closely for any drops, because their head, literally drops, into the pelvis and it can startle them. The fluid that comes out is carefully watched, the care providers watch to make sure there is no color in the waters - it they are not 'clear', they may be light or dark brown or green, or yellow, it can indicates the baby has meconium (had a poo) in the birth sack. It is more common for baby to have a poo when they over the due dates, or when they are a bit stressed, usually from the labor.

The procedure is fast, and you do not feel anything; the sensation is usually similar to if you have peed or wet the bed. This is very effective in giving you much stronger contractions straight away, as the head puts pressure on the cervix. Usually, when there is meconium in the amniotic water, a Paediatrician is called ahead of delivery to come in the room for delivery to ensure there is no stimulation to the baby in case when they take the first breath, they can ingest some of the meconium fluids into their lungs. I have often seen when the baby comes out wailing, the Paediatrician waves goodbye and leaves the room. However, it is extremely serious that if the baby gets any of the amniotic fluid with meconium in the lungs, they could have serious repercussions. So the Paediatrician will monitor the baby and is needed put a tiny catheter into the baby's throat or stomach to suck out any unwanted fluids and tend to all of their needs if this occurs.

Episiotomy: These are *not* routinely done in my part of the birthing world. I *only* see them done when the baby is stressed and needs to be delivered *quickly*. The care provider has already tried to stretch the perineum by putting warm water pads on the perineum and stretching the tissues with gel. They use a very small and sharp pair of scissors. They choose the spot to make a small cut. The fear is that a tear can be much bigger than a guided cut and a hand placed at the perineum to ensure not too fast of a delivery.

Care providers want this also, but if needed, they will try to repair the area as well as possible, as if there was no tearing. It is common that first-time pushing people can have tight tissues. With a warm compress and guidance, we try to encourage you to gently push your baby through.

You are going to the Operating Room: Your labor may not be progressing, meaning your cervix is not dilating to 10 cm, which means your body is not responding and/or you are not tolerating labor, or the baby is not tolerating labor. There are many many reasons why you are leaving the delivery suite:

- The baby's heart rate is low or high.
- Other signs that the baby is not tolerating labor.
- Signs that you are not tolerating labor.
- You have a high temperature.
- The baby is not going to be born vaginally.
- Labor has stalled. Your cervix is not progressing, even after the membrane is broken.
- The amniotic bag ruptured for a long time.
- The cervix is not dilating.
- Fetal distress - baby is showing signs they are no longer tolerating labor.
- Fetal distress - baby has been holding their cord or is wrapped in the cord.

I have written about *what* happens when someone goes into the operating room for delivery in the *Procedures chapter.*

If you are in the OR to deliver a baby, here are some tips:

- Bring your phone to take pictures or a small camera.
- With permission, you can take in a speaker for music.
- The environment is sterile, cool and bright.
- The staff is professional and efficient.

- They work under pressure every day.
- They are confident; they have done the procedure many times.
- If you go in for a forceps delivery, you will need to push the placenta out.
- If it is a Caesarean Section delivery, they will make sure the entire placenta is removed.
- While the Doctors finish the procedure, you may have your baby on your chest.
- If you are too tired from exhaustion, you may nap.
- If you nap, the partner can cuddle the baby.
- The lying down position is difficult to hold the baby.
- People often experience shaking (like shivering) from the medications.
- When the baby is born and cries, they are allowed to go straight to you for a cuddle.
- If doctors expect the baby may not thrive at delivery, there may be a crew of Paediatricians, doctors and nurses in the OR that will tend to your baby.
- When the baby cries and sounds healthy, the Paediatricians will leave the operating room.
- If the baby needs some attention at delivery, they will go straight to the Paediatrician in the room and have the baby checked.
- If something serious is suspected, there may be a crew of baby doctors and nurses to attend the baby immediately.
- If needed, your baby will be taken to the NICU (neonatal intensive care unit).
- APGAR Scores are done for the baby (explained in chapter BORN).
- You will have had a long labor, possibly with an epidural and the drugs you have had in the delivery suite, in additional drugs the Anesthetist administers for your procedure.

- The Obstetrician will ensure that all repairs are done, and when you are ready to go to the recovery area, both you and the baby to have one-on-one care.
- Paediatricians are asked into every birthing suite for delivery, and if the baby is crying loud and moving around, the Paediatricians and Nurses from the NICU leave the room.
- Partners are encouraged to go with the baby to watch the exam and put the first diaper on the baby. The baby station at the back of the operating room can do many tests or help the baby to breathe easier or if suction is needed or oxygen is needed.
- Paediatrician, Care Provider or Obstetrician or Midwife can do the 1-hour baby check.
- The baby check is head to toe; make sure all their body parts, toes and fingers are counted. Babies are measured head to toe, head circumference and then weighed.
- If you are in the operating room because it is suspected that the baby may have ingested meconium, they will put a tub down the baby to suction any meconium.

If the baby needs special care, they will be taken to the NICU for more testing or extra care, as needed. The partner is usually allowed to follow the baby to the NICU, and the birthing person will follow when they come out of the recovery room.

Author's Note: Meeting up with a multip client at the hospital, who is in active labor. They have a vaginal exam and are 3 cm. Our hospital is very busy, the client needs to be at least 4 cm to be admitted, we stay in the assessment room. I get my clients active, bouncing on a ball or dancing. Their bodies become *very* active and they start too feeling 'pushy', I call for the nurse and the client has another vaginal exam, they are 9 cm and trying to push. We have to run down the hall to a delivery suite, and they can deliver within a hand full of pushes. Sometimes we have a baby in the assessment room.

Fun Facts:

- Labor and the outcome of delivery are *Never* the same or predictable from one to the next pregnancy. There are huge variations in how labor starts, and the progress from labor to delivery can be different. Each different human grows in your belly or the possibility of the birthing parent with a different partner or a different surrogate. Outcomes are never predictable.
- It does not matter the size of your hips. It is the size of your pelvis, which is impossible to know until you have delivered. I have seen people with tiny and narrow hips have a fast labor and delivery. These people are more likely to have their baby at home, or on the side of the road, in their car.
- Complications will be taken care of, do not worry about them beforehand.
- There may be many changes and exceptions in the moment. Believe and trust your team of care providers and helpers to do what is best for the baby and yourself.
- Your heart expands with the second (or subsequent) just as easily as the first baby.
- Your question to yourself is, Can I love this one as much as the first baby?
- The second baby looks so small, or the first baby looks so big.

"Mother's job is to dilate

Baby's job is to rotate."

Unknown Author

Chapter 25: Born

Baby is Here!

BIRTH ~ ***The moment the baby is born and takes their first breath and cries, you will let out a sigh of relief (I hear it all the time)***

Third stage ~ Delivery of Placenta: You have just pushed strong and long and *Birthed* your baby into this world. You watch with anticipation as the care provider lifts your baby up and rests them on your chest to cuddle. All your focus shifts to seeing and meeting your sweet baby for the first time, and the first cuddle is spectacular! When you start to talk to your baby, they will look up at you, the voice they know and connect your voice to your face. The pain from the crazy and intense contractions stops when the baby delivers.

I have been telling people for years that meeting your baby is the single, most important day of your life!

If you are interested, ask to see the placenta, it is really quite fascinating, the care provider will show you the inside of the sac, where your baby swished around, then the outside of the placenta and the 'Tree of Life" where all the veins that nourished your baby are very pronounced, this is definitely worth a picture.

Umbilical Cord: It has two arteries that carry carbon dioxide rich blood and waste away from the baby to the placenta to be purified and one vein that carries oxygen nutrient-rich blood from the placenta to the baby. This is how your baby receives 'food' and oxygen in your uterus, and then waste products are moved away. The cord can be either long or short and is a fairly small tube that looks like a large rubber band. It is attached at one end, where your baby's belly button will be, and the cord's end naturally dries, shrivels, and then falls off. The other end of the cord is attached to the placenta (soon to be delivered). Clients have often asked me if their baby will have an 'innie or an 'outie', I can only say, you will not find out until the cord falls off.

Author's Fun Fact: The cord can be very long, up to several feet. This is a bit of a toy for babies in utero; they get themselves wrapped up in the cord. I have seen the cord around their neck several times. Those births end up in the operating room because the heart rate had many decelerations, meaning the baby's heart rate would have fluctuated. Or I have seen it wrapped around the foot several times (like the image of the baby at the end of this chapter), or the baby will come out and have their hand clenched around the cord.

Many care providers practice delayed cord cutting, where the cord stops pulsing, usually by two minutes. Your baby will be placed on your upper chest/tummy area. Delaying the cut gives the cord blood a chance to move into the baby's body, and the care provider can 'milk' the blood towards the baby's body, then cut. There are times that the care providers must cut it immediately, for instance, when the baby is not breathing properly and needs quick attention from a Paediatrician.

When the cord has stopped pulsing, the care provider will ask either of the parents or a helper if they want to cut the cord. Otherwise, they will cut it themselves. I have had the privilege of cutting the cord many times. Often the partner or the birthing person cut the cord, but it is definitely okay to decline this procedure; the care provider will gladly cut the cord for you.

They clamp near the baby's belly and another clamp about 3 cm away from the baby. With scissors, someone will cut the umbilical cord. The cord is large, rubbery, and thick like an elastic band; a few times cutting are necessary to finalize the cut, and there may be some cord blood that drops onto your tummy and is wiped away. I mention this incase the person cutting is not good at seeing blood.

Before you go home, you will be given lots of instruction on keeping the cut cord, now a stump with a clamp on it, to stay clean and dry at the base with a cotton swab. At home, it will dry up and turn a dark brown or dark red and will shrivel up and drop off. This should happen within the first 7 - 12 days. Care providers may advise to only sponge bath and not bathe your infant in a tub until the cord comes off on its own. When changing a diaper, try to remember to put the cord up and on the outside of the diaper.

*Please note that if there is any yellow or white discharge, redness, swelling or a few drops of blood, call your doctor straight away just to make sure everything is healing properly.

At delivery, you were given an injection of oxytocin, and you were most likely oblivious to the fact. The placenta starts to separate from the wall of the uterus and you may be asked to give a few more pushes to help with the delivery of the placenta. It is usually very easy to push the placenta out because there are no bones, and the placenta is not very big compared to the size of your baby. It should come fairly easy with a few strong pushes and you are now an expert at pushing. The wait until the placenta is delivered typically takes from 5 to 15 minutes, but it can take up to 30 minutes.

Contractions stop when the baby and the placenta have been delivered, and you will still feel a more gentle tightening as the uterus tries to contract to its normal size. You most likely will be focused on your baby and ignore most everything else that is still happening in the delivery suite. If the placenta has not been delivered within fifteen or more minutes, you might be given more medication, *or* you can try to release your own natural oxytocin to help. You can start by having a few long kisses with your partner, rolling your nipples and, best of all, having the baby suckle on your nipple. In addition, do more of the Spleen 6 pressure points.

The placenta may move down itself, and you will only need a few gentle pushes, but sometimes you will be asked to push hard to help deliver the placenta. Your health care provider will examine the placenta to ensure it is intact and that there are no remaining fragments that might be left in the uterus. If this is the case and some part is left behind, then your uterus will not shrink back to normal, and this can lead to bleeding and infection. If the process lasts much longer or the care providers suspect there is some placenta that is left inside, they will advise you are going to the operating room for help to remove it.

Many people do not realize they are still having gentle tightenings because they are oblivious to what is going on around the delivery suite, especially down where baby came out. You will continue to have mild and less painful contractions that are close together. This helps your uterus to contract and gently get back to its normal size.

If the delivery was straightforward, the care provider would have put your baby onto your chest for an hour of skin-to-skin snuggling, both of you covered with a warm blanket. This is a great time for you and a designated person to take pictures of you and your partner staring at your new baby. Getting all of the first reactions of the baby meeting you, everything in the first hour of the baby's life is amazing. There is nothing better than meeting your new baby and you will likely feel a great sense of relief that baby is finally here. While cuddling baby in your arms, many babies will smell and try to wriggle themselves toward the nipple. Cherish every moment!

Here is why **Skin to Skin** within minutes of birth is very beneficial for you and your baby:

- Looking at each other - baby to parent.
- To keep the baby warm.
- Bonding starts at delivery.
- The baby puts your voice and face together.
- The baby and parents are now a family.

- The baby can smell and will move toward the breast to suckle.

If your baby is premature, it may be challenging for them to take the nipple into their mouth, as their mouth is tiny and/or they may not have the strength to suck effectively. They most likely will go to the NICU for a full check because it is imperative for the baby to have calories; they may need to have a feeding tube that will be inserted down into their stomach to ensure the baby gets what they need to thrive and grow.

Author's Note: I love to watch the baby at delivery and the first cuddle, when clients are talking to their baby, and the way the baby looks up at the parents quizzically. They are literally putting a *face to the voice.* Seeing each other for the first time is magical. I always try to get as many pictures of the new family as possible.

Born in the Caul (en caul) is when the baby is born in the bag of waters, it means your bag of waters did not break at delivery, and the Care Provider will most likely have to break the sack by putting a finger through the sack. This is rare but an amazing birth to watch! Many years ago, it was believed to be a mystical event, and people feared the baby and parent because it was so unique. I personally have seen these a handful of times, and to say they're magical is an understatement!

The first hour after your baby is born is a beehive of busyness. Many things happen that you may not be aware of. Your care provider uses this time to evaluate how the baby responds when born. When the baby is born, did they cry or scream at delivery? If so, you will be given your baby to cuddle skin-to-skin straight away. The baby has passed the first test of their life, called the APGAR score given when they are delivered.

This is a visual and touch score given to your baby upon delivery and again 5 minutes after delivery. The care provider that delivers your baby is watching for their skin color - heart rate - reflex irritability - muscle tone - breathing rate, and effort, with five categories that are each given a top score of 2 for each category. 10 out of 10 being the best score.

Most babies score between 8 - 10, or if the baby has had a difficult delivery, they may have a lower score. If the score is 6 or less, they will need immediate attention from the paediatricians and possibly have to go to the NICU.

Apgar Sign	**Score = 0**	**Score = 1**	**Score = 2**
Appearance (skin color)	Bluish gray or pale all over	Normal color (but hands and feet are bluish)	Normal color all over (hands and feet are pink)
Pulse (heartrate)	Absent (no pulse)	Below 100 beats per min.	Normal (above 100 beats per min.)
Grimace (reflex irritability)	Absent (no response to simulation)	Facial movement only (grimace) with stimulation	Pulls away, sneezes, coughs, or cries with stimulation
Activity (muscle tone)	No movement, floppy tone	Arms & legs flexed with little movement	Active, spontaneous movement

Respiration (breathing rate & effort)	Absent (no breathing	Slow or irregular breathing, weak cry	Normal rate and effort, good cry

If there is a specific reason to have a paediatrician at the delivery, the baby will go straight to the bassinet at the back of the room for a thorough check from the doctor. Possibly there was meconium in the amniotic fluid, and the baby might ingest some of the fluid at delivery. Or the baby has been showing signs of distress with a high or low heart rate before delivery, the doctor will do a full *baby check* as soon as the baby is delivered.

The Perineum: After delivery, your care provider will assess your perineum (the area where the baby came out) to determine whether you need a repair from a tear. The majority of people often need some repair, and it can be a very small one that needs one or two stitches or more, which might take 5 - 10 minutes, depending on the difficulty. Your care provider will give the area some freezing, and then they will not rush this part as it is very intricate to put things back together the same as it was. If you have an epidural, you may have good or some coverage, but many people still may need some local anesthetic, which is injected into the area where the stitches will go. An option for people without an epidural is to try nitrous oxide - the gas during the procedure. The care provider will do a needle test; they touch your skin, where they will be stitching, and if needed, they will give you more anesthetic in the area.

If the severity or 'degree' of the tear, it can take up to half an hour for the repair. When the repair is done, your care provider will explain to you how the repair went, whether it was difficult or easy, whether it was a first-degree or up to a fourth-degree tear. They will say it came together nicely or they will advise you need to be careful, and you will be given instructions, on how to take care of this area. The stitches will disintegrate, you do not have to have them taken out.

Intact Perineum: The goal is always for you to have an Intact Perineum; it means no tear, and it can be very hard to achieve! With a first baby, the push can be very long, and when crowning, to allow the tissues to stretch, a warm compress on the perineum is helpful, it softens and helps stretch tissues. Once your tissues have stretched, with subsequent babies, you may achieve this the next time.

When done the nurse will clean the area, including fresh linen underneath you, then put some ice on the perineum for approximately ten minutes, this helps with the swelling of the area, from your pushing. You will stay there to cuddle your baby for approximately one hour. You and your partner are usually oblivious to most of what is going on, because you are cuddling and talking to your baby.

Your nurse should put a small plastic bag of ice wrapped in a face cloth, to put onto your perineum, or you can have a couple of sanitary pads with Witch Hazel (pre frozen), to put onto your perineum for ten minutes at a time, you should only have to apply two or three times. This will help calm the swelling around the bruised tissues in that area from the long hours of staining to push and you may have hemorrhoids from having to push for a long time or if you had an Instrumental delivery or a tear at the perineum.

When you are back at home, put some Witch Hazel on your sanitary napkin but not frozen as you did in the hospital. Place the pad in your underwear to help heal a tear where the stitches are, or if you had a cesarean section, put it onto the incision after a week, or if forceps delivery, put the witch hazel afterwards on your perineum (where the stitches are). This product helps to heal cuts and bruises faster than most other products, but does not sting your skin or tissues.

Several checks for you while you hold the baby. They take your blood pressure and redo this for the first hour. At delivery, your nurse will have asked for your consent to have an injection of Oxytocin on your outer hip as the baby's head is delivering. This is precautionary, and it will help give the uterus some extra strength to expel the placenta within the first 15 to 30 minutes after the baby delivers. When it is time for you to push your placenta out, it is often fairly easy and comes out within a couple of minutes; it is not like pushing your baby out. Your uterus may have become tired after a long labor or a long pushing stage. The nurse or care providers will be very diligent in pushing on your fundus to make sure it is retracting and becoming firm. It is very uncomfortable to have them press on your abdomen, but it is very important in helping your uterus contract and expel any blood clots. If they are not successful in getting all of the blood clots out, or a part of the placenta is left inside, they will know because your uterus is not firming up and you are still bleeding (this would indicate a retained placenta).

The Obstetrician may be called to the delivery suite if they believe that part of the placenta is not delivered at the appropriate time and/or you are still bleeding too much. If you have an epidural or want to try without medication (it is very painful), they will put a hand into the vagina and try to extract the clot(s) and any remaining placenta still inside. However, if your uterus is not firming up and you are still bleeding, then you will be taken to the operating room for a D & C called a dilation and curettage. This is where the lower narrow part of the uterus is dilated, and the uterine lining is scraped with a curettage (a curette is a tiny spoon-shaped instrument) to remove any placenta tissue. In the operating room you will be given pain relief, if you do not already have an epidural that is working well. This does not take too long and is very successful in getting everything out. The other parent will be able to stay with the baby until you are back to your post partum room.

Bleeding after delivery is normal and can have mucous, tissue and blood that the womb sheds. Normal bleeding can last 24 to 36 days. If there is any heavy bleeding or you pass a lot of large blood clots anytime in the first 24 hours, and even after you are back at home, you need to call your Doctor or go back to the hospital. You may be having a post partum haemorrhage. The fundus should be around your belly button after delivery, then it should start to decrease, approximately 1 cm every 24 hours. At one week post partum your fundus should be at your pubic bone.

If later on at home and any part of the placenta was left in the uterus, you can have very serious complications. Watch for any indications that might include a fever, foul smelling discharge, heavy bleeding, pain or pieces of tissue coming out of the vagina. Tell your care provider straight away and they will ask you to go to the hospital or into their office.

If the placenta has been delivered and your uterus is firm, the nurse will be taking your blood pressure every fifteen minutes, and watching your general health for the first hour.

Then you will be asked to get up to void your bladder at one hour after delivery. You can take this moment to wash up, possibly shower and then get back to your bed and have cuddle time with baby.

Author's Story: I was at a birth where the partner asked if they could cut off a tiny piece of the placenta and eat it. The person had a huge curiosity of *what things tasted like* and wanted permission to try it, I now know placenta has no flavor (and yes watching it made some of us cringe).

Why you might have a Hemorrhage:

- Long labor
- Short labor but very intense labor

- Uterine infection
- Uterine fibroids
- Placental abruption
- Placenta previa
- Distended uterus (twins or more delivered)
- Induction or augment of labor with oxytocin
- Delivery in OR: vacuum, forceps or cesarean section

Author's Note: Some people want to take the placenta home to put in their garden. I have heard that a garden can grow very lush with pieces of placenta underneath the roots in the ground.

Some people want to have the placenta encapsulated. You will have hired the person that will do this process for you. Your partner should contact the person, as soon as you have delivered and ask them to come and pick up the placenta as soon as possible. You should have everything necessary at the hospital with you, for the transport of the placenta. The placenta should be put in a plastic bag and then stored in a small container that holds both the ice and the placenta, you will need to keep the placenta cool until someone comes to pick it up from you. The placenta can not be stored in a hospital fridge.

Author's Note: There does not seem to be enough definitive evidence that ingesting these capsules works in the way they are promoted (I do not have an opinion on this process).

There is another fabulous idea, but you must be prepared and bring supplies to the hospital. You will need several pieces of white paper just after delivery and supplies at the ready for someone to help with this project. Your designated person will place the 'vein' side of the placenta onto the paper, then put the paper aside to dry. When the sheet(s) are dry, have a large manila envelope to bring it home in. This can go into a picture frame or into your baby's birth book. They are stunning! The vein side will look like the 'Tree of Life'.

A member of your health care team will massage your abdomen many times in the first couple of hours, this helps the uterus contract and decreases the possibility of bleeding and helps your uterus continue to return to its normal size.

Baby Facts: This is a big transition time for a baby; you may notice the following, so ask your care providers before you start to worry; they can explain further.

- Baby at delivery has 'bluish' hands and feet. This is normal, and it can take a few days for the baby to have a full circulation of their extremities. The skin on their body and face tends to have a rosier complexion. When they cry, their face can appear quite red; this is normal
- Baby's breathing can be irregular, then followed by a short period where they hold their breath, then you hear a deep shuttering breath. This can be a bit disturbing but know it is common.
- Baby may have a lot of mucous from their mouth or their nose, they are clearing what was in their lungs and nasal passages, and separately, they may have hiccups. Tilt the baby's head back and, lower their body, rub their back to help bring up any mucous. Wait a few seconds, and then bring them back to a normal upright position.
- Baby's head may look a bit odd, coming through the birth canal. Their head does some molding, and it will return to its natural shape within a couple of days. There are two soft spots on babies' heads, a large diamond shape on the top of the head, and it may take up to eighteen months to completely fuse. Then the smaller triangle at the back of the head should take two to six months to fuse.
- The membranes covering the fontanels are thick and tough, so brushing or washing the scalp will not hurt the baby. Common sense would be 'not to push into this area'.

- Try not to bundle the baby too tightly. They do like to wiggle. They may prefer to have their arms out of the blanket, or some babies prefer the security of arms bundled inside the blanket. Your baby will usually dictate their preference, so do not worry too much about this. Your baby may fuss more, not having their way. What is important is you should tuck the blanket under their back, arms in or out.

Feeding the baby after delivery: It can be very difficult in the first hour while laying on the delivery bed because *you are not* in an ideal position to feed the baby. You have decided on chest or bottle feeding for the first feeding after delivery. You are often laying still while having a repair done to your perineum, but babies are very intuitive. They know to wiggle their way and find the nipple and suckle. If needed, have someone help you to put the baby in a position close to the nipple and see what your baby does. It is so sweet to watch! Have someone put a warm blanket from the hospital warmers over the birthing person and baby to keep them snuggled up and warm.

Baby is not 'hungry' at delivery; they instinctually find the nipple and try to latch and suckle.

Once they suckle, they want to go to the nipple often, and it will signal to your brain that it is time to start producing milk. This ensures that the baby has enough for their nutritional needs, which should *come in* sometime in the next three days or more. Colostrum is the first 'milk' that you have in the chest. It is golden yellow, thick and sticky. I tell clients it is like 'Astronaut' food (the small packages of concentrated food they eat). Your baby will get a small amount of colostrum in the first few days, which is perfect because their tummy at birth is the size of a cherry; it explains why the baby wants to suckle or 'eat' every three hours. Colostrum changes over the first few days into mature milk, that is usually a murky white and not too dense. The colostrum satisfies the baby but also helps to cleanse the meconium, the first couple of blackish or dark brown bowel movements that are in their system.

Latching is unique to you and baby, with each different baby you may have, they will latch in their own way and in their own time. There can be many reasons why a baby is slow to the nipple, but they usually try within the first 24 hours. *Have patience!*

Do not be discouraged with the first feeding after baby is delivered, they are often very tired, as you are. On the 3rd day of birth, your milk should 'come in' or it is called 'mature milk'. Most importantly for feeding a baby, we need to have patience for when you try to put baby to the nipple, you are both learning how to achieve a good latch. You will be able to ask doctors and nurses in the post partum ward, everyone will have many chest feeding tips and they are happy to help and advise.

Author's Tip: Take all of the advise that you are given by hospital staff, family and friends. If it does not work today, keep the knowledge and as baby gets a few days or weeks older, try the advise again. Baby grows quickly and their brain is learning just as fast.

The one-hour baby check: This is usually done in the delivery suite, in a warmed bassinet. The baby will be checked head to toe by the care provider, or if a paediatrician is in the room, they will do this exam. They check the baby's reflexes and make sure all their parts, their throat, eyes, ears, anus and everything is there; sometimes they find out it works perfectly well because the baby has a bowel movement or pee's on the care provider. The head circumference and length of the baby are measured, then, that special moment you find out how much your baby weighs, they will put the baby on a scale, and this is a very important picture-worthy moment. Baby is brought back to the warmer, and I encourage the partner to put the first diaper on the baby (you may have to ask the care provider before they go ahead and put the diaper on the baby). This is a meaningful moment for the parent, especially when they have never done it before. It is easy, really, and the most important parts of diapering are to make sure the clamped cord is up and above the diaper, and always make sure that if there is a penis, it must be facing down so as not to have a wet baby.

Author's Tip: When you are about to take the diaper off a baby that has a penis, do so very gingerly, and have another diaper handy. That quick whoosh of cold air can make for a fountain, and the baby will immediately pee straight up in the air or towards the baby's head or the wall behind them. Also, make sure the diaper is secure around the leg, but not too tight. If it is too loose, you will find poo all over the area where your baby is lying.

The first couple of times baby has a bowel movement, it is called meconium, and it is blackish and slimy. It has been recommended you use a water resistant cream on their bottom where the meconium or urine may cover. It makes for a much easier wipe, meconium is very sticky on baby's skin. Their skin is sensitive and can become raw very quickly from all of the wiping.

The disposable diaper has tabs and they should be on the bottom side, you place baby's bottom on the diaper and the tabs open up and with the other half of diaper comes between the legs and tabs are attached across the tummy area of the diaper.

It may be necessary to quickly take the soiled diaper away as you put the new one under the baby's bottom. Sometimes when the diaper is very soiled fold over the top half of diaper leaving it under baby, proceed to clean baby's bottom and then slide a new diaper under baby's bottom and take away the soiled one at the same time. It sounds difficult, and it is, but with all the practice you will get, you will perfect it quickly. Sorry, but in the beginning I would be lying if I said, changing diapers was easy. You have to find the best way for you to take away and put a clean one, all without your baby soiling the new diaper, themselves or you. Yes they can soil more business as you put the new one down. Expect 10 - 12 diaper changes in an average days and this is also a learning moment for the partner who may not have done this before, and more pictures of that!

Author's Tip: I encourage the partner/new parent to talk to their baby. They will look up at you (the voice they know) and will stop crying, and your baby will grasp your finger when you put your finger into your baby's hand. A very magical moment!

Important: *Skin-to-Skin is important and improves chest feeding success*

Frequent and early feeding or hand expressing helps stimulate milk production.

The goal in the first 24 hours is 6 or more feeds.

The baby may not appear interested, *yet, they may be as tired as you.*

The goal in the second 24 hours and beyond is 8 or more active feedings.

The baby may appear fussy and/or cluster feed.

All of the above helps to stimulate milk production.

When the baby is put to the nipple, it helps relieve the fulness and discomfort of a full breast and helps prevent engorgement but keep in mind that if too full, the baby will pull off because they have gotten a gush of milk.

Decreases newborn crying and stress.

Stabilizes heart rate, respiration rate and temperature.

Improves newborn immunity and decreases the risk of infection.

Assists in developing the parents' confidence.

Decreases security risks.

Provides soothing to baby during procedures such as administration of Vitamin K needle and newborn screening for the baby.

After delivery, there will be some routine tests in the first 24 hours of your baby's life that are hospital protocols and routinely given. If you have forgotten why you might have wanted to decline, discuss this with your care providers, they can explain the procedure and give you their advice.

- Erythromycin, eye ointment treatment, from the baby coming through the birth canal. This is put in the baby's eye within the first hour of delivery. It is done to prevent eye infections caused by the possibility that chlamydia and gonorrhea are in the birth canal, leading to possible blindness.
- Vitamin K injection is recommended for all newborns and is given to a baby within the first hour old. This helps to supplement the low level of vitamin K, which can lead to serious bleeding problems. This injection is given in the baby's left thigh when they are cuddled up with a parent.
- A bilirubin screening blood test is to measure for high bilirubin levels, which can cause jaundice in the first few days of their life. This appears two to four days after the baby's delivery, and then it should start to decrease and go away when the baby is two weeks old. You will notice a faint yellow color on their skin and in the whites of their eyes. Your baby may have testing to measure their bilirubin levels at hospital. This is done by taking a small sample of blood from the baby's heel. If levels are high, baby may need treatment to prevent any serious problems. The baby would be treated in hospital with phototherapy by putting them under special blue light which penetrates the skin and destroys the bilirubin.

- Hearing screen test, with a small rubber probe - into the baby's ear to check the baby's hearing. This is for early detection of problems of hearing if treatment might be needed. This is in place to help prevent speech and language delay when your baby is older.
- Newborn Screening tests or PKU testing for metabolic disorders that could cause lifetime mental disability if not identified and treated soon. This is given approximately 24 hours after delivery. While you are holding your baby, this is usually given by a nurse, and they will prick the baby's heel for a drop of blood. The results will confirm whether the baby does or does not have any of the 24 rare but treatable conditions. This early identification and care can be managed when treated early.
- Kangaroo care: This is good for the partner after delivery, in case there is a repair or the birthing person has to go to the OR for bleeding and other times. For the person holding and cuddling baby skin-to-skin and have someone with a warm blanket/sheet from the hospital warmer, you lean forward with the baby in your arms, have the helper fold the ends of the blanket behind you, and then you sit back. This makes a sweet cocoon for cuddling with both you and your baby.

Within an hour after a vaginal delivery, your nurse will want you to get out of bed to try to void your bladder. This may not be possible if you had an epidural and if your legs are still restricted from supporting you to stand. When you do go to the washroom, the nurse will give you small squirt bottles that are filled with warm water to rinse the perineum. Your nurse may allow you to have a shower and then get into a clean hospital gown and back to baby for more cuddling, feeding or possibly a nap.

Your nurse and care providers will explain about perineal wash and sitz baths for your tender tissues 'down below' when voiding. Some hospitals have a sitz bath that can be used in the hospital and then taken home at discharge. They will talk about stool softeners because it is common to have hemorrhoids from the pushing and give you guidance about how to take care of *that* area. For your stay at the hospital, you will be given a small packet of ibuprofen for pain management after delivery and will be advised how often to take them.

A summary of delivery, you and the baby are physically separated at birth, but their energy and emotional systems are still intricately interconnected with you.

What about those hormones! You grow an organ, the placenta, then after labor, it is expelled from your body. Your hormone levels will drop dramatically and begin a months-long process of recalibration, from growing and birthing a baby to now nursing a baby and helping your body recover. Hormones start to shift rapidly, from pregnancy mode, to chest-feeding mode (if that is your choice). There are endorphins swirling around inside for about forty-eight hours, and then they start to leave your body. The progesterone and estrogen levels are decreasing fast, it is like our body is flushing itself of the 'make a baby hormones' to 'we need to produce milk for baby hormones.'

Between 48 hours and 2 weeks, postpartum may start to be obvious, and it is very normal to be weepy and emotional, more commonly known as the baby blues; this may be the start of a time called post partum depression. Sometimes, hormone imbalances, autoimmune disorders, isolation and lack of support can look like depression. I will talk more about postpartum depression in the next chapter.

Thank your team of care providers. They work hard during their long shifts. They can see a variety of birth scenarios, some trauma and other times fun and exciting moments, all the while helping people during a single work day. They are human also, with a life at home that steps in their way, but you will never expect that they process 'their stuff' and put it on a shelf, so they can come to work and help the next birthing person. Every new day for you at the hospital, you may have a change of staff, delivery nurses, then, postpartum nurses. They are very special people. Please respect them and talk kindly to your team.

Ask your team about your birth journey and ask any and all questions regarding your labor. Sometimes the 'way' our baby was delivered can cause you worry, frustration, or anger. Later on when you get home, you may want to thank them. The doctor should come in the next day, but the nurse may go off shift and not be back for the next few days. Before being discharged from the hospital, try to glean as much information about your baby's delivery as possible. Midwives and doulas can talk to you afterward at a postpartum appointment to fill in some of the gaps that you most likely will forget fairly fast.

How long is a Hospital stay? For the first baby, you usually stay in the hospital for 24 hours or up to three days, depending on how you deliver. If you had a fairly easy and short delivery, with no or little complications, you might be able to go home within the first 24 hours. If complications occur, and especially if you deliver in the operating room for a Cesarean section or Forceps, you may be encouraged to stay three nights at the hospital.

If you had a second or third (or more) baby, and knowing your first delivery was fairly quick and uncomplicated, you may be able to leave the hospital after six hours of delivery **if** the baby, and you are both healthy; otherwise, you will need to stay longer. After you are discharged from the hospital and go home, you should have one more appointment with the person that delivered your baby. Your postpartum care will be transferred back to your regular doctor. Your baby will be followed up for six weeks with the midwife or doctor whom you had your prenatal care with. If needed and if your doctor does not take newborn babies, then you may have to look for a paediatrician as the baby grows.

For a birth that is difficult or where the baby requires special care with a Paediatrician in the NICU ‘neonatal intensive care unit’, your baby may have to stay at the hospital for several days or weeks. Depending on the hospital, you may be able to stay at the hospital for the first days, or you will have to commute from home daily to be with your baby.

Contact your postpartum nanny or postpartum doula or family members to tell them *when* you will be leaving the hospital and set up times to come to your home and help you.

Savor this special time with your baby. Your preparation, pain and effort have paid off. Revel in the miracle of birth.

The baby’s first bath in the hospital is not recommended. It is suggested to delay a bath until 24 hours after delivery or, for cultural reasons, to wait at least 6 hours. Preferably you should wait until you are at home because it is easier and with more access to your baby’s bathtub and counter space. In hospitals and for practicality, there is very restricted space for bathing a baby. More importantly, babies can not regulate their body temperature and can become cold and easily develop hypothermia and have some minor stress. An early bath can make some babies more likely to have a drop in their blood sugar levels. Your baby is not born dirty! They came from a sterile environment.

Some Fun Facts:

- Baby’s eyes will change color and take up to six months to come into their true color.
- Baby will have a reddish-purple look to extremities. This is normal and, in a few days, will be gone once the circulation gets up to speed and makes a change.
- Baby’s skin color may be paler at birth and can take up to six months or longer to fully come into its natural tone.

- Lanugo is the fine and soft hair that covers the body at birth; it may take three or four months to go away.
- Vernix, on some babies' skin, is a natural moisturizer and is usually left alone to soak back into their skin. Another thought if the baby has a lot, you can help by gently rubbing it into your baby's skin or onto your skin.
- I have seen *so much* vernix on baby's face that the care provider had to wipe it from their face, so the parent could see their face. Most people feel that it is beneficial to allow the vernix to be absorbed back into the skin naturally.

My Number One Tip - Sleep when Baby Sleeps!

Bonding with the baby by being skin-to-skin and early chest feeding are the most important things to accomplish in the first day or two of the baby's life. Listen to your gut and your heart; they will never steer you wrong in raising your baby.

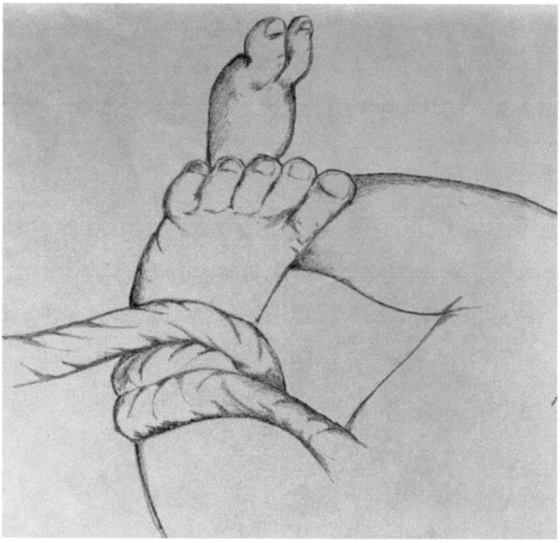

You have delivered your baby, the excitement starts now!

Congratulations, and I wish you much love in your life with your new baby(ies)

Born Still

Many people find out that they are pregnant after no or little tries. Other people have had difficulty getting pregnant and found help to become pregnant by having long IVF treatments, or they found the perfect surrogate; there are many options. No one goes into pregnancy thinking it will not have the best outcome possible - having a healthy baby. But…sometimes keeping a baby healthy in utero is difficult; they come too early. The care providers and parents have done all they can for a healthy pregnancy, but some babies don't *stay* when they are born. It may be that you knew ahead of time, or it happens that the baby passes at delivery or soon afterward.

Your reaction to a loss will affect you physically, mentally, emotionally and spiritually.

You may feel denial, disbelief, confusion, anger at yourself or others, guilt and blame. It is intense and cuts to the core of your soul. There are many intense emotions and a sense of nothingness. You should have brought home your baby, and yet you are left to sadness, depression, isolation, and trying to figure out if you will ever get back to you.

There is no easy way to talk to the parents when this happens to a baby(s) at delivery. I have been with clients and separately with family at the passing of their baby(s). This is an extremely sad experience and is beyond difficult, but helping them arrive and then ensuring the parents get as much time as possible with their baby is essential.

It is especially important to honor their time here. It may be unthinkable to hold and touch your baby skin-to-skin, but it should be encouraged for both parents to have as long of a time as it is necessary for you to say goodbye. Have someone take pictures of you and your partner with your baby. You do not need to look at pictures now, but pictures can be stored away for later or forever. Having someone bring in a hand & foot impression kit to make an imprint of the baby's hands and feet will make a very fond memory.

Talk to everyone that was at the labor and delivery about circumstances around the birth and passing. Write notes or record the conversation with the nurse or doctor. This grieving process can take from six months up to several years, but this trauma may never leave you. Hopefully, you can find gentle counseling to help both parents to grieve. From my observation, it is also essential for the other parent (that did not deliver) to be given the time and counseling needed as well. They can feel left out while they are suffering. If you can journal, like you did when you were first pregnant, with mementos (the card with the birth and delivery particulars, time and date of birth) and come back to them when you are ready, it can help you.

Author's Story: It was excruciating for all of us in the delivery suite when the birthing person looked up at us (knowing their baby would not live) and asked, "Did the baby take a breath?"

If your baby is born still or silent, I am so sorry for your loss. You may not feel like you can look at or hold this angel. But I know from personal family experience that it is very important to be given as much time as needed to cuddle, touch, hold your sweet baby, and yes, have someone take pictures. You may not want to look at the pictures for a long time, but they will be there when you decide, *you can look ~~*

Chapter 26: Quick Guide & Resources for Newborns

How often should I feed baby? It will depend on whether you feed with human milk or formula. Formula is heavier and will fill baby's tummy faster, a good judge of whether your baby is full, they stop drinking, if they take too much, they will throw it up. Please refer to Dr Jack Newman's chapter on Feeding Baby.

First week they should feed every 3 hours approximately, 24 hours per day. The range can be less time if they have a heavier feed, (formula is a heavy product) but more often for human milk.

Baby's tummy at birth is the size of a cherry, by day 2 a walnut, at one week an apricot, then by one month their tummy is the size of a large chicken egg.

Your baby will lose on average 7% of their birth weight in the first 3 days. From there on they should gain back 20 - 35 grams per day, and regain their birth weight at 10 to 14 days. Your Care Provider will weight your baby often to ensure they are growing at an acceptable weight in a certain time frame, and are thriving. For instance if baby loses 10% of their birth weight, in the first few days, they may ask you to supplement. So if you are Chest feeding, they would ask you to supplement with formula. After day 4 they should gain 20 to 35 grams per day, then regain their birth weight by day 10 - 14.

Storing Human Milk

Where	Temperature	Time
At room temperature	66 - 72 F 19 - 22 C	10 hours
In a Fridge	32 - 39 F 0 - 4 C	8 days
Freezer compartment inside a Fridge	Temperature will vary	2 weeks
Freezer compartment with a separate door	Temperature will vary	3-4 weeks
Separate Deep Freeze	0 (zero) F -19 C	6 months or longer

Baby has Gas, Constipation or Reflux: After your baby has eaten, to help relieve any gas that accumulates, try some of the following suggestions. If you wait too long, more than a half hour, your baby will tell you they are uncomfortable and start to cry or wiggle about in pain.

+ Have baby slightly angled back and supported on something, like a pillow, try to bring baby's knees up to their chest and back down again, gently repeating a few times.

+ Gently rub or make circles on their back, (I do not believe that you have to smack their back), they are so delicate, gentle pats on the back works wonders.

Baby Poo the first day or two, soiled diapers should be black or dark green and thick like tar, it is called meconium. Often with the first diaper and until meconium stops, people will put vaseline or diaper cream on baby's bottom to prevent it from sticking to their soft bottom and causing a raw skin rash these poos can last two to four days. Then as movements transition, from black to dark green or brown, the sticky consistency softens a bit, it changes over a few days to a week, usually when baby is getting into a good eating pattern. Then they should be at least 3 large and soft yellow diapers. Formula will be brown and stinky. Human milk looks like curds, and has no smell.

By the end of the first week, if you are chest feeding, the color can be bright yellow and watery, sometimes looks seedy or similar in looks to cottage cheese. If baby is being formula feed, their poo will be yellow brown, green brown or brown, and thick and firm, similar to peanut butter. If a combination of formula and chest milk, then the color may be brown or dark yellow poo. When baby starts to eat, infant foods their poo changes to browner, and becomes smelly.

As baby gets older and is eating baby foods, and if you notice changes in their poo, becoming a bit like diarrhea or very loose, or hard dark brown, similar to marbles or tiny logs, it may indicate that they are having a food intolerance; infection; or an allergy, it is best to seek more information from Baby's care provider, as they can become dehydrated and ill.

Pee At delivery, your newborn baby is put on your tummy, and they may pee and/or poo. They can 'go' many times in a day, and have 4 - 8 wet diapers a day. Tell your baby's doctor when they are not 'going' as often as they should. For wet diapers, there will be at least one for the first day of life, then increase one extra wet diaper for each day, until day 5, when they should be having 6 diapers per day. The color should be clear or pale yellow.

Hungry Babies give very clear cues in the first few months and once learned it will save you and baby from much stress and frustration. Babies are very in the moment, they need to be feed *now* or their diaper needs a change, or they are over tired. When they are left too long and have started crying, it is very difficult to console them and bring them back to calm. Early cues that Baby is hungry will be, putting their fingers or hand in their mouth and sucking or chewing motions. They will open their mouth and with their tongue, reach out and turn their head as if looking for the nipple to root.

IF a baby has to wait too long they get frustrated and will cry loudly, arch their back and it can be very hard to settle them, and have them go to the nipple. They need to be calmed first.

Consoling the Baby: Wrap or bundle the baby in a light blanket, sit on your exercise ball (from pregnancy), cuddle your baby and start to gently bounce on the ball. Then start to talk, sing or hum to your baby, at a greater level - as they are crying, enough for them to hear you, but not being too overpowering. You will know you have it right because they will stop crying, and listen to you. Keep bouncing until they are settled, and then take care of their needs.

La Leche League Canada. www.lalecheleaguecanada.ca or www.llli.org

Low Milk Production by Diana West. www.lowmilksupply.org

NEVER - Ever shake a baby to settle them; they *do not respond* to being shaken out of their crying fit. You can easily shake and damage their brain. There is a time, usually in the early evenings when they seem to be restless and can not settle into a nap, even after feeding or having cuddles. This has nothing to do with you or what you have or have not done. They are tired and ‘beside themselves,’ and nothing but patience will win. This is a good time to suggest someone else help to rock them or bounce on the ball with them and for you go and take a break. It can be frustrating when trying to soothe them and then you become anxious, your baby can pick up any anxiety in the room, and they do not know what it is or how to process these feelings.

For more information, I would encourage you to take a look at this website dedicated to describing what PURPLE Crying is, http://www.dontshake.ca

P is Peak of Crying. Your baby may cry more each week, the most in month 2, then less in months 3 – 5.

U is Unexpected Crying can come and go and you do not know why.

R is Resists Soothing; your baby may not stop crying no matter what you try.

P is Pain-Like Face Crying; babies may look like they are in pain, even if they are not.

L is Long Lasting Crying can last as much as 5 hours a day or more.

E is Evening; your baby may cry more in the late afternoon and evening.

This group recommends 'Three Action Steps' on how to respond to crying in order to reduce crying as much as possible and to prevent shaking and abuse.

- Carry, comfort, walk and talk to the infant.
- If the crying is too frustrating, it is okay to walk away but place the baby with someone else.
- Never shake or hurt an infant.

SIDS, Sudden Infant Death Syndrome: They say this information should be shared with **anyone** that takes care of your baby regarding safer sleep practices. For more information, go to the SIDS fact sheet in this book. For full information on SIDS and safe sleep, please visit. ***www.Canada.ca*** For information on baby sleep products, search the "Is Your Child Safe?" series.

Post-Partum Resources If you have any concerns about your baby, call your care provider, but if it is an emergency, call 911 or go to the hospital.

Postpartum ***www.postpartum.net***

Chapter 27: Fourth Trimester!? Post Partum

Welcome to *The Fourth Trimester!? ~ Post Partum*

You thought there were only three trimesters?

"You need dedication to have a baby.

You only have to live in the moment with your baby."

P & TJ, wise advice from first-time parents of a 3-week-old.

Babies do not come with a *How Too Book;* you will know in your heart how to raise them.

In the first few months, specifically the first six weeks, there is no real preparation for *you.* You will be expected to switch gears quickly now that you are at home with a newborn; your life has now changed forever. Each day is new and different, you will be constantly learning to navigate your days and nights and experience all the wonderful things that your baby and their routine are all about, and you will start to understand what your *new normal* is going to look like. Your baby will be constantly learning and experiencing all the wonderful things that you and members of the family teach them by *being with them.*

Your birth journey will have been unique and different from all others, and you may have journeyed through fertility drugs, IVF, surrogacy and adoption to find your baby, or you may have experienced pregnancy and delivery. Especially when you have help becoming pregnant or someone else carries your baby. I hear that people can have issues bonding with the baby. Please take to heart that when you look at this tiny person, they ONLY see the parent holding them. You loved them enough to start this journey, and your baby will pick up on your anxiety. It may be beneficial to seek guidance from someone and to talk about your feelings sooner than later. For now, your world has changed forever. The bond with your baby is truly life-changing. The journey is part of the magic!

There will be doctor appointments for the baby to ensure they are gaining weight at a normal rate and thriving. Then you will see your care provider to check that stitches are healing and you are recovering nicely from your delivery. You may feel that you cry often, or you are emotional for no reason. You may be irritable, impatient, desire to have everything perfect, have low self-esteem or lack of confidence because, as new parents, you may tend to overthink, worry and judge yourself too much! Be open about how you are feeling, your thoughts or concerns and talk to your doctor, family and friends about what is going on in your head.

Having concern for your new baby and feeling anxious are common in the first year. Actually, you will never stop worrying about your children all their life. It is common that people worry when they become a new parent. Some thoughts in your head might be;

- Am I doing the right things for my baby?
- Will my baby stop breathing?
- Am I feeding my baby enough?
- When they cry, will I know how to soothe them?
- Why do they not sleep very long?
- When will I get more than 2 hours of sleep?
- I feel so isolated from everyone and everything.
- When will I find time for myself?
- Why do I feel anxiety and stress? Where does that come from?
- How long will it take to get my life and/or body back?
- What if I do not know how to take care of a baby as they grow?
- Can I afford this?

- I think I am way out of my comfort zone
- Will I find a new normal?

After some time and introspection, you will say this was the start of the best and most amazing time and the most depressing and sleep-deprived time in your life! You may feel your world has turned upside down; it has! You doubt yourself and have no idea about what your baby wants or what their needs are at any given moment of the day. You have become a family, or your family has grown.

Most likely, you will have an incredible and intense *Love* for your baby, and you will be exhausted, confused and frustrated all at the same time. For most people, our body releases oxytocin, when you cuddle the baby or feed them, look at them, it can flood us with feelings of *being in love* with your baby, and it starts a unique bonding between you and them. Your new reality into parenthood started when you were excited that you got pregnant or your labor started! If this was your first labor, it might have taken up to 30 hours to get to 10 cm dilated. When you were told to start pushing, you dug deep and found the energy needed, which most likely took from one to four hours. But you did it! Or, for many reasons, you might have needed some help with delivery, and that went down a different path than expected, possibly a cesarean section and, with that, a longer recovery. Now after meeting your baby, you will feed them and tend to all their needs, feeling unprepared and totally exhausted!

Your new normal will include sleeping when the baby sleeps and eating when possible; so please be good to yourself and sleep when the baby sleeps!

Check in with yourself to ensure you are doing well at home. Now that you're no longer pregnant, common things can be hard to cope with. Your body will take some time to change back to your normal size and shape, and it will be similar to when your body changed when you started these nine months of being pregnant. This can impact your emotions and mental health and the way you look at your new life:

- How are you truly feeling? Be honest with yourself
- Do you just want to have a good cry?
- Are you chest-feeding and waiting for your milk to come in?
- How come you can not get enough sleep? When will this ever end?
- Feelings of being out of control with your life.
- Feeling that you need some time to yourself.
- Everyone in the home, especially you, needs self-care.
- How are you supposed to recover from the delivery of your baby?

If you have any concerns about yourself or your baby, call your care provider, but if it is an emergency, call 911 or go to the hospital. It may be nothing, but better to have answers than to fumble through the early days with your baby postpartum.

Taking Care of Yourself: For most people, this is not the time to worry about getting their body into the same or similar shape and condition that they were in before getting pregnant. It is enough to start gently by lifting the baby, some gentle exercises, doing Kegels while feeding the baby, or taking the baby outside for fresh air and a gentle walk. You may need to wait for up to six weeks if you have had a caesarean section. Realistically your time will be focused on your baby and on learning all their cues and habits, and trying to set up a routine. Chest feeding is supposed to help you to lose weight and help you to fit back into pre-pregnancy clothes faster. However, not everyone can or wants to chest feed, and depending on how much weight you put on during your pregnancy, it may take a bit longer. Either way, your body has changed because of the pregnancy and delivery, and you will, at some point, come back to a new normal. Your pregnancy was 40 weeks in the making. Allow yourself the same time for your hormones to calm down and get you back to a pre-pregnancy state. In the first month, your goal is to feed both you and baby on a regular basis (feeding you may be harder) and do not be concerned that your baby only sleeps for three hours at a time. They will get into a longer sleep pattern at around week six.

A trick for you when having a tub or shower is to take your baby into the bathroom so you can have a shower or tub while your baby sits in a secure car seat or later on in a bouncy chair that is placed on the floor, they will listen to the water running or when you are drying your hair with a hairdryer may fall asleep, they like to listen to 'white noise'.

Sitz bathes: Often, you are given a small bowl to rinse your perineum, and you can bring it home, and you should continue to use this or start when you get home. There are stores that specialize in perineal washes, or Homeopathic herbs or Arnica or Witch Hazel, any of these in the sitz bath. Witch Hazel and Arnica products are most effective when used on your sanitary napkin and put directly on the repair of either the perineum or the tummy cut from a cesarean section. It will calm tissues and will help heal this area faster. These products may not come with instructions, but they are gentle and very effective in healing soft tissue damage, for example, bruises or cuts.

A regular bowel movement may be difficult and trying may be just that, many times the hospital staff will give you stool softeners in the hospital. Sometimes it can be recommended, you continue using them, as needed when you get home. You most likely will get back to your normal diet routine. Your body has gone through so much in a short time frame.

Post-Partum Checkup: You should schedule one during an appointment with your care provider. They will make sure any repair from the delivery is healing properly. This is a good time to explain how you are feeling physically and how your mental health is, or if you have any lingering concerns about the delivery, let them know. You can ask questions about your labor and delivery. You might be upset about an emergency procedure, a cesarean section or forceps. Did they give you enough time and explanation in the delivery suite beforehand? Now when is it fresh on everyone's mind to talk or discuss your lingering questions? The doctor (if not your regular doctor) will transfer your care back to your general practitioner. Some questions you might have:

- Ask about birth control.
- Do you have any bleeding or clots?
- Do you have Haemorrhoids? How best to manage them?
- How your repair from your birth is healing: c-section incision, perineum tear?
- How are you feeling, your mood, your thoughts? Do you have any depression?
- Do you have any other concerns about yourself or the baby?
- Do you have any feeding concerns so far, either chest or bottle feeding?
- How having had a caesarean section is impacting your care for other children at home.
- Are there any tips they can give you?

Fun Fact - You can get pregnant while breast feeding, it is not a form of contraception.

Baby and their schedule: The following will start within the first hour after delivery. This usually happens every three to four hours, your baby has their own random routine, they are used to sleeping and then moving about in your tummy, and will now be learning a new routine, (that will change and evolve over the next few months and years).

Starting at birth and for the first six weeks, you can expect 1 to 2 hours of sleep at a time, because your baby will be on their own schedule of being awake, wanting to feed, needing to be burped, (it is very important to get any air out of their tummy) a diaper change or two, wanting cuddle time with you, they may want to feed a bit more or just the 'nibbling' at the nipple, so they can be close to you. This process may take 1.5 - 2 hrs, then they sleep an 1 - 1.5 hours and wake, to start again. This is a normal baby's routine.

After a bit of time, the baby will want to feed every three hours (or so), and that can take a full hour. It is essential to have a designated place where you can feed the baby and have diaper changes, and for cuddling and soothing your baby back to sleep. They may need several diaper changes as they can 'go again' after the first diaper change. They may spit up, and you will need to change their clothes. They may not want to settle for a nap right away, but they adore it when you cuddle and sing to them. Sometimes they want extra cuddling, which makes it hard to put them in their bassinet because they enjoy the warm embrace and being close to you (as much as you enjoy them). This can take several hours, then it is repeated again. This routine will repeat all day and night and is very exhausting for you. Sleep deprivation is going to be the new normal for you in the next several months. There is no real preparation for what is to come.

You will need support, and it can come in a variety of ways. Now that you are home and settling in, start using your calendars and signs. The Post Partum Calendar is for your family and friends that have volunteered to help during the first six weeks or more. The saying "It Takes a Village" has never meant more than at this time. Signs for the front door and doorbell, posters and lists that you made in the 3rd Trimester, it is imperative that you get as much rest every time the baby naps. When the baby sleeps, you must sleep or rest! If you have not practiced resting or taking naps in the last few months, you need to try napping when the baby does; it is harder than you think. You will want to sleep when the baby does, but the reality is that you are so excited to have the baby in front of you, or anxious that the baby may stop breathing, or the big question, will I wake up when they need me and the questions and concerns can be endless. If you have not practiced napping during pregnancy, start now. Do you remember the relaxing tips for labor, anything that will help you to nap or take a break when the baby naps? There is no best scenario for getting through this time, and it may be that keeping visitors to a minimum and immersing yourself with baby and the new routine only allow people that are there to help you and baby, no visiting.

As a new parent and after time when baby has a routine, your baby will go into their own room, when that happens we seem to have 'super hero' hearing, because you will be able to hear your baby, in their own room. The smallest whimper or noise from a hungry baby, will get you out of bed.

It will surprise you how you can not believe they are here in front of you, all those tiny little parts, arms and legs everything about baby is exquisite. It can be tough waiting for them to look at you and smile or reach out to you, have patience this will all come in a bit of time.

Have family or friends come and help, and bring cooked meals, or cook for you in your home, help tidy around your home, allow you to take a bath or nap. After you feed your tummy, remember your mind and soul, need attention. You might have feelings that you are not in control of your environment, or you are unhappy or depressed? You need to have some personal time to meditate, read, relax, listen to music, sit in nature, anything that makes you feel calm and happy. Go walking with baby bundled up in a stroller, as weather permits, the fresh air is good for you both, and this gentle form of exercise will help your body, get back into pre-pregnancy shape.

Think of the next few months, as a time to get to know your baby, with no other obligations than feeding you and your baby. Try to sleep or rest when baby does, leave household tidying or cooking to your partner or family and friends.

Your body feels different; You are responsible for a baby(s).

They did not come with an instruction book!

Your life will never be the same! But you are so in love with your baby!

Be kind to yourself. We can be our own worst enemy. Your baby did not come with a *How To* Manual for a reason because you and your baby are uniquely joined for life. Sometimes the ‘way’ our baby was delivered can cause us worry or have frustration, or lingering anger. Talk to your care provider and get more answers about your birth journey.

Many cultures, offer family care, where they invite the new parent and baby to come and stay in their home, or they come to your home, for six weeks or more. Clients talk about how it really makes a difference for them, because they receive knowledge and advice from family; tricks for how to cope with baby, while family help you adjust to your baby’s needs and learn their routine. They help by cooking, tidying, watching baby while you rest and recover from your labor and much more, but most important the bonding of grandparent, parents and baby is priceless.

I was so fortunate to have my Mum come and stay with me for all my babies.

There are many options, if family is not available you can hire Nanny’s or Post Partum Doulas to help with baby in your home for several hours a day, or live in support that stays for the first 6 weeks (or longer) in your home. They offer services such as cooking, cleaning the home, laundry, being with baby during the night for feedings and changing diapers while you get some sleep. Doing some errands, the list of what is offered is varied. It would be advised to interview and hire someone before baby was born, however if you have just decided you need help, there will be someone that will be available to help out, seek and ask. The duration for help varies and will depend on what you can afford, for a couple of weeks or months, and several hours at a time or full 8 hour day or night.

Etiquette for visiting a newborn and their parents;

- Visit baby only if you have been invited. Never arrive unannounced.
- First thing upon arriving at the home, wash your hands.
- If you are coming for a visit, never come to the home when you are not well, not even a cough or sniffle. Do not arrive with strong perfume or aftershave.
- Do not arrive straight from a workout.
- Keep your visit short unless you are there to help cook or clean.
- Always ask permission before picking up the baby.
- Do not kiss or snuggle the baby without permission.
- Take pictures with permission from the parent.
- Never post pictures of a baby on social media without permission!
- Do not expect to be entertained; your host is tired.
- Expect to make the tea and bring food and cookies for everyone in the home.
- Know when to give the baby back to the parent.
- Do not comment on the appearance of the parent.
- Do not comment on the condition of the home, unless you are offering to clean.
- Never give unsolicited advice; only when they ask for it.
- Offer to help the tired parents in any way needed.

First six weeks with the baby. Here is a list of tips to help navigate your newborn. Always ask the baby doctor for advice or for more information with the following (as needed):

Umbilical Cord Care: the clamp that was put on the umbilical cord before the care provider cut the cord. It will take one to two weeks for the end of the cord to dry up and then naturally fall off. It is important to keep the cord dry and clean by taking a small gauze pad or a tissue with a tiny drip of water on it to clean the area (if needed) around the tummy. Dab at the base of the cord and tummy very gently, and do not pull on the drying cord, even if there is only the last thread. (It is recommended that you do not bathe the baby in a tub of water until the stump of the cord has fallen off) it is best to sponge bath the baby at this time. Watch the cord if the stump is smelly or there is some redness or swelling or looks tender on the skin; it could be infected. If your baby's stump does not fall off in 4 weeks, call your baby's provider. There may be another problem that needs attention.

Gooey eye: The baby's tear ducts can be blocked, one or both. They may have some pale yellow watery discharge (as if they were crying) from the corner of their eye that will dry up. Sometimes an infection develops if the fluid is not cleared properly from the eye. You can put a drop or two of chest milk on the corner of the eye using a sterile/clean cloth. Wipe below the eye and gently massage in an upward direction from the nose to the inner corner of the eye a few times a day to help clear any build-up. Or consult with your care provider.

If the baby is fussy and trying to sleep, white noise can be helpful, for example, gentle music, rain or running water or hairdryer or vacuum sounds. There are many downloadable sounds from your cell phone or other devices. If you listen to music while pregnant, let the baby listen to the same music they got used to, it will be very comforting. Sometimes they may need to fuss for a bit but will go back to sleep. They will learn that when the room is bright, they can eat and they have play time with you, but when the room is dark, it is time for feeding and going back to sleep.

Room temperature: If you are comfortable in the room, baby should also be comfortable. If baby has a onesie or a sleeper on and wrapped in a receiving blanket or light blanket they should be comfortable. Bundling baby up, you may over heat your baby, and that is not safe for baby.

Teach baby to sleep through noise during the day hours. Have the room filled with daylight, and regular sounds of household activities, people talking, television, music playing, running the dishwasher, vacuuming, (preferably not too distracting or loud) They will get used to having sounds in the room, and you will be able to take them anywhere for visits or shopping and they will still nap.

At home ~ bathing baby: Baby is not dirty; they do not *need* to have a bath at the hospital, but you may want to bathe your baby when you are home. Bathing your baby might be easier if both parents participate in giving the baby a bath until you are both comfortable bathing them on your own. Set up a place in your bathroom or a kitchen counter, then make sure you have all the essentials needed for your baby's bath at hand. It helps if you have easy access to a water facet. Put enough warm water in the small baby tub, just enough that baby will be immersed up to their waist. This will make holding the baby and washing them easier.

Start by holding baby in your arm, (wrapped in a towel) just above the tub then with the other arm, drizzle warm water over their head (not the face) with a small cup, trying not to get the water in their eyes. Wipe the face, then you can dry their head, by gently wiping the head with a clean towel, (always wash and dry the head first) Now you can put baby into the water and gently wipe all the creases on their body, for example under their arm pits, under their chin, and most importantly is to give their bottom time to soak in a bath, especially if they have a diaper rash. A baby bath tub is a perfect size for baby to fit in and the bath includes a place for baby to lay on, resting on their back in a reclined position. It is not necessary to use products on their skin or hair, especially anything with scent, they naturally smell heavenly, but it is not necessary for their hygiene. Your baby does not need a bath per se, they are clean, however when they are older and play outside daily bathes are recommended, but that is a still a long while away.

When baby is a bit older, and you are comfortable and have the other parent at home, have one of you sit in a filled bath tub, with legs bent at the knee, have the other person bring baby to the person in the tub. Baby will face you laying on their back against your legs and looking at you. You can now bathe your baby and they are being entertained.

Babies love to wiggle in the water, and you should keep one hand on baby while they are in the tub at all times. The baby will tell you they have had enough tub time; they will start to cry. Take them out and dry them off you will have another try again soon. When you take baby out of the tub dry the baby's bottom and put a diaper on them (it prevents getting the counter space from having a messy pee or poo) then continue drying them off and dress them. Bathing is a time for play and they will engage with you over time, as they learn.

Have handy at least two towels, two face cloths, a couple of diapers, diaper cream for the baby's bottom. Two outfits for baby to wear, for when tub time is over.

If the baby is fussy now, wait ~ they will learn to enjoy tub time soon enough.

Author's bathing tip I learned this from personal experience, when you are over-equipped, you never have to pick up a wet baby and take them to go get more diapers or a dry and clean outfit. Here are a few things that make being prepared necessary;

- Babies love to do their business (pee or poo) as you take them out of the tub.
- Baby's clothes get wet while baby is in the tub splashing (they are usually in an infant tub on the counter).
- While dressing the baby, they may take this moment to throw up.
- Take your cell phone in the bathroom with you in case someone is trying to call you.
- This task of bathing the baby can take anywhere from a half hour or longer.
- NEVER leave a baby in a tub or water of any depth at any time.

Diaper Rash: Try to prevent your baby's bottom from getting too raw. Once it starts, it is hard to get back to soft skin. This often happens when a soiled diaper is left too long on your baby's bottom, and can become a red rash with open sores very quickly.

Air dry a baby's bottom by leaving it un-diapered, open to the air in the room or place with a hair dryer on a low setting close to their bottom (not too close to their bottom to burn them). Dry their bottom with a soft clean tissue or cloth if they will allow you to touch their skin, and with a lot of diaper rash cream, slather on their bottom and put their diaper on. Use a light cream with zinc oxide. It is perfect for leaving on their skin that makes a protective coat to help relieve diaper rash. Baby can be very cranky because of this and cry constantly. The best prevention, keep the baby's bottom dry and protected.

Baby's Skin may be dry and or flakey in the first couple of weeks. It is not going to stay like that. If it bothers you, you can use organic and unscented oil, for instance, almond oil or olive oil and only small amounts. Baby acne or blotchy red 'rash' will disappear very quickly by not putting anything on the baby. A cradle cap can be present on the forehead and/or scalp, and it can often be flaky. You can apply a small amount of non-scented olive oil to the area, and with a small comb and gently, after a few hours of the oil being on, comb it out.

Trim the Baby's Nails: People are often surprised that their newborn baby has long fingernails. To try and trim nails, first wait until your baby is sleeping. This way, they will not notice and fuss with their hands. There are tiny clippers for newborns, or you can try filing the nail. Many people bite the nail with their teeth.

Author's Tip for the bassinette, where your baby is sleeping, either or both parents wear a t-shirt for several days to have your scent transfer to the t-shirt, then put the shirt on the baby's mattress, and then you lie baby down, and they can smell 'you' and will know you are close.

If the baby shows signs of not feeling well, the first thing is to take their temperature. Normal newborn temperature ranges from 36.5 to 37.5 degrees Celsius. Take their temperature under their armpit (as they get older, there are new recommendations about rectal or by mouth check with your care provider). It can be difficult holding them still while waiting for a proper reading, so have someone else help you, it makes it much easier. Times that you should call is when baby is not feeding well, is lethargic, has a fever of 38 c or 100.4 F degrees, or baby has poor muscle tone and is floppy, OR if the cord was pulled off too soon, it may start to bleed, dab the blood drops and if the bleed continues, call your care provider.

Anytime you are concerned for your baby, either call your Care Provider or there may be an infants emergency number to call and ask for advise.

Colick, what does that mean? A baby communicates with us by crying, and they make gestures with their hands to their mouth if they are hungry. I have heard people say that the baby must be colicky, because they are fussy and crying. I am really not sure colick is a 'thing'. I know that most babies have a period of time in the late afternoon and early evening when they tend to be fussy, cry louder and more intensely and do not stop crying for no obvious reason. It can make for a stressful time, not knowing what your baby wants, take a moment and consider the following:

- Is the baby hungry again because they are going through a growth spurt?
- Did you eat something that went through your milk that has upset your baby's gut, for instance did you eat onions, that would aggravate their tummy?
- Do they need to have a burp? They may have baby 'indigestion.'
- Did you have chocolate, and now you can not sleep because the small amount of caffeine is going through their body?
- Are they having a 'moment' and are inconsolable?
- Would they prefer to have more cuddle time?
- Are they constipated?
- Are they bored and want someone to be with them, just when you are doing something, like preparing dinner?
- You have no idea about the temperament of this small person, and it may take a some time still, to get to know them better.
- Is there too much stimulation in the room? TV, music, lights, too many people etc.?
- Swaddle baby or put baby into a baby wearing pouch and cuddle them up.
- Do they want to be in a baby swing, go for a walk or stroller or go on a car ride?
- They might just be tired and not know what they need or want, so they cry.

You are seeing a tiny piece of their personality and who they will become as an adult.

Post Partum check-up for Baby: Check-up appointments for the baby for their first six weeks will be done by the person that delivered your baby and at their clinic. They watch the baby's general health and check to see if the baby is gaining weight weekly and if they are responding as a baby should. Questions will be how often the baby feeds, how often does your baby pees and poops, and what its color is. You will know the baby is thriving with chestfeeding by the fact that they are gaining weight regularly.

Ask about the baby's routine for sleeping and other routines, and if you have any concerns about the baby. The baby is then discharged from their care, and you will need to find a doctor that takes care of your baby's needs (it can be a Paediatrician or general practitioner, depending on where you live).

It is normal to feel stressed, anxious, nervous, upset, arguing with someone, or if you are talking loudly or aggressively. The baby can pick up all of this negative energy, but not knowing what it is or why it is in the room, they become confused with the energy, and they can feel anxious themselves. They become cranky or fussy and will cry. My advice, take a couple of cleansing breaths, focus on your baby, pick them up and let everything in the room stop and slide away from your mind. They will become calmer themselves as they emulate you.

Feeding your baby: Their body is growing fast, they have a tiny stomach, and they need to be fed every couple of hours, whether you chest feed or bottle feed or both. I love that people try to chest feed, I believe it gives babies the best start in life, but I have had clients that physiologically can not produce enough milk to satisfy a baby's tummy and for them to thrive and grow. This is unfortunate, but thankfully, we have the formula. In the first few months, your milk or formula is all they need. Never give baby water because there are no calories in water, and they need all the calories, especially in the first few months, to thrive. Feeding a baby can be stressful and very time-consuming. Using bottles can be a lot more work. The bottles, the nipples for the bottle and soothers all have to be sterilized in the first few months.

At the 3rd day, your milk has probably ‘come in’, or some say ‘matured’, and latching is (hopefully) getting better, so feed baby on demand. In the first week, if your baby sleeps more than 4 - 5 hrs, wake them to feed. It is important for the baby to eat every 3 - 4 hrs in order to grow. If babies do not get enough to eat, they become lethargic, which can indicate latching issues or something else. But you should seek help from a care provider (baby not eating is not healthy).

When your milk comes in, your breasts may become engorged. If this happens put *green cold* cabbage leaves (not red, as it will stain your clothes and skin) or cold packs (a frozen face cloth) directly on your breast (inside the bra) to help relieve the pressure and hard feeling. In a warm shower you can hand express and massage the firm ducts. If you want to save the milk, hand express into a container for your baby or if you are not home, hand express into a sink.

If this hard feeling or pressure is not relieved within 12 hours, call for help!! Your care provider will help or refer you to someone who is a breast feeding expert. Don’t let things escalate, it is important to get help sooner than later. If breast feeding results in sore nipples or there is a latching problem, you need help. I suggest a nipple shield for certain latching issues but have someone find the true reason first. Breast feeding issues can easily escalates to mastitis, you will need to have a prescribed medication to resolve this painful problem.

Breast milk works by ‘supply and demand’. The more the baby sucks at the breast, the more milk you produce. Try not to introduce formula, as your supply will decrease. Pump and give baby expressed milk as a supplement, and ASK for help! *Never* give a newborn water. There are no calories in water. Review Dr. Newman’s chapter or go to their website.

Chest feeding the baby: You may be wondering what food you can eat. Many people tell me they miss eating Sushi; they crave it, and it is very often their first meal at the hospital after delivery. Once home, you can pretty much have whatever you want. However, if you are chestfeeding, you are now eating for two. Eating healthy is very important because your baby gets the same food as you. The spices in your food, some of which will come from your milk. I see many babies usually do not even notice. They only know that everything is new, so they are experiencing many different flavors. I wonder and tend to believe that when Baby is exposed to many flavors through human milk, they learn to tolerate and enjoy all flavors and foods later in life. I am not sure that there is any serious research on this, but 'food for thought'?

Possible foods that may help to increase milk production, is truly a tough one to know if it really works. I have seen people try all the foods and drinks that should have increased milk production but not make a different. Some people simply will not produce enough for an infant to grow and thrive, at an expected amount of weight in the first month or two. If what you eat works, then great! Most people will try most anything as they navigate eating for baby and what is being suggested for them to try eating. Here is a list of suggested foods that are expected to increase milk production, feel free to research and try (I am not an expert): Fennel, Carrots, Beets, Yams, dark green leafy Vegetables, Oats or Oat milk, Millet, Barley, Rice, Ginger, Garlic, Chick Peas, Mung Beans, Nuts cashews, almonds, macadamia nuts, Sesame seeds. Herbs, Fenugreek and Blessed Thistle. Lean meat and poultry.

When you are chestfeeding, some foods that you eat can make their way through to the natural milk, which can make the baby have an upset tummy, or they become gassy, cranky or will stay wide awake. This may be because of certain foods that you have eaten. For example, if you eat onions, the baby may have an upset tummy and be cranky for a few hours, or if you have chocolate or caffeinated tea or coffee, they are more likely to stay awake longer, which results in the baby becoming cranky because they are overtired because of the caffeine. Try no caffeinated beverages. Simply put, they eat what you eat. When clients talk about the baby's tummy being upset, I ask them to think back over the last 24 hours, and remember what they ate, because there might have been something that upset the baby's tummy. I would suggest that you take it out of your diet and see if the baby's tummy calms down or if it makes a difference. Wait for a few days before you have that food again, and watch closely how the baby reacts. If their tummy is fine, then put that food back into your meal.

Early on, your baby should be having 8 feeding in a 24-hour period, which will space out as they and their tummy grow bigger. Allow them to have the nipple more often, as long as they want to suckle. They will never overeat at this time in their life, their tummy is still small, and they will spit up if they happen to get too much. Do not fret, and try to be patient with all feedings, both you and baby will have a routine soon. You are both learning.

Author's Tip: Asking the other parent to share feedings by taking one of the nightly feedings is especially nice for that parent. It gives the baby some special bonding time with both parents. More importantly, it gives *you* precious sleep time or time to do something for yourself. Most often, the baby will take a 'once in a while bottle' from the other parent without disturbing their routine of chestfeeding. Their preferred place to feed will be with the lactating parent because of the closeness to that parent, skin to skin. Both parents can and should be doing skin-to-skin while feeding the baby.

If you are concerned about whether you might not be producing enough milk and you wonder if you should supplement with formula, this change-up can often only confuse the baby. Firstly, ask your care provider and confirm with them that you have enough milk. You need to confirm that you are, in fact, producing enough and baby is growing and putting on weight weekly.

Author's Tip: There may be many reasons surrounding bottle or formula, or that you can not or do not want to chest feed, the next best thing will be formula feeding. It is not my place to be promoting or endorsing anything regarding how to feed your baby and especially any products involved. There is much advice from care providers and friends or family. Talk to your postpartum care provider before buying formula. Firstly you may not need it at all, but it is best to get a recommendation on which formula to buy. Note: I have had clients buy the A+ formula with extra Iron in it, only to have their baby cranky because their gut can not digest it well.

Fun Fact: Putting the baby to the nipple often will ensure more milk production, BUT it is important to know that some people physiologically can not and will not be able to make enough milk to fill the baby's tummy and have them thrive.

The most important thing on your mind is feeding your baby. Dr. Jack Newman has all the answers, and if you have not spent too much time in this chapter, then do it now! Feeding your baby may be the biggest reason for stress in the first few weeks.

I am so grateful that Dr. Jack Newman has given you this full chapter, for this book. The chapter is filled with everything to do with feeding your baby. Dr. Newman and the clinic is highly respected. They have worked in Toronto, Canada for years, and the chapter references their website, which will help you to find all answers regarding feeding your baby. Enjoy everyone!

As my favorite Chest Feeding Guru, Dr. Jack Newman, says, "It Gets Better!!"

Lactation Cookies recipe:

- 1 cup butter
- 1 cup sugar
- 1 cup brown sugar
- 4 tablespoons water
- 2 tablespoons flaxseed meal*
- 2 large eggs
- 1 teaspoon vanilla
- 2 cups flour
- 1 teaspoon baking soda
- 1 teaspoon salt
- 3 cups oats, thick cut if you can get them
- 1 cup or more chocolate chips
- 2 tablespoons of brewers yeast** (be generous)
- Preheat oven to 375 degrees F.

Mix together 2 tablespoons of flaxseed meal and water, set aside for 3-5 minutes.

Cream (beat well) butter and sugar. Add eggs one at a time, and mix well. Stir the flaxseed mixture and add vanilla to the butter mix. Beat until blended.

Sift together dry ingredients, except oats and chips. Add to butter mixture. Stir in oats, then chips. Scoop or drop onto the baking sheet, preferably lined with parchment paper. The dough is a little crumbly, so it helps to use a scoop.

Bake for 8-12 minutes, depending on the size of the cookies.

Serves: 6 dozen cookies

This is from a Midwife, Linda (I do not know her last name), in Vancouver, Canada, that claims to increase milk supply. I will leave it up to you to try or not.

Have a primary place to feed your baby. Your chair, in the place you will feed the baby, has been set with everything you need for feedings. One that has very good support for your back is comfortable and where your feet rest on the floor (or use a stool or box for your feet as needed). Have a table on one or both sides, so you can put everything you might need while you feed the baby. A place for your sealed water bottle, tissue or a cloth for spit ups and tissue, a snack for yourself, possibly an apple or a granola bar in a wrapper, a baby 'feeding pillow' that wraps around your tummy to help hold and support baby when they are small, then cushions for when baby is bigger, a cell phone (as needed) a remote control that you can turn tv or radio on or possibly a magazine or book, while they have a feeding, and a blanket to cover you and baby (if needed) if the room is chilly at night, be close to a change table that you can change a diaper, (with all of the required supplies). Then anything else you believe might make this time go by (a feeding can take thirty to sixty minutes).

You can download apps on your cell phone or tablet/iPad that you can track the feedings, time how long they are, and time when you started the feed, so you know when the next feed should be and how much the baby drank from a bottle, when the baby had a dirty or wet diaper. It may sound like a silly thing to have to do, but be prepared, in the first few months, it will be a life saver. I can guarantee you will forget any and all information regarding how many times that feeding and diaper changes happened in a week. The reason is, your Care Provider will be asking about the baby and what goes in and what comes our, at all check-ups and you will have all the information you need to show them.

Football or Cross Cradle: There are two specific ways to hold a baby when we feed baby at the chest. Sit straight up in a supportive chair, with your feet on solid ground (so they do not dangle). Have your baby on the feeding pillow or pillows that support the baby to lay on, so their mouth will be directly at the same height as your nipple.

The Cross cradle hold is when the baby is close to your left side at your chest, put the baby's lower arm (their right arm) under your breast, ensuring they get closer to your nipple. Have a receiving blanket handy so you can tuck the blanket around the baby's left hand that is flying about near their mouth and your nipple. This secures their hand and keeps them from putting their hand near their mouth and your nipple. You will support the baby's head with your right hand, the left-hand cups the breast, and you will squeeze above and below the breast to make a 'sandwich' type formation. The baby will try to open their mouth to grasp the nipple.

The Football hold is when the baby is held like a football in your left arm, tucked close to your left side, and your hand holding behind the the baby's head, and then the baby will be going to latch onto the left breast. I may not have given a very good explanation of these holds, but Dr. Newman's chapter has lovely visuals for holding the baby and how to grasp the breast.

Feeding Cues for Baby It's been said to *Watch the Cues, Not the Clock!*

Early cues means "I am hungry" When the baby starts to stir and waken, and makes noises, they may root with their hand (putting a hand near the mouth) for something, turn their head, and try to put a fist or finger into their mouth.

Mid cues means "I'm really hungry". The baby stretches and they increase their physical movements and put their hand to their mouth.

Late cues means "I need food now!" and they will start crying. They will have some agitated movements, and their face can turn red from trying to tell you they have some tummy discomfort from being hungry.

Calm/soothe the baby first, then feed the baby. A crying baby will not settle to eat, you must cuddle and calm your baby so they come out of their crying outburst, and then they will take the nipple. If they have not settled down and start at the nipple, they will gulp, and because of the fast injection of milk, they may throw that up.

Babies just cry. It is the only way of the baby has any exercise at this young age. I am not so sure about that. l know that this is the only way to get your attention. It is their form of communicating with anyone in the room. The obvious reasons are that they are tired or over-tired, or they are hungry, and the longer you take to get to them some milk makes them cry louder. Sometimes they are overstimulated in a room with too many people, bright lights or the noise from tv, or music is too loud, and it becomes overwhelming for them. They may want to be held and cuddled or just want your attention without people moving about, or someone is not holding them properly and are giggling them about, or they may be bored, and they will cry to alert you they want YOU.

If they are not hungry, then they may want to have a soother, often people confuse them as being hungry, but they are not; they want the action of sucking. They did this in the birth sack, all the time, with a hand or finger. It is a form of self-soothing for them. They may be too cold or too warm where they are laying. They may have a full diaper or are truly in pain, possibly because they are constipated or other possibilities.

When you go to them when they are very new, they learn that they can rely on you to take care of their needs. It helps you to learn their cues sooner and why and what they need. Do not be worried about how long it will take you to understand them, all their habits and preferences will come in time. They are communicating with you, and you will find the path there.

Learning routines This whole time to feed baby, burp, diaper, calm and sooth to sleep may take you two to three hours. Then the rotation will start again, and you haven't eaten or slept or had a bathroom break. This routine for feeding the baby is done approximately every three hours, in the beginning, and until your baby is bigger. Feeding can take approximately one hour to chest feed. Bottle feeding may be less time, followed by gently trying to burp baby by rubbing or patting their back. There will be at least one diaper change, then the baby may 'throw up'. You will need to change the baby's outfit. Then you get precious cuddle time with your baby, settle them, and put them in their bed for a nap. The rotation will start again in about two to three hours, depending on how long they sleep.

When both parents help with the feeding, especially in the middle of the night feeding, it is a unique and fabulous time for both parents to have a bonding time with the baby. It also gives the parent that feeds the baby most often, to get some extra sleep over the night, while the other parent gives the baby a bottle in the middle of the night. Even if they only do one or two feedings per week, it is very beneficial for everyone. For one parent, it is easy to have feelings of being frustrated and depressed and feeling like they are left out, that parent wishing they could be more hands-on with the baby. If you are chest feeding, they may have to wait until you have a good feeding routine. Then, you can pump your milk and save it in a bottle for midnight feeds.

Even if the other parent takes the baby for a diaper change, then a cuddle and puts the baby back to bed. Work out how many nights the partner can take a feeding during the middle of the night and try to make it a routine. Many people complain that living on 2 to 3 hours of sleep is exhausting, and it is! The extra time to sleep will make a huge difference in how that person can cope during the day and the energy they regain, making it more manageable getting through their day and taking care of the baby and the family.

When one parent shows the other parent how to be more hands-on with the baby, helping with the baby's bath and sharing other baby duties, shared tasks allow more time for the primary parent to have some much-needed time for themselves. When bottles are given, or you choose to do one bottle feeding for your partner, for this sole reason, they can do the middle of the night feeding (and skin-to-skin). This allows you more sleep, and they get a chance to feed, diaper, and cuddle baby to sleep. They get all the same important bonding moments with the baby, which are essential for both parents. These moments release oxytocin from our brains, which makes everyone, feel better. Everyone is learning about each other with this new family member, and you will find out that your baby is born with habits and a mind of their own. It is so beneficial when the baby gets their basic needs meet from both parents; it also solidifies the family unit faster.

It is beneficial for you to take care of yourself in this early time, to eat and rest, and have time in the tub, nap or relaxation.

Holding baby: When you pick up the baby, put one hand behind their neck and head to support the weight of the head. Your other hand goes under their bottom (rump), and you bring the baby to your chest or the fold of your arm. Baby will wiggle and move, so be careful that they do not wiggle out of your hands. Bring them close to you to snuggle, feed, or play. Babies are very floppy for the first several months or so, but they will gain strength in the muscles of their neck, make sure you support your baby very well for this entire time.

Burping baby: When holding the baby to burp them, use the same holding techniques as above, but I would advise in the beginning for you to sit down. Baby will come to your chest, or often people hold the baby on their knee, the baby must always be secure in your hands. With one hand, you can *gently* pat the baby's back or make circle motions on their back. You will find the best way to pat the burps out of the baby's tummy. This is essential when bottle-feeding babies because when they suck on the nipple of the bottle, they will bring in air. When the baby is chest fed, there is much less or no air brought into their tummy, so do not expect as big of a burp with chest feeding. However, it is a must that you bring up burps after every feed. The air or gas in their tummy will make for a very cranky baby.

The craniosacral Therapy procedure is described as light touch therapy that has been shown to be effective in supporting the central nervous system and releasing restrictions through out the body. After delivery, it will help your baby's body to self-correct and heal naturally from being in a precarious position in the uterus. Specifically when baby's head has been tilted in Utero and upside down for several weeks, and trying to maneuver their head further into the pelvis. This can get their head stuck, it can strain the muscles in their neck and become stretched on one side and tighten on the other side, then during labor and trying to come through the birth canal. Baby can strain their neck muscles on one side, and this can make it painful and difficult for baby as they will prefer one side over the other, making it difficult for chest feeding on both sides.

This technique will help relieve the tightness that exists in their head, neck and mouth and can enable them to feed more efficiently, laying on both their left and right side. When born, this is not visible, but many times the baby may have a difficult time resting their head to one side or the other for feeding. They appear to not want to feed or are not happy feeding while laying on one side but are happy on the other side. If not treated it can make your baby fussy and/or cranky from the discomfort while feeding and also baby has difficulty sleeping or resting in your arms, on one side. The amount of milk baby drinks can be compromised if they do not feed well on 'one' side.

Some reasons your baby *or you* could benefit from having Craniosacral would be:

- Did you have a long and difficult labor?
- Did you have a cesarean section, forceps or vacuum delivery?
- Was the baby's head engaged for a long time?
- If you notice the baby is very fussy for no reason.
- Baby will be happier when the strain in their neck is gone.
- You will have difficulty feeding the baby.
- Does the baby cry inconsolably or have trouble sleeping?

During your appointment with a craniosacral practitioner, the procedure is done in a quiet setting with the baby on a massage table, lying down (you sitting in a chair beside them). There is no manipulation of the neck or spine as in chiropractic procedures, it is similar to acupressure, but with a very delicate touch, the practitioner will find tension in the area that needs to be released.

Practitioners have told me securing an appointment within the first week or two of delivery is most beneficial for new babies, especially because *you* are compromised with chest feeding and you are trying to establish a feeding routine with baby. The procedure is a gentle touch using their hand on baby, at the head and neck. One or two appointments should be enough.

Find a practitioner before you deliver in your area and add their contact information to your list of Post Partum phone number list.

Author's Note: Craniosacral therapy for one of my children. They were around 12 years old at the time and had a groin injury from playing hockey. I watched how the therapist worked. It was simple touch in the exact affected spots on the body. My child actually fell asleep during the procedure and was cured of the pain after only a couple of appointments.

Massage for babies: Different modalities talk about the effects of touch on the body to release tension in the body. Babies can be calmed very quickly with a *gentle* touch to parts of their body. Here are a few that are very effective:

- Stroke the forehead, beginning between the eyebrow and moving upwards to the hairline.
- Press the point between the eyebrows very lightly.
- Beginning at the temple, lightly massaging in an arc around the back of the ear and ending at the base of the ear.
- The shoulders and down the spine and the pressure points Bladder 32, Gall Bladder 21.
- At the bottom of the foot, with your thumb, gently press KID1 below the toes and middle of the foot and on the heel.

Touch a newborn baby, and bonding happens straight away when they are placed on your skin for the first cuddle. They recognize your voice and look up to see what your face looks like as they listen to your familiar voice. This is where they feel safe and cared for, and secure.

Post Partum checkup for Yourself: During an appointment with your care provider, make sure any repair is healing properly. This is the time to explain how you are physically and if you have any mental health issues or if you have concerns about the delivery. You can ask questions about your labor and delivery, whether you are upset about an emergency procedure, a cesarean section or forceps, did they give you enough time and explanation, are you sad or confused about the baby's delivery. After this appointment, they will transfer your care back to your general practitioner. Some questions you might have for your doctor:

- Any bleeding or clots?
- Hemorrhoids.
- How your repair from your birth is coming along c-section incision, perineum tear.

- How are you feeling, your mood, your thoughts? Is there any depression?
- Any problem sleeping?
- Do you have any concerns about yourself, physically or mentally?
- Do you have chest feeding concerns?
- Are you worried about the baby?
- Ask about birth control.
- How having a caesarean section is impacting your other children at home?

Fun Fact: You can get pregnant while breastfeeding; it is not a form of contraception.

Food and what can you eat now; this applies to anyone that is going to chest feed. If you are formula feeding, you can eat everything and anything you want. Many people tell me they have craved Sushi, and it is most often what their first meal is after delivery. If you are chest feeding, you are still eating for two, although you can pretty much have whatever you want. Eating healthy is still very important, as your baby gets the same as you, and we want them to gain an average amount of weight weekly.

The spices in your food will come through your milk, and your baby usually does not notice, except they may be aware that it tastes a bit different at different feedings, which is fine. They do not really seem to be fussed with it. Sometimes babies can have upset tummies, or are gassy, or cranky, or they stay wide awake. This is because of certain foods that you have eaten. For example, if you eat onions, they may have an upset tummy, or if you have chocolate or caffeinated tea or coffee, they may stay wide awake and become cranky because the caffeine keeps them awake, and they get cranky. Chocolate and some Energy drinks have more caffeine than we realize, which is not good for a growing baby. If you are chestfeeding, you may want to give up or reduce Coffee and Black tea and switch to herbal tea until you wean them. Simply, they eat what you eat!

If the baby has an upset tummy, think back through the last 24 hours and try to remember what you have eaten that might have caused the upset. Then take it out of your diet and see if it makes a difference with the baby's tummy. If their tummy settles down, it would be suggested to wait for some time, possibly a week or so, before you re-introduce it back into your diet. So enjoy your food again. If their tummy is still upset, then you should talk to their care provider. It could be from something else.

After you feed your tummy, remember your mind and soul need attention. You need to have some personal time to meditate, read, and relax while the baby sleeps. You can try to have a nap also, or just rest on the couch, have a snack, have a tub, or do anything that makes you relax. Listen to your heart, have others help you around your home and through recovery from your delivery, you will learn new routines for the baby. The first three months are for cocooning with the baby and learning all about their routine. Take this time to enjoy being a new parent.

Try listening to your favorite and relaxing music, drawing or painting or coloring or writing your thoughts of sadness or whatever crosses else is in your mind. Talk to people about what you are feeling inside, good or bad. Sit in nature as often as possible. After your baby goes to sleep, sit and enjoy 5 to 10 minutes, just sit and reflect, then do something for yourself. Have your partner, family or a friend look after the baby while you have a shower, a tub or a nap.

Sleep When Baby sleeps! The downfall of most new parents is they take the time when the baby sleeps to tidy or cook or do some 'chores' that are really of no consequence. Your primary responsibility is to be ready for the baby when they wake up. We can only survive the early weeks and months by delegating everything in your home to others.

Now is the time to have help from people making and bringing you healthy food items. A healthy diet and lots of water will ensure that you recover faster. Stocked freezer with pre-made meals, done weeks before your due date. Have a generous supply of healthy foods in your cupboards. You should have finished general household shopping several weeks in advance of the due date. Allowing your family and friends to drop off fresh items that you normally eat. If you are stocked up with items, you will be prepared if your baby delivers early, and you take the pressure off of meal planning when you are farther along in the pregnancy.

So how do I get sleep! Have your place to rest or sleep, ready to lay on. Start by turning off all things that make noise, phone, tv, and telephone, and make your room as quiet as possible. Hopefully, you will want to listen to White Noise or such as the sound of rain, the ocean or bird sounds. Choose your favorites. Your baby will definitely enjoy this kind of listening while they sleep, and it can be very soothing for you. Darken the room and cozy down with a comfortable blanket. If it is hard to sleep with the light of day, use an eye cover. Be good to you! When you are tired, leave everything in your home for later. It will still be there, but most importantly, this is your time out! Being aware and then preparing ahead of time, you will get through it better than most. You will still go through this sleep deprivation period, which can last 6 weeks to a couple of months, depending on when the baby starts to sleep longer during the nights.

Author's Note: New parents that can not sleep because they are worried about their baby, if that escalates and you do not get any sleep, it can add to your anxiety levels, and that can cause some postpartum depression, which can have devastating consequences if not taken care of by professionals. Please read more in the PPD chapter (postpartum depression)

Exercise Ball for After Feeding and/or a Crying Baby: The exercise ball was very helpful during your pregnancy to get the baby in a good position in your pelvis, and it is also very helpful after delivery. First, figure out if the baby is crying because of a dirty diaper, is hungry, tired or has an upset tummy, or you simply do not know why. Possibly, they are in a purple crying phase. Babies are very clever beings, they can sense your anxiety, and it will make them fussy. The exercise ball can be very soothing and relaxes babies when they are tired or cranky, and it will settle a baby almost every time.

Either parent or anyone that is in the home can sit on the ball, with really good support close by, so in the middle of the night, you do not fall over while bouncing on the ball. Wrap baby in a light blanket and cuddle them, this gives them a similar feeling from when they were in the uterus, and you hold them close to your chest so they can hear your heartbeat. With one hand supporting the head and the other hand holding under the baby's bottom, you bounce up and down. Start humming or singing to the baby with a calm voice that is just a bit louder than their cry. Your baby will stop crying so they can listen to your voice, forgetting why they were crying. Bouncing long enough will put them to sleep. I say 'long enough' because it can take them some time if they are fussy before they can fall asleep. If there is actual pain from a burp or the need to have a bowel movement (then nothing is going to happen). You will most likely have to rub their back to help get a burp out. If the baby is hungry or has a fussy belly, they will not settle down until the problem is resolved.

An alternative is to rock on the baby feeding chair (if it is a rocker), which is another great place to help the baby to fall asleep faster. If their bassinet rocks, give a gentle rock of their bed and put on some white noise. No matter the reason, you slowly calm them, and the rhythmic bouncing will help them fall asleep.

- Babies tend to be fussy in the early evening.

- When you are successful at soothing them to sleep, gently place baby in their bassinet, then more quietly tip-toe out of the room.
- Bed Time is always a glorious time of the day or night, bedtime for your baby.
- When the baby is very new, I have told many people to wear a t-shirt for several days so your scent is on the t-shirt, then put it down where the baby will lay. They will smell you, and the baby usually settles faster.

The only things you will be doing in the first few weeks are feeding your baby, changing the baby, and helping the baby to sleep. YOU must find time to eat, sleep and have bathroom breaks for you!

Author's Tips: Remember to Breathe and Believe! These are very important words to use when you think of pregnancy, labor and baby, maybe in life. I believe this baby is here because you are the perfect parents for them. So any time you doubt yourself or want to give up, please breathe! Then take another look at the beautiful baby, who is looking back at you and falling more in love with you. It can melt your heart.

- Ask for Help: Make sure that you can have at least one or more people that you can talk openly to about your concerns and feelings regarding how your postpartum time is. Ask for help from these people that are close, and they can guide you to the help you may need if you are having any postpartum thoughts or issues.
- Affirmations all around the house 'You *can* do this!' ~ 'I Love myself and my Baby' ~ 'Look at what I made' ~ 'I am an amazing Parent!'
- While feeding the baby, they will want to hold on to your finger. If you lift your hand to move, they will want the finger back.

- Baby Talk ~ you will come up with your own baby talk. Babies make us become different people, and we change in sweet ways. Lots of cute and silly talk, whether you talk or sing to your baby, is fun, and as they get older, they really enjoy it!
- Reading books is super fun. Even at a very early age, they can look at pictures as you talk about the image on the page. They really like to hear your voice.

Author's Tip: During the night hours, when you come to get the baby for a feeding, keep the room lights very low or have a night light on. Keep stimulation to a minimum. The Exercise Ball that you used for pregnancy to get the baby into an ideal position is perfect to settle them after any feeding or to stop them from crying. Babies are very clever beings, they sense your anxiety, and it can make them fussy. So when you are tired and want your sleep, get them settled, and you will have more time for yourself.

The baby will have several growth spurts. The first one is at 2 - 3 weeks after being born. They grow, and their brain develops more. The important growth spurt is at 6 weeks, which brings some much-needed change. They understand that a dark room is a night, and when they have shorter feeds and longer sleeps at night, this is when you will get a bit more sleep. A bright room is a time to be up and awake, they become more engaged with you during the day, and they are interested in looking at things, like a mobile, or at your face. It is a magical time! This is also a time of patience, while routines are random and quick but will change for the better.

All you need to do during a growth spurt is allow the baby to feed when they want, which will change and be more often, every hour or two, they are cluster feeding. It may take a few days for the human milk supply to increase, but during the growth spurt, they will be totally satisfied in their tummy. However, when the growth spurt is over, you will have an abundance. When the baby is not eating as much, the growth spurt is finishing. At the start and end of this, there may be an over abundance of milk. As the baby goes back to their regular feeding, you could save the excess milk by expressing and pumping the extra milk and freezing it. This is an opportunity to safe the milk, so the other parent gets a chance to give the baby a bottle for that middle-of-the-night feeding.

Baby has many growth spurts in the first year of life:

- The first is at 2 - 3 weeks
- 6 weeks
- 3 months
- 4 months
- 6 months
- 9 months

A new baby feeds all the time; they have a tiny tummy and are hungry often. They will cluster feed at different times, especially when they are about to start a growth spurt. If you are chestfeeding, this signals for more milk production, and it is essential to have the baby to the nipple as often as they want. They love the closeness of being near your body, and they can hear your heart beat and smell 'you'. This builds love and attachment by being near you. A growth spurt is when a baby's body grows and also their brain develops, and they will have many more all their life.

Important signs that you might notice when a growth spurt is coming, are the baby starts to cluster feed; they seem to want to eat more often. This signals your brain to produce more. If you are a first-time parent at the two to three-week growth spurt, and feedings are established, it can make you question if you are not producing enough milk, which you are, and your baby will start eating more for several days, then the growth spurt slows, and your body will slow down milk production, but your breasts may feel very full. Breasts during and especially after this time may take several days from the start to end to come back to a regular flow of milk. Your baby may seem to be fussy at the nipple. By pulling off or unlatching often, they are getting too much at a time. For those few days of cluster feeding, your production can be over whelming as they get a big amount at a time.

I suggest when you have that *full feeling,* and you are home, you can express some into a container and give it to baby later on, Or if you are not home and/or you do not have your baby with you, go into a bathroom and into a sink or toilet stall, and squeeze of a bit of milk to release the pressure. If the breast stays too full, it can clog the milk ducts, you may feel the breast becomes so full, and it feels hard in some places (along where a plugged milk duct is), and the breast may feel warm. This may indicate some infection.

You should massage the breast where you feel lumps; these are in the breast sinuses that carry the milk to the nipple. Y*ou must massage the lumps!* This is done by using the knuckles or ball of your hand, starting at the top of the breast and, in a downward motion towards the nipple, massage the lump down.

Put cold (from the fridge or freezer) green cabbage (not red, this will stain your skin and a bra) leaves inside your bra directly onto the skin to will help relieve some pressure and to calm the warm breast. If this persists, it can turn into mastitis, and you will need anti-biotics to help reduce the infection and inflammation. It is recommended that *when* you feel something is not right with your breasts, contact your doctor.

The growth spurt at six weeks is where there is a fairly significant brain development, and that is when the baby learns that a room with natural light is day time, and they are supposed to stay up and play. More importantly that when it is dark, it is night time, and then they tend to start to sleep longer than the three or four hours they have been accustomed to. Giving you more time for your sleep.

Your Uterus should feel firm and will shrink over time in the first few weeks. If this is your second or more baby, after the pain of the uterus contracting, you will feel stronger pains than with the first, especially if you are chestfeeding the baby. IF any of the following is happening, you must call your care provider straight away or go to the hospital. This may last one to six weeks postpartum.

- Your tummy feels especially tender, and you have a fever.
- If you pass large clots up to the size of a small orange.

And if you are worried, you can take a picture of the clot and send it to and tell your care provider. Check your fundus to make sure it is firm, and if not, vigorously massage it. Get exact instructions from your care provider after you have talked to them, and they have diagnosed exactly what you need.

Pelvic Floor Health has its own chapter. If you need this support and instruction for your pelvic floor exercises or if it is now time to do your Kegels, I am happy to offer a chapter on Pelvic Health written for you by the self-professed *pelvic health evangelist* known as The Vagina Coach, Kim Vopni. I also enjoyed reading Kim Vopni's other published book 'Prepare To Push'.

Relaxation to calm, regroup and ground yourself is important to stay positive as you go about your exhausting postpartum routine. If you have some favorite practices that will take a few minutes or more at a time, please start. Playing music can set the tone of the day or moment, it relaxes you and your baby, it can be a big part of your recovery, and your baby has gotten used to your music for the last several months. I recommend clients take at least ten minutes to sit in quiet once a day or more, maybe with a cup of non-caffeinated tea. It is very grounding and allows you to carry on with baby duties. You do not get the opportunity to do much of anything, in the first 12 weeks, because of the baby's needs, but you need to calm your mind and relax into parenthood because your baby can pick up on your feelings, and it can be confusing for them. They may become cranky or fussy or cry when anyone in the house is stressed out. They thrive on peaceful and calm energy, so stay calm, try to relax, ground yourselves and be positive; you can accomplish a lot. After having your baby, these moments feel far and few between, but they did help to relax and calm yourself while you prepared for delivery. It took you nine months to grow a baby in your tummy, and your body needs that much time or more to get back to something that is the same or similar to what you looked like then. (This is very subjective, with too many factors for how to get 'you' back to pre-pregnancy).

Exercise: I say the word *exercise* loosely. Getting started with some kind of exercise, albeit lifting your legs up off the bed several times with each leg before you get up, might be a start. If you have the okay to get back into your regular exercise routine, then have fun. It is very easy to put babies near, so they can see you, possibly doing yoga or other stretch activities, and you can talk to them. Exercising has been proven to relieve stress, and with a new baby, there may be stress and some Post Partum depression that may cause a lot of anxiety for you. With your new life and no set routine as yet, daily coping can be frustrating.

Buy and use a baby-wearing pouch, which is a secured body wrap for your baby. When they are small, it is easier to wear, as they get older, they may get too heavy for you to walk around in a pouch, and then changing to a stroller will be more comfortable for you and your baby. Baby will learn to love the walks as they watch everything, I always liked that the fresh air helped them to fall asleep, and when taking them home, you gently move them into their crib to sleep longer. But mind your spine has taken all the weight of the baby for a long time, and your posture is not as good as it was nine months ago. Go slow with any form of exercise and self-help for you to get back to you.

- You need to rebuild your mind, your body, muscles.
- A repair from delivery.
- Walk - go outside - be in nature.
- Learn to breathe for life, slow and gentle - long and deep - bringing in the energy – releasing.
- Inside yoga, pilates, stretch.
- Build your core.
- Mind your back when you place or lift the baby into their bed.
- Use your Ball - while soothing baby on a ball, be aware of your posture - use this moment to hold in muscles & sit straight on the ball.
- Stretch every part of your whole body, head - arms - legs - shoulders - stomach and back.
- Be gentle and mindful of all parts of your body.

Many people will not have stopped doing their regular routines, but if you are starting back into a routine, this will help your body to come back to something close to before you got pregnant. It can take some people years to get back into shape, for others, this is your normal routine, and results may be faster. Your body will have changed with the delivery. Since everyone is so different, one may never get back to pre-pregnancy. No matter how you recover from your pregnancy, please do not be wrapped up in getting your body back to what it was before pregnancy. There is a smaller percentage of people that get their original body back, most people see subtle changes, and this will be your new normal. It makes sense that with everything that changed in your body and the birthing experience, there will be changes.

Give Yourself a Year: I hope you have support in this big change of a year. Allow yourself and your body to get back to the new 'you' until you have another baby or grow old. Your hormones need time to settle into a new normal. The weight should come off by doing exercise and eating healthy, and keeping hydrated. Staying mentally healthy by finding a small bit of time each day for yourself, at least 10 minutes or more if you can, where you have a cup of tea, meditate, sit in a tub, or whatever allows you to stop and BE and enjoy YOU. This is not the time to be Super Person and try to do and finish things. Don't be afraid to ask everyone or anyone for help if you need it. Try to put encouraging and positive notes all around your home to give you encouragement when you need it most.

If you or your partner suggests that you may be having post partum issues, read about this in post partum depression chapter and consider that you may need to talk to someone about how they can help you!

Incorporate any movement and stretch your muscles that can relax and release your muscles. Social media and tv can keep you going with any exercise, or start easy with yoga, simple stretching on the floor on a mat, or lunge at the bottom of the stairs for release in your legs; there are many different exercises at any time of the day or night that will be convenient for you, in the comfort of your home. Of course, if you have had a cesarean section, you should wait until your care provider has given you the okay to exercise.

- You need to rebuild your mind ~ your body ~ and muscles ~ and repair from the delivery.
- Walk ~ go outside ~ watch and be in nature.
- Breathe slow and gentle ~ long and deep ~ bringing in positive energy.
- Stretch every part of your whole body head ~ arms ~ legs ~ shoulders ~ stomach ~ back.
- Be gentle and mindful of all parts of your body.

I speak too many that might be staying at home, that when you go out, the fresh air and movement will be beneficial to you. Many people will not have stopped doing their regular routines, but starting back into a routine will help your body come back to something close to before you got pregnant. It can take some people years to get back into shape. To others, this is your normal routine, and you should recover faster. Your body will have changed with the delivery. Since everyone is so different, you may never get back to the pre-baby weight, and others may only take a couple of months. Start small, and don't over-exert yourself. Your body has just gone through a huge change. Not only does your body accommodate a baby, but your hormones need a year to get back to pre pregnancy.

No matter how you recover from your pregnancy, please do not be wrapped up in getting your body back to what it was before pregnancy. There is a smaller percentage of people that get their original body back. Most of us see subtle changes, but there should not be any expectations in the first year or two because *your expectations may be hard to fulfill*. It makes sense that with everything that changed in your body and the birthing experience, we will see change. As a mature woman, I have noticed that with every new decade, the body has subtle changes that happen all by itself.

Introduction to solid food for Baby after being feed milk exclusively for several or more months because chest milk or formula was all baby needed. In the early months, we should not give an infant water, there are no calories in water, but when they are well established at eating regular foods, then water is a good option for the baby. When your Doctor gives you the okay to introduce solids, the recommended first foods may be pablum or infant cereal. After a bit, they will transition to puree foods. The doctor will advise how much your baby should have per 'meal' (it is really a few tablespoons). This can be mixed with a bit of chest milk or formula for extra calories or water. The amount is small to start, a couple of **tiny** spoons full. The baby must be able to sit upright in a high chair on their own. Then baby will have to learn how to swallow pablum. Usually, it is a very messy time as they are learning, but a feeling of accomplishment, both by them and you, that baby is learning and growing.

Store-bought puree is definitely more convenient, but it comes with extra ingredients to keep it from spoiling. You may want to puree food yourself so you know that they are getting only fresh ingredients, without preservatives and sugar. I like the thought of home made puree food that is not sweet; when you give a baby sweeter foods, you may create a baby that has a fondness for sweets which can make it hard to get them to eat all varieties of food groups. For example, yams, potatoes, peas, and carrots are good starters, then adding fruits into their diet like bananas, mangoes, and pears. But once they taste the fruit, they get fussy with the other more bland foods.

It is easy to get ideas from the internet. There is a plethora of recipes for different age groups, starting around 4 months with cereal or pablums. The ingredients are explained, how to prepare, and how to store in a freezer or fridge and storing by using small ice cube trays, as babies eat a small amount of food, even though they slop most of the food on themselves or the table tray. Then transitioning them into finger food, they will have to be old enough to sit in a high chair without wobbling, and they are usually very interested in wanting to feed themselves; they have been watching you. They will also learn how to swallow more than liquid. Also recommended by doctors is to give a single ingredient type of food at a time. It could be mashed yam, then a few days later, mashed protein foods.

During the family meal, the baby will be interested in what you are eating, and you might find they want what you are eating. Please have your camera handy near the dinner table; pictures of the baby trying all first foods is a picture must-have! You are starting a huge ritual of memories for your family, where you can have many laughs and fun times. As they get a bit older, they may want to have solid pieces of food that they can hold in their hands. They need to be supervised in the beginning so they do not put something into their mouth and gag or swallow too big of a piece of food. While teething, cold pieces of food will feel good on their gums. There are also many teething chew toys that go in the freezer and are used cold.

Playing with baby: It is not so much play time in the first few weeks or months, but talking to the baby, singing to the baby, and rocking the baby, are about as much stimulation a baby needs. Do not expect babies to reach for their toys in the first weeks; it may be several months. As the baby grows and their neck becomes stronger, you can do more with them. They absolutely love when you get close to their face. Talking and making funny faces is a simple exercise for them to focus on you. As they focus better, they will be able to imitate the faces you make, like sticking your tongue out, smiling, pointing a finger or waving.

There are many visual toys that are made for infants, and they will enjoy watching these. They may not yet reach for their toys, and it may take some time before they start to reach and discover their hands and feet.

Cuddle and dance around the room, sing, read books, put the baby in a stroller or use 'baby wearing' type pouches and go for walks, point out things in nature and show your baby all that is close to them. The fresh air will usually put the baby to sleep. A *tiny* bit of sun on the baby is a very good way to absorb vitamin D.

Tummy time: Put your baby on their tummy on a blanket on the floor in a secure and clean space. You should always be present and beside your baby. You can start by doing it a couple of times per day and for a couple of minutes at a time. Your baby will fuss if they are not comfortable. When they are not happy, leave it and try again for another day. Tummy time will help them develop muscles in their neck and body. Put baby on their tummy several times a day. Start for a few minutes and gently increase as they tolerate the position. You can get on the floor with them. Never leave them alone, especially when the baby has fallen asleep on the floor during tummy time.

Milestones: When you might expect your baby to do the following, but know that not all babies follow the same time frame, these are just average times that they may be able to:

- lift their head, usually around two or three months.
- roll over at four months.
- reach for toys at four to five months.
- start to bounce their legs (when held) at six months.
- pull themselves up (in the crib or at coffee tables) between seven to twelve months.
- stand by nine to twelve months.

This will all lead to crawling and the first steps! I hope you document all of these milestones because you will forget when they did any of these things (From personal experience).

Author's story: My sister and I flew to a family funeral, we took her baby, she had mentioned that her baby was not crawling yet. In the bedroom we shared, I put my nephew on the floor, and got down onto the floor in front of the baby, then I dangled a red liquorish in front of the baby. Well, let's just say the baby learned how to crawl. I am not saying, you feed an infant candy, I actually can not remember if they tasted the candy or not. But it worked, and from then on, they were mobile.

When or if you notice the baby has a flat head or a small patch on the back of the head that has no hair when they lay in the crib, alternate putting the baby with their head facing left and then the next day facing right, it should help with equal time on both sides.

Balloons: I saw a picture of a baby with a huge smile, laying on their back on a blanket on the floor. The parent had four different colored balloons with a ribbon tied to each balloon, and the ribbons were gently tied to the ankles and wrists of the baby. The baby was looking at the balloons bop about as they moved their feet and arms, looking very interested in the balloons.

*Please use caution if you do this. Supervision is needed in the event the balloon pops and your baby tries to put it in their mouth. You could have them hanging from the ceiling. Just saying!

Travel or Flying with the Baby: I have always thought that it was easy to travel with a baby. When they are young, they can be unpredictable on a plane and can make everyone that sits near babies or young children leery, knowing they can cry or be fussy most of the trip. The pressure in our ears is difficult when the plane takes off or landing; for a baby, it is also confusing and very uncomfortable. They can become fussy and cry for long periods of time with the pain. Giving the baby a bottle or chest feeding or a soother is very successful when the plane is taking off or descending into the airport. It helps baby's ears to pop from the air pressure in the cabin of the plane, and they cry less.

When they are very young, from newborn to 6 months, they sleep much of the time. Ask the airline carrier if they have bassinets they can offer for the baby. You may have to book specific seating and most likely have to pay for the extra seat for the baby. Ask if you can bring a car seat that will fit onto the plane seat. You can use a baby-wearing carrier on your body, and the baby should be able to sleep most of the way. Take a couple of plastic sealable bags for dirty diapers. Bring their favorite blanket and/or plush toys.

Choosing Day Care and Schools: It may be the last thing on your mind, but in many bigger cities, it has already become difficult to find a daycare center and private schools that you want your child to attend, because there are long waits. You should consider and decide where you might want to place your child, so you can have your unborn baby on a list.

This is from a past client, who is a very sweet person. I was her Doula, and she decided to make a career change and become a Doula herself. Jen posted this online, and it really resonated with me. I wish I had been that clever.

Today, I sent my sweetie to her bedroom to look for her belly button so I could put the dishes away without her climbing into the dishwasher. Am I the meanest mum?

If you are looking for a Doula in Toronto, Ontario, Canada, Look up the delightful and talented Jen LeClair:

jen@mamabeardoulacare.com

Fun Facts:

- When the baby is older, and they can hold onto a bottle or a popsicle, take your chest milk and freeze it in a popsicle tray; you can make a 'milk'scicle.
- Giving birth and becoming a parent are two of the biggest life-altering events in your life.
- Babies don't come with a *Manual* because "you and your baby are uniquely joined for life".
- Listen to your heart and gut; you already have all the answers to guide and raise this baby to adulthood.
- When we calm our minds and relax into parenthood, our stress levels can be relaxed. As a baby can feel your stress levels, it can also be calmed when you are relaxed and loving toward them.

- There is no ‘right’ way to raise a baby into adulthood, BUT your way.
- Love your baby and *yourself.*
- Document everything! Milestones should be journaled, and many pictures should be taken. These tiny little people will be standing in front of you one day, asking to drive your car. Life goes by way too fast!
- You are responsible for a human being that did not come with an instruction booklet!
- Take what you learn from family, friends, professionals and this book to come to the best 'way' of navigating your birth and raising your child.
- Do not worry about teaching them to talk to you - too fast. They will learn to say the words that you say. For instance, they see the reaction a swear word gets and will repeat those words.
- When they get older, they *talk back!*
- Your life will never be the same again.
- You are SO in Love with your baby.
- Take this baby and go with love and kindness, knowing that they are here to be your child and you, their parent.
- After 9 months of being pregnant and a month or two with a newborn, you will be exhausted! Learn to sleep or rest. Meditation is a very good way to relax, any form that works best for you.

I need help are 3 magical words that may make a huge difference in your daily routine.

Remember, ***Breathing and Believing*** is more important than ever. Use the techniques from this book for pregnancy, labor and life now with your baby. Try not to doubt yourself, and do not give up. Breathe and take another look at your beautiful baby, the one staring at you. Who is falling more in love, you or them? Learn to relax and allow your heart and gut to make some decisions for you, not your critical mind.

My Experience in raising human beings. I wanted them to grow and be sustainable in this world, to become part of society and live happily and successfully on their own. When they were ready and I had taught them enough, I helped them to move out of the family home. One of my children came back for a visit and asked sincerely, "Do you know how much toilet paper costs?!" It made me smile, and I responded, "Yes, yes I do". So thankful and proud that he was understanding adult life and is still excited to be on his own.

Labor ~ Birth and Beyond:

Raising your baby will come with challenges for you, both mentally and physically. Complications will be taken care of, don't worry about them beforehand. Your baby will become *the* most important person in your life.

I always believed there was more than one way to do something, and most times, there are a plethora of ways, *especially* during labor and birth.

You will experience and grow with this baby and become someone that understands a more exciting purpose in life, being a *Parent.*

Chapter 28: PPD - Post Partum Depression

Post Partum Depression ~ PPD is definitely real! Congratulations, you have a new baby(ies). Your birth and delivery journey matters and how you define the experience will impact your recovery. Your perception of your birthing experience may leave you wondering about many things that occurred during labor and the baby's birth. You may have felt trauma from the experience of having a diversion or different delivery than the one you perceived, your wish for a 'natural birth' that changed. You may be wondering why and what happened while I was laboring?

- You do not fully understand why your labor diverted course.
- You delivered in a delivery suite with 'help'.
- You had a vacuum delivery.
- You delivered in the operating room.
- You had a very difficult and long labor or delivery.
- You had a fast labor that was overwhelming.
- You had a repair of the perineum (no matter how severe).
- You had an emergency cesarean section.
- You had forceps delivery and the more severe repair.
- You had to change your birth wishes.
- How do you feel about your labor and birth? Do you feel your body or the system failed you by not having the birth you expected?
- How are you coping with the pain from any of the procedures that you were required to have during labor?
- How are you coping with the emotional side of the birthing process? Is there sadness or depression?

Each different baby you birth, and the unique experience during that birth process affects us in different ways. With your new reality and life, you should be given tender care to heal and recover from, especially if you had to let go of the exceptions that you had for this birth. It is common that most people take up to the first year post partum, where their hormones return to pre-pregnancy. Unfortunately, many people are not aware of or do not take advice from loved ones, believing they do not need any help. It should be considered part of your postpartum care for your mental health. Talking with your care provider is essential for your self-preservation; they can refer you to a specialist for postpartum issues.

As a new parent (meaning either or both parents), it is common for you to be exhausted and feel out of your element or isolated; the responsibility alone is frightening. You have a tiny baby that you are responsible for keeping healthy, let alone thinking about raising. Your emotions and feelings can be debilitating, and you may find yourself sliding into a bit of a hole; this may be the start of postpartum depression and/or anxiety which can make you feel like 'you are crumbling inside your world'. When family mentions that they have concerns about you crying often, being irritable and/or impatient, or a desire to have everything in your world perfect or having low self-esteem or lack of confidence, listen to them and reach out to your doctor for help. Family and friends are also good to talk with, but professionals are experts in finding you proper care and the tools you need to help *you.* Postpartum flips your life sideways and upside down. It doesn't differentiate between parents; it affects everyone with a newborn in different ways. It is real.

This is something I wish no one had to experience, but with the pleura of hormones and (often) drugs used to manage your labor, over the course of long or fast deliveries, any and all can leave us in a state of confusion. I believe we can get through this time postpartum by asking for help. I wish for you to be proud of yourself, considering everything you had to go through to deliver this baby!

PPD can affect people in many ways, and an extreme can take on a silent and deadly form. If you are not feeling those 'love feelings' people talk about, you may already have some form of postpartum depression; please talk to someone straight away. People having struggles with their daily routine and taking care of their baby can change into a destructive mode where the baby and/or themselves are harmed.

The tools your care provider gives you can help you to succeed faster in your postpartum time. Techniques that allow you to become more confident and learn and trust yourselves with parenting instincts. Be kind to yourself; you may be your own worst enemy. Ask for help!

Sometimes the 'way' we deliver our baby can cause worry, frustration or anger. It is important to talk to all care providers about the delivery and your birth journey as soon after delivery as possible.

Hormones: When you became pregnant, your hormones changed to accommodate all of the developments of the fetus, growing a placenta and the birth sac that cocooned and grew your baby inside. Now that baby is here, your hormones will fluctuate for up to a full twelve months while your body gets back to pre-pregnancy. Your emotions will take you on a new journey that feels like you are on a roller coaster ride, partly because you are so tired and confused with a sprinkle of stress. You doubt yourself as a new parent while trying to learn what the baby wants, their habits and schedule as your days and nights flit by.

Postpartum depression can be extremely detrimental to a new family, it can be mild to severe, but it should never be taken lightly. Many times you are in denial and believe that you are just tired and doing fine. You may not realize you are having mood swings that can vacillate from mild to extreme. The reality and responsibility of being a new parent, learning your baby's routine during this time, is a huge lifestyle change. Your baby was in a warm dark environment where they could simply suck a finger or thumb and move around at their leisure. Now your baby is learning from you how to fill their belly, find a different sleep pattern, and understand the people that are attached to the voice they know so well. You spend all of your time consumed with the baby and their needs and feeding them, keeping them clean, and comforting them to sleep, learning their personality, while your need for food and sleep takes a back seat.

It can happen to both parents; you may both have difficulties and feelings of frustration, being overwhelmed and exhausted while adjusting to the time parents dedicate to their baby and their very different routines. Possibly you are not coping with the simple and easy tasks because you have a tough time sleeping and you are not eating properly, or possibly you are cranky to those around you because you believe you are the only one that can look after your baby. Family may be asking if you are okay or need help, but you ignore them in your quest to be a perfect parent.

Every person will go through a similar time in the first couple of weeks postpartum with their baby. Your biggest obstacle will be sleep deprivation. For your own self-preservation, try to delegate household chores and watch other children. Lack of sleep can run you down, and with hormones that are trying to settle and get back to pre-pregnancy, it may take a year. Many clients tell me all the time, "I just can't sleep"! All you need in the beginning is to love up this baby - feed your baby - and get sleep.

It can make you feel like things are over the top. This is when you should consider that you need some help.

When YOU are in the throws of depression, it tricks your brain into thinking that you are tired, but outwardly people notice many changes in your routine and how you react to them. Being paranoid or having fear and doubts can play around in your brain. If your loved ones ask you to go to your doctor for a visit, please listen to them.

You can have hormonal changes affecting how you perceive life, and depression can set in, making it hard to cope with the needs of your baby. When severe, people can have suicidal thoughts, and you may be having *depressing* thoughts. Suicide is real and something for everyone that might see something is not right to do the best thing - tell the care provider.

Allow them to ask the questions and get the correct help for the post partum person.

You may not yet be quite aware of and should consider talking about postpartum depression.

Knowing your baby will be okay.

You are having problems as you try to chest feed.

Baby has their own schedule, and it can take months to figure it out, then it changes as they grow.

Your days are consumed with baby's routine; feed, change diaper, change clothes, burp, cuddle, and try to soothe baby so you can put them to sleep.

You are fully immersed in looking after the baby and not asking for help.

All of this can take up most of your time in the 24-hour day, leaving you exhausted, hungry and cranky! Hopefully, you are not taking that understood emotions out on your partner.

You just want to feel 'normal'; you want to have a warm meal, spend time in a tub or shower, and Sleep!

I have seen many people worry about their new baby so much that they can not settle and relax or get sleep themselves. Others worry in case the baby stops breathing. Meanwhile, they themselves can not sleep.

Formula must be made, and if the baby is crying for a bottle, it can make for a stressful time.

Your body size and shape may also take up to a year to look the same or similar as it once was. There may be other professionals that can help with exercise and advise.

INCLUSIVE w partner:

Being able to include the other parent will make a huge difference for both parents. If you allow your partner to hold and feed, especially a bottle, in the middle of the night, you get a longer portion of sleep. It can make a huge difference to you for the extra hours, but more importantly, the partner is involved in having more baby bonding time. It does not even have to be every night, but maybe 2 nights over the weekend.

Cuddle and change diapers; you will have time that you can do some of the things that are truly for you and special, like going to the washroom or having a bath. It is so okay to ask for help from the partner first and family, then even other close friends and a postpartum doula.

Unfortunately, the other parent can have a postpartum depression for different reasons:

Their reality and their life has also changed.

They see a partner that is very different.

They may be concerned that they are now the sole income provider.

They see you exhausted but not allowing them to help with the baby or small chores or meal preparation.

If you do not trust them, you are giving up a good resource, having them learn about and bond with their baby.

When you say no too many times, it can be confusing and frustrating for them.

I believe when both parents are aware of the team effort, meaning that both parents, together, raise and love and nourish this baby, the satisfaction and better well-rounded this small person becomes. They will always have the knowledge in their heart that both parents loved and took care of them.

So please try to communicate with each other; you are the reason this baby is staring at you. Take time to talk, sing, cuddle, and raise this baby together as much as possible.

Their body and hormones have gone through a huge change for 9 months, and it can take up to a year to get back to your pre-pregnancy body. Unfortunately, your body has changed forever, yes, you may be able to get back to a pre-pregnant weight and size, but inside, we do not see. The silent changes come strong for both parents, and many people have a hard time knowing when they have PPD post partum depression.

Inclusion, knowing that both parents should be considered, their role in life has changed.

The demand from the baby can be overwhelming; it can make either parent left feeling powerless to control the daily routine. The realization that baby comes first, or one parent is now responsible for a family; one person will not be working and how will that change the finances; the 'couple's' physical and intimate relationship will be different; is the partner feeling inadequate or left out of the baby's needs in the first six months; does the parent taking care of baby, not seem to be too interested in the partner;

The most important thing, is to acknowledge your concerns with each other. Knowing that everyone is sleep-deprived, hormones can be spiking or crashing. Try to have an open conversation with other people (family, friends or professionals) that you can trust and glean some wisdom about managing through this very intense time and the most exciting time in your life - your baby.

Babies are high maintenance; they need 24/7 attention for the first year.

Being angry with each other certainly does not make anything easier; it can bring more separation.

This postpartum time should be an exercise in caring for the baby and each other.

A tender cuddle; a hug; a gentle massage or sending them to have a spa treatment, or nice comments to each other can make a tough and long day feel not so bad.

Get help! Make sure you have people that can come and do for you both, even if it is giving you a few hours while you take a nap or have a meal without having to worry that the baby in the other room needs something.

Look for groups that have had babies - you can learn so much from others that have gone through or are going through the same as you. I know there are a lot of 'online' groups that talk about babies and give tips - during the middle of the night., or join a group and take the time to go out and talk/gather. Even other PPD groups, when we know that things we thing about and feel, but are told that it passes soon enough. Be strong and get the support you should have.

PPD does end, and life will be a bit easier. Until your baby goes through something else - changes - grows - parenthood is never-ending, and that is also okay.

They may be the next president of a country. In the early days home with your baby, you can easily become exhausted, with the extras, like doctor appointments for either you and/or your baby. Remembering to eat? Or have a shower or go to the toilet? Please do not tell me you got any house cleaning done! Or did you get a moment to have a warm meal? You went shopping, when and how?

When both parents get to take care of the baby's needs and wants, you grow together as a loving family unit. It is so important for the baby when both parents are involved in the daily routines, the baby learns about what family means, and they become more secure, happy adults.

Mixed with sleep deprivation, everyone experiences this.

Connect with others and/or support groups: There is something to be said about family and friends and ancient wisdom, especially in pregnancy and postpartum. Feeding your baby for an hour in the middle of the night can be lonely, but there are many other new parents looking for support or guidance or just someone to text with. People from your pregnancy group or other sources with similar birth experiences, a C-Section or chest feeding tips, or just a "Hi, how are tonight?" There are many support groups where you may receive good advice or a quick answer to something bothering you, which can be very comforting, especially for first-time parents.

You must learn to relax and allow your heart and gut to make some decisions for you, not your critical mind. Your body and mind can be the single defining dictator when you are out of postpartum. When we can wrap our heads around what is needed for our self-preservation, and we manage to get that for ourselves - we succeed faster in our postpartum time.

Allow yourself to have as much help as possible so that you become confident and learn to trust yourself with your parenting instincts. Postpartum is a time that our life is flipped sideways and around. It does not differentiate between either sex parents or biological parents.

Postpartum affects everyone with a newborn, and in different ways. It is real. Always be kind to yourself. We can be our own worst enemies. There is no manual for a reason, “this baby and you” are so uniquely joined for life.

This can start both the best and amazing time and the most depressing and sleep deprived time in your life. You may feel your world has turned upside down, you doubt yourself and have no idea about, what your baby wants and or what their needs are.

Concern and feeling anxious are common in the first year. If you feel you often cry for no reason, are irritable, impatient, desire to have everything perfect, have no patience, have low self-esteem or lack of confidence.

Purple Crying or Shaken Baby Syndrome: There are times, usually in the evening time, when babies tend to be fussy. There seems to be no reason why the baby is crying. You have fed the baby, bathed them and then have a clean diaper rocked and cuddled baby.

It has been reported that babies are being shaken, sometimes to death.

The shaking does nothing but makes the baby cry more. Added to your frustration with not having a solution for the baby, it is best to GET help. Tell someone that you would like help. If you are having thoughts or shaking your baby, stop! There will be serious and irreversible damage to the baby and its brain. It can also cause death.

Seek help, tell someone friend, family partner care provider.

On the internet - find support groups that have had a similar experience, i.e., C-Section or Breastfeeding tips. Depressing thoughts, or postpartum, although no one believes they have postpartum depression.

If you have a C-Section, try to find online groups where you can find some other people that have gone through the same experience. They will have some good basic advice - especially when you are in the middle of the night and want to find an answer. OR just to have someone else to talk with. Having a long labor and then a c-section can cause some issues of their own - to do with depression - you may feel like you failed to naturally birth your baby. This is something I wish no one had to experience; please be proud that you had this baby! The tough part comes when they get older and can talk back. For now, you love up this baby - feed your baby - and get sleep.

Put new post-it notes up on the mirrors and fridge like before.

Self Care; What are your needs - as you recover from your labor and delivery?

How can we not get totally run down?

Need for Sleep.

Feed your baby - that means you have to be healthy.

Take 10 minutes (or longer) to yourself per day. Have a cup of tea. Sit outside or Quietly in your home.

Help from others. i.e., schedule - see my schedule.

Allow family and friends to bring you meals, clean your home, run errands, and take other children to play dates - appt – school.

Recovering from Birth.

Your Emotions - Exhaustion - Feelings of being lost or helpless.

Please talk to your care provider about your birth. You and your baby will have checks in the first 24 - 48 hours after birth. Many people have had either slight or massive changes to their birth plans, in addition to some trauma. This subject is very internal, and I come across this with my clients often. Somewhere in your life, you have had a trauma that has impacted you, and you have surpassed it, dealt with it and moved on with your life.

Birth and the way you are spoken to or treated; the way you felt when you felt you were not in control of your birth decisions. This can all make a huge impact on your mental health recovery postpartum. Make a list of questions you want answered about your delivery. It helps to talk about it sooner than later. Care providers attend many births, and their memory of your delivery may become harder to recall as time passes. Get your answers when it is fresh for you both.

After spending so much time with all care providers that navigated your pregnancy and labor, there seems to be difficulty getting help postpartum. We definitely need more postpartum care providers. Some issues can come up that all seem to stem from past trauma, birth trauma and postpartum hormones. It will take approximately one year and longer to fully get your body's hormones back to where they were before you got pregnant. The journey is made faster and easier if you have people you trust, can talk to, and listen to when they advise you to seek professional advice. I refer to the Post Partum Depression or Baby Blues. This topic is definitely out of my scope of practice. However, if a trusted family member or friend asks you to go to see someone, please do as they ask. I have had postpartum clients that get themselves into a depression that can only be rectified by professional help. Good family and friends may be a huge help.

People that get this debilitating time are real; your hormones take up to a year to get back to normal. Even the partners can have a form of PPD.

It can be severe to mild, and the length of time is hard to tell. It is best dealt with by a professional.

Talk to your care provider about anything that seems not normal for you. Or talk to family members -good friends - try to get some sleep and help to manage better.

- When a new parent asks for help, we need to help and nurture the person so that person can nurture the baby.
- I do not wish this ppd experience, but with the pleura of hormones and (often) drugs used to manage your labor, over the course of long or fast deliveries, any and all, can leave us in a state of confusion. I believe by asking for help, we can get through this time post-partum time easier.
- My wish for you is to be proud of yourself, considering everything you had to go through to deliver this baby!

Chapter 29: SIDS - Sudden Infant Fact Sheet

This information is from the Canadian government website, informing anyone that will be taking care of your baby. **For the full document of information on SIDS - Sudden Infant Death Syndrome and safe sleep and more topics, like baby sleep products and more, go to www.Canada.ca.**

Let everyone know; parents, all caregivers, including grandparents, family members, child care providers, babysitters and friends, how they can help keep babies safe by following the steps for safe sleep and for every sleep, nap time and night time, at home, in childcare settings and when traveling.

SIDS is when a baby that seems healthy, dies suddenly in their sleep, and the cause can not be explained. The reasons for what causes SIDS is unknown, and so it can not be prevented. Other deaths that happen during sleep time can be prevented, such as when a baby accidentally suffocates because of their sleep space.

There are many steps to help lower SIDS during your infant's sleep time. Always place your baby on their back to sleep, every time. The environment should be smoke-free. Their sleep space should be a firm, flat surface with a tightly tucked-in sheet. They should be in a crib, cradle or bassinet in the same room as you sleep for the first six months.

Swaddling is sometimes used to calm babies, but it can also be a risk. Babies can get tangled or covered in the blanket if it comes loose or can roll onto their tummy while still swaddled.

These are the risks of suffocation:

- If you swaddle your baby, be sure to do it safely.
- Use a lightweight blanket.
- Make sure it stays well away from the baby's nose and mouth.
- Wrap your baby so they can still move their hips and legs.
- Overheating increases your baby's risk of SIDS.
- It is safest for babies when they sleep in simple, fitted sleepwear, like a sleeper. It should keep your baby comfortable at room temperature, so they do not get too hot.

Keep the room at a comfortable temperature. If it is comfortable for you, it will be comfortable for your baby too. Babies do not need a hat when indoors, as it can make them too hot. Babies do not need blankets when they sleep. When babies move their arms and legs, they can make the blanket cover their head, this can cause them to overheat or suffocate. If you use a blanket for your baby, make sure it is thin and lightweight OR use sleep sacks instead of a blanket. If you use a sleep sack, make sure it is the right size for your baby, if it is too big, your baby can slip down inside the sack, which can make your baby overheat or suffocate. If it is too tight, your baby may not be able to move their hips and legs freely, which can be dangerous, especially if they roll onto their tummy.

Babywearing and using baby slings and carriers is popular, and babies often fall asleep while being carried in them. If you use one, be sure to use it safely. Babies, especially those who are less than 4 months old or who were born prematurely or with a medical condition, have poor neck control and are at a higher risk of suffocation.

- Keep your baby visible at all times.
- Make sure your baby is in an upright position.
- You should be able to see your baby's face; make sure it is not pressed into your body, your clothes or the carrier.
- Check your baby often and watch for overheating.

For more information, visit Canada.ca (search for - baby sling and carrier safety).

Room sharing helps your baby sleep safely and lowers the risk of SIDS.

Room sharing means placing your baby to sleep in their own safe sleep space, a crib, cradle or bassinet, which is placed in your room next to your bed.

Room sharing is recommended for your baby's first 6 months, the time when the risk of SIDS is the highest.

Room sharing makes it easier to breastfeed and check on your baby at night.

Room sharing is not the same as bed-sharing.

Understanding the risks of bed-sharing.

- Bed sharing is when a baby sleeps with an adult or other child, on the same sleep surface, such as an adult bed, sofa or armchair.
- Bed-sharing increases a baby's risk of SIDS and suffocation. Some parents end up bed-sharing with their baby, even though they do not plan to. It is important to understand the risks and know the situations that make bed-sharing especially unsafe for babies, so you can take steps to avoid them:

Babies that share a sleep surface with someone else have a higher risk of SIDS and suffocation because:

- The baby can get trapped between the sleep surface and the wall/side, bed frame, or the body of the adult or other child.

- The adult or other child can roll over onto the baby, or soft bedding (pillows, comforters, blankets) can cover the baby's face or head, which can make them overheat or suffocate.

In-bed sleeping products, like baby nests or pods, do not keep your baby safe when bed-sharing. The padded sides increase the baby's risk of suffocation.

These situations put babies at especially high risk when bed-sharing:

- The baby is less than 4 months old or was born preterm or with low birth weight.
- The person bed sharing with the baby has taken alcohol or drugs.
- The person bed sharing with the baby has taken medication that makes them tired or harder to wake up.
- The baby's parent smoked during pregnancy, or the person bed sharing with the baby is a smoker, or if there is smoking in the household.
- The sleep surface is soft; sleeping with a baby on a sofa, armchair, air mattress, waterbed or bed with a mattress topper is very unsafe.
- There is more than one other person (or a pet) bed sharing with the baby.
- There is loose bedding, pillows, blankets and other objects near the baby.

If you bed share (even if you did not plan to), be sure to follow the other steps for safe sleep, including:

- Always put your baby on their back.
- Make sure the sleep surface is firm and flat, with no gaps where the baby can get trapped.

- Keep all soft, loose bedding or other objects well away from the baby.
- Dress your baby so they do not overheat.

For more information, talk to your baby's health care provider or your local public health department.

Not recommended for sleep:

- Bedside sleepers that attach to an adult bed, baby can get trapped in the space between the bed and the bed-side sleeper
- A baby nest or a pod is a portable pad with soft padded sides, and other soft products like nursing pillows are not recommended for sleep.
- Sleep surfaces that are not flat, like inclined sleepers, hammocks or crib wedges, should not be used.
- High chairs, baby swings, bouncers, strollers and car seats are not for babies to sleep in. The baby's head can fall forward and can make it hard to breathe.
- Do not leave the baby to sleep in a snowsuit, raincoat, jacket or other outerwear. When inside, they run a risk of suffocation or overheating.

Author's Note

Author's Quotes:

All my life, I believed there was more than one way to do something.

And most times, there are a plethora of ways,

Especially during Labor and Birth

~~

Always be kind to your wee baby angel. They may have come here unexpectedly or after a long time of waiting. This baby can feel your emotions and hear your words in utero. What if, in 30 years, this baby that you are carrying inside your womb may head the government in your country, cook your meal in your favorite restaurant, or be drilling a cavity in your mouth. It is up to us to love unconditionally, nurture and guide our babies to be the best they can be.

Try to enjoy your pregnancy, the birth and your baby.

~~

Your life and future is about to change forever, and meeting your baby will be the single most important day of your life. They complete your life and open you up to a love that you cannot get anywhere else.

~~

Being excited and terrified is an understatement, but falling in love immediately with your baby, is inevitable.

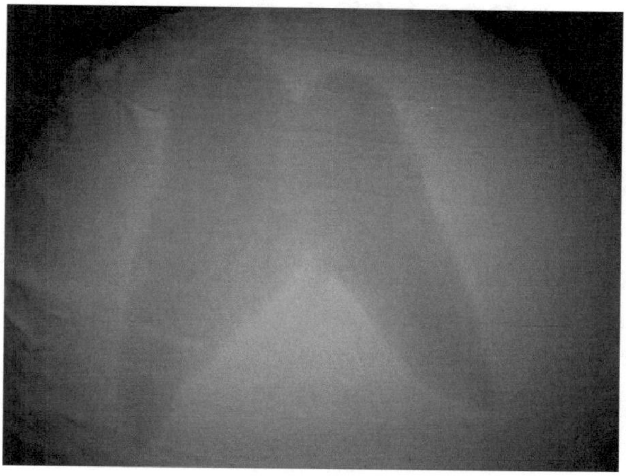

This is a picture I took at a birth. The client had been bouncing on an exercise ball with a white bed sheet on the ball. When they got up, this mark from the amniotic fluid was there, I thought it looked like ANGEL WINGS!

My wish for you is a safe and uneventful labor and that you hold your healthy baby at the end of labor.

About the Author

Kim has raised 5 children. All are now thriving adults whom she proudly believes are her best accomplishments in life. Kim lives a quiet life with her husband, hands in the dirt and making gardens grow. Being a Reiki Master, Kim also practises the calming ways of being in the moment and looking with positivity to the future.

At some point, Kim plans to start writing children's books, so please look for those in the future.

https://mydoula.ca/

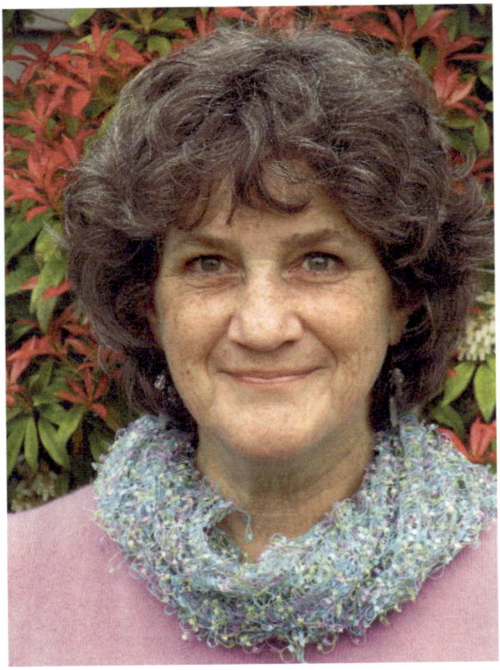

Made in the USA
Las Vegas, NV
03 November 2026

57424296R00249